Progress in Inflammation Research

Volume 92

This book series addresses all key topical aspects of basic research, therapy and its clinical implications in the field of inflammatory diseases. It provides a unique reference source for academic and industrial biomedical researchers, drug development personnel, immunologists, rheumatologists, cardiologists, allergologists and many other relevant clinical disciplines. Each publication supplies regular scientific updates on newest developments and allow providing access to state-of-the-art techniques and technologies.

The series gathers knowledge from leading authorities on the multiple facets of inflammation research, making it a valuable asset for advanced students in biomedical sciences, early career investigators and for professionals in both basic and translational research and in the clinic. Each volume comprises a carefully selected collection of high-quality review articles on the respective field of expertise. They also introduce new investigators to the most pertinent aspects of inflammatory disease and allow established investigators to understand fundamental ideas, concepts and data on sub-fields that they may not normally follow.

Thus chapters should not comprise extensive data reviews nor provide a means for authors to present new data that would normally be published in peer-reviewed journals. Instead, the chapters should provide a concise overview and guide to the most pertinent and important literature, thus reflecting a conceptual approach rather than a complete review of the particular field of research. Moreover, each chapter should be intelligible for less experienced researchers or even newcomers to the fields of pathology, mechanisms and therapy of inflammatory disease. To this end, authors should consider introducing PhD students or postdocs who are new to the laboratory to the major concepts and the most critical literature in their chosen field of research.

Bruce K. Rubin • Masaharu Shinkai
Editors

Macrolides as Immunomodulatory Agents

Springer

Editors
Bruce K. Rubin
School of Medicine
Virginia Commonwealth University
Richmond, VA, USA

Masaharu Shinkai
Clinical Trial Develop & Research Center
Tokyo Shinagawa Hospital
Tokyo, Japan

ISSN 1422-7746 ISSN 2296-4525 (electronic)
Progress in Inflammation Research
ISBN 978-3-031-42858-6 ISBN 978-3-031-42859-3 (eBook)
https://doi.org/10.1007/978-3-031-42859-3

This Springer imprint is published by the registered company Springer Nature Switzerland AG
The registered company address is: Gewerbestrasse 11, 6330 Cham, Switzerland

Paper in this product is recyclable.

Preface: A Brief History of the Macrolide Antibiotics

Macrolides are a class of bacteriostatic antibiotics containing a large macrocyclic lactone ring, generally 14- ,15-, or 16-membered in size, with one or more deoxysugars (e.g., cladinose) attached. They bind to the 50S subunit of the bacterial ribosome inhibiting bacterial protein synthesis and thus growth and reproduction. The most commonly used macrolide antibiotics are the 14-membered erythromycin, clarithromycin, and roxithromycin and the 15-membered azalide, azithromycin.

The first macrolide identified was erythromycin. Dr. Abelardo Aguilar was a physician and pharmaceutical representative working at Eli Lilly Company in the Philippine island of Iloilo. In 1952, he was doing independent research to attempt to identify novel antibiotics and he found that some soil from the Molo cemetery had reproducible antibacterial activity. He sent some soil samples to Eli Lilly where erythromycin was isolated from a strain of *Streptomyces erythreus,* which produced erythromycin as a metabolic product (1). Commercially, the company launched the product in 1952 under the brand name Ilosone to honor the discovery of Iloilo.

Although erythromycin and a similar compound, troleandomycin, had excellent antibacterial activity, their relatively poor bioavailability, unpredictable pharmacokinetics, and low stability in the acidic pH of the stomach, as well as uncomfortable gastrointestinal side effects prompted early searches for new derivatives with improved properties. Of note, troleandomycin (no longer sold) is a CYP3A4 inhibitor affecting drug metabolism and its use caused hepatic dysfunction. Taking advantage of erythromycin's binding to the gastrointestinal motilin receptor, it is now used as a prokinetic for some patients with delayed gastric emptying.

The antibiotic clarithromycin was invented by scientists at the Japanese drug company Taisho Pharmaceutical in the 1970s as a result of efforts to overcome the acid instability of erythromycin (2). Hoechst Marion Roussel in France synthesized roxithromycin (3), and azithromycin was synthesized by PLIVA in Croatia (4). Clarithromycin and azithromycin are highly marketed worldwide.

Early studies suggesting the immunomodulatory properties of these antibiotics reach back to the late 1950s when erythromycin and especially troleandomycin were observed to be "steroid-sparing" agents when used for patients with asthma who required regular systemic corticosteroids for disease control (5). However, it was in the early 1980s when Miazawa and Kudo in Japan first exploited these properties for the therapy of diffuse panbronchiolitis (6) as detailed in a later chapter by Taniuchi and Azuma.

Much has happened in the 40 years since this discovery with greater understanding of the potential immunomodulatory mechanisms and effective use, in particular for neutrophil-dominated inflammation. We bring much of this information together in this book.

Richmond, USA Bruce K. Rubin

References

[1] https://www.thenewstoday.info/2005/05/03/iloilonews3.htm
[2] Morimoto S, Nagate T, Sugita K, Ono T, Numata K, Miyachi J, Misawa Y, Yamada K, Omura S. Chemical modification of erythromycins. III. In vitro and in vivo antibacterial activities of new semisynthetic 6-O-methylerythromycins A, TE-031 (clarithromycin) and TE-032. J Antibiot (Tokyo) 1990;43(3):295-305.
[3] Chantot JF, Bryskier A, Gasc JC. Antibacterial activity of roxithromycin: a laboratory evaluation. J Antibiot (Tokyo). 1986;39(5):660-8
[4] Retsema J, Girard A, Schelkly W, Manousos M, Anderson M, Bright G, Borovoy R, Brennan L, Mason R. Spectrum and mode of action of azithromycin (CP-62,993), a new 15-membered-ring macrolide with improved potency against gram-negative organisms. Antimicrob Agents Chemother 1987;31(12): 1939-47
[5] Kaplan MA and Golden M. The use of triacetyloleandomycin in chronic infectious asthma. Antibiotic Annual 1958-1959. New York, Interscience Publishers. pp 273-276
[6] Kudoh S. Applying lessons learned in the treatment of diffuse panbronchiolitis to other chronic inflammatory diseases. Am J Med 2004; 117 (Suppl 9A):12S–19S

Contents

Part I Mechanisms of Action and Novel Macrolides

Macrolides and Diseases Associated with Loss of Epithelial Barrier Integrity 3
Clive P. Page, Fridrik R. Gardarsson, Jennifer A. Kricker, Thorarinn Gudjonsson, Virginia Norris, and Michael J. Parnham

Macrolides and Inflammatory Cells, Signaling, and Mediators 25
Mitsuko Kondo

Part II Clinical Use for Airway Disease

Macrolides as Immunomodulatory Agents 45
Namiko Taniuchi and Arata Azuma

Macrolides and Cystic Fibrosis 59
Rishi Pabary, Adam Jaffe, and Andrew Bush

Non-CF Bronchiectasis 93
Dustin Mills, Anne B. Chang, and Julie M. Marchant

Macrolide Use in Chronic Obstructive Pulmonary Disease 115
Iwein Gyselinck and Wim Janssens

Macrolides and Asthma Therapy 149
Krishna Undela, Adil Adatia, Brian H. Rowe, and Giovanni Ferrara

Macrolides and Interstitial Lung Diseases 161
Yu Hara and Takeshi Kaneko

Macrolides in Acute Respiratory Distress Syndrome and Acute Lung Injury 177
Kodai Kawamura

Azithromycin for Other Lung Diseases: Lung Transplantation and Sarcoidosis 195
Geert M. Verleden and Stijn E. Verleden

Macrolides for Rhinosinusitis and Nasal Polyps 207
Isao Suzaki

Part III Clinical Use for Other Diseases

Macrolides for Cancer 223
Masahiro Shinoda

Macrolides in Chronic Skin Disorders 255
Yozo Ishiuji

Macrolide Use in Preschool-Aged Children with Acute or Recurrent Respiratory Tract Illnesses with Wheezing 271
Lauren D. Benton and Fernando D. Martinez

Macrolides and Immunomodulation: Today and the Future 283
Masaharu Shinkai

Part I
Mechanisms of Action and Novel Macrolides

Macrolides and Diseases Associated with Loss of Epithelial Barrier Integrity

Clive P. Page, Fridrik R. Gardarsson, Jennifer A. Kricker, Thorarinn Gudjonsson, Virginia Norris, and Michael J. Parnham

Abstract *In addition to the antiinflammatory/immunoregulatory actions of macrolide antibiotics, more recent investigations indicate the potential barrier-protective effects of these drugs on the epithelium.* This chapter builds on and expands the chapters on the cytoprotective effects of macrolides, on airway epithelial cells, and on mucoregulatory effects of this drug class on the respiratory mucosa, which were published in 2005 in a previous PIR volume on Antibiotics as antiinflammatory and immunoregulatory agents. Birkhäuser Basel, Basel, 2005 (75); Takeyama K, in: Antibiotics as antiinflammatory and immunomodulatory agents [Internet]. Birkhäuser Basel, Basel, 2005; 96). We consider here the accumulated clinical literature on the subject, including more recent publications since the last PIR review, which particularly concern azithromycin and its efficacy in the treatment of patients with asthma and chronic obstructive pulmonary disease (COPD). We also mention possible effects of barrier-protective macrolides on the dermal and gut epithelium, suggesting their potential for efficacy in the treatment of skin and gut diseases associated with epithelial barrier injury.

Keywords Epithelial integrity · Barrier function · Epithelial cells · Barrier failure · Nonantibiotic macrolides · Azithromycin

---

C. P. Page
Sackler Institute of Pulmonary Pharmacology, King's College London, London, UK

F. R. Gardarsson · J. A. Kricker · V. Norris
EpiEndo Pharmaceuticals, Reykjavik, Iceland

T. Gudjonsson
University of Iceland, Faculty of Medicine and Landspitali, University Hospital, Reykjavik, Iceland

M. J. Parnham (✉)
EpiEndo Pharmaceuticals, Reykjavik, Iceland

Faculty of Chemistry, Biochemistry and Pharmacy, Goethe University Frankfurt am Main, Frankfurt am Main, Germany
e-mail: mjp@epiendo.com

B. K. Rubin, M. Shinkai (eds.), *Macrolides as Immunomodulatory Agents*, Progress in Inflammation Research 92, https://doi.org/10.1007/978-3-031-42859-3_1

1 Introduction

Since 2000, azithromycin has become the main macrolide investigated for pharmacological effects beyond antibiosis. Its demonstrated efficacy now covers the treatment of patients with asthma and chronic obstructive pulmonary disease (COPD) [1–4], patients exposed to various airborne viral infections [5–7], and other diseases associated with loss of epithelial barrier integrity.

This current review will consider the characteristics of the epithelial barrier and the in vivo and in vitro evidence for the effects of macrolides on epithelium that may contribute to their clinical efficacy in a range of diseases known to be associated with epithelial dysfunction, including those in the skin, as well as data suggesting their potential for efficacy in the gut. A novel class of modified macrolides or so-called "Barriolides" exemplified by EP395, an azithromycin-related macrolide with reduced antimicrobial resistance potential, that recently entered early clinical development targeting chronic airway disease (CAD), will also be discussed [6].

2 Epithelial Barrier Failure, a Common Pathophysiological Feature of Various Chronic Inflammatory Diseases

Epithelial integrity and barrier failure are emerging as fundamental determining factors for health and disease in a range of organs [8]. While the major focus in diseases involving injury to the epithelium has been placed on the involvement of inflammatory cells and the vascular endothelium in the past, more recently, the concept of epithelial barrier dysfunction as the basis for disease progression has been proposed, particularly by Akdis and his colleagues in their recent treatise on the epithelial barrier hypothesis [9]. Others, such as Georas and colleagues in the USA, have conducted research in patients with asthma to address a "barrier failure" hypothesis [10, 11]. Loss of epithelial integrity or barrier failure is now recognized as a feature of a number of chronic inflammatory diseases including COPD, asthma, cystic fibrosis (CF), dermatitis, inflammatory bowel disease (IBD), and diseases associated with lung injury such as acute respiratory distress syndrome (ARDS) and sepsis, and is postulated as the underlying defect responsible for infective exacerbations, poor resolution and fibrosis [9].

The increasing interest in the epithelial integrity paradigm both in academia and the pharmaceutical industry is indicated by the growing number of patents and publications appearing in this field over the last five decades (Fig. 1). Furthermore, several pharma and biotech companies are now developing drug classes targeting the epithelium for the treatment of a range of disorders [12].

This relatively recent introduction of agents developed based on epithelial pharmacology and the use of endpoints investigating barrier integrity in inflammation research programs has been aided by recent advances in our understanding of epithelial biology (discussed below). The stem cell revolution of the nineties with

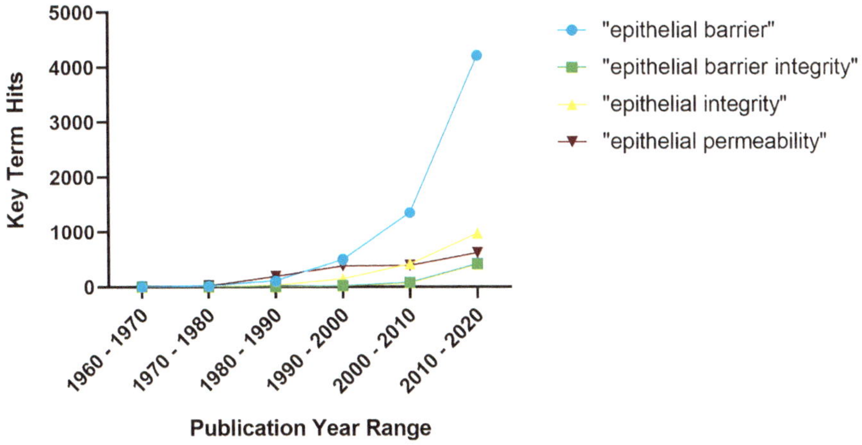

Fig. 1 Evident increase in epithelial terms by decade in publications cited in PubMed

its transformative effects on tissue culture technology and organoid development coupled with the equally transformative effects that genomics, as well as other omics, have had in recent years on analytical capabilities on all fronts of biology research has also impacted investigations of epithelial cell biology. In the last 20 years, modern epithelial cell culture systems have created ways that did not exist before to detect and analyze the epithelial pharmacology of test compounds independently of immune cell pharmacology, antibiotic potency, or any other nonepithelial effects in laboratory settings.

2.1 *Epithelial Homeostasis, Remodeling, and Barrier Failure*

All epithelial tissues share unifying structural and functional features like hexagonal orientation and ongoing cellular renewal, as well as their undisrupted continuity, which provides separation between the external environment and the body's interior tissues, acting as a contiguous surface for all organs and a lining for other tissues.

The epithelium is generally capable of remodeling itself and is often the first line of defense against the external environment. It is widely distributed and is the key surface lining in organs such as the airways, skin, and the gastrointestinal tract, whereby its varying architecture reflects its different functions. Apical to basolateral polarity, as in the upper airways and in the gastrointestinal tract, and the stratified squamous epithelium of the skin are pivotal to the barrier function of the epithelium and its organ-specific functions.

2.1.1 Airway Epithelium

In the respiratory tract, the epithelium changes from being pseudostratified in the upper airways to cuboidal in the lower bronchioles and simple squamous epithelium in the alveoli (Fig. 2). The pseudostratified epithelium is responsible for the mucociliary clearing of particles and infectious agents. Goblet cells produce mucus which entraps infectious/hazardous agents and ciliated cells produce a thin periciliary fluid, which with the help of the beating cilia, move the mucus up the respiratory tract to be expelled through the mouth or nose. Macrolide antibiotics such as azithromycin are well known to inhibit the secretion of mucus by the airway epithelium [13, 14]. Basal cells are responsible for the renewal of both ciliated and goblet cells in the trachea and large bronchi [15]. In the lower bronchi, the epithelium has a simple cuboidal structure, with club cells replacing the basal cells as the stem or progenitor cells [16]. The bronchioles open into the air-filled alveoli that are composed of a thin layer of alveolar type 1 cells with cuboidal type 2 cells distributed in between. Whereas the type 1 alveolar cells are responsible for the gas exchange, type 2 cells produce surfactants to prevent the alveoli collapsing. They are also the progenitor cells for new type 1 cells [17]. The epithelial barrier is generated by the ability of epithelial cells to form tight contact to each other via various adhesion proteins, most notably the tight junction complexes. Tight junctions formed by epithelial cells regulate the paracellular flux and infiltration of leukocytes, and are also important in generating apical-basal polarity by controlling the distribution of phospholipids and transmembrane proteins within the semi-fluid cell membrane [18]. The tight junctions are formed by a variety of adhesion molecules, including transmembrane proteins, claudins, occludins, and junctional adhesion molecules (JAM), which are linked to the actin cytoskeleton through scaffold proteins, most notably, zonula occludens (ZO-1 to −3), cingulin, and afadin [19]. These, in turn, are regulated by cytokines, which cause junction modifications during inflammation. Together with numerous other proteins involved in cell signaling, they form the intracellular tight junction plaques [20]. As discussed below in sect. 2.2, azithromycin has been shown to modify airway epithelial tight junction molecule expression.

Loss of epithelial integrity/barrier failure also increases during aging. Indeed, aging results in reduced lung function which makes the elderly more vulnerable to chronic lung diseases. Aging reduces the mucociliary clearance, thus weakening the epithelial barrier, which makes older people more prone to infections such as pneumonia [21]. Recently, Angelidis et al. used single cell transcriptomic and mass-spectrometry proteomics to quantify changes in 30 lung cell types in young and old mice. They demonstrated significant changes in gene regulation and cellular remodeling that may affect the epithelial barrier [22]. Several respiratory diseases affect the epithelial barrier including COPD, CF, and asthma with cigarette smoking and other types of oxidant pollution being the main causes of COPD. Cigarette smoking facilitates goblet cell hyperplasia and disrupts tight junctions resulting in

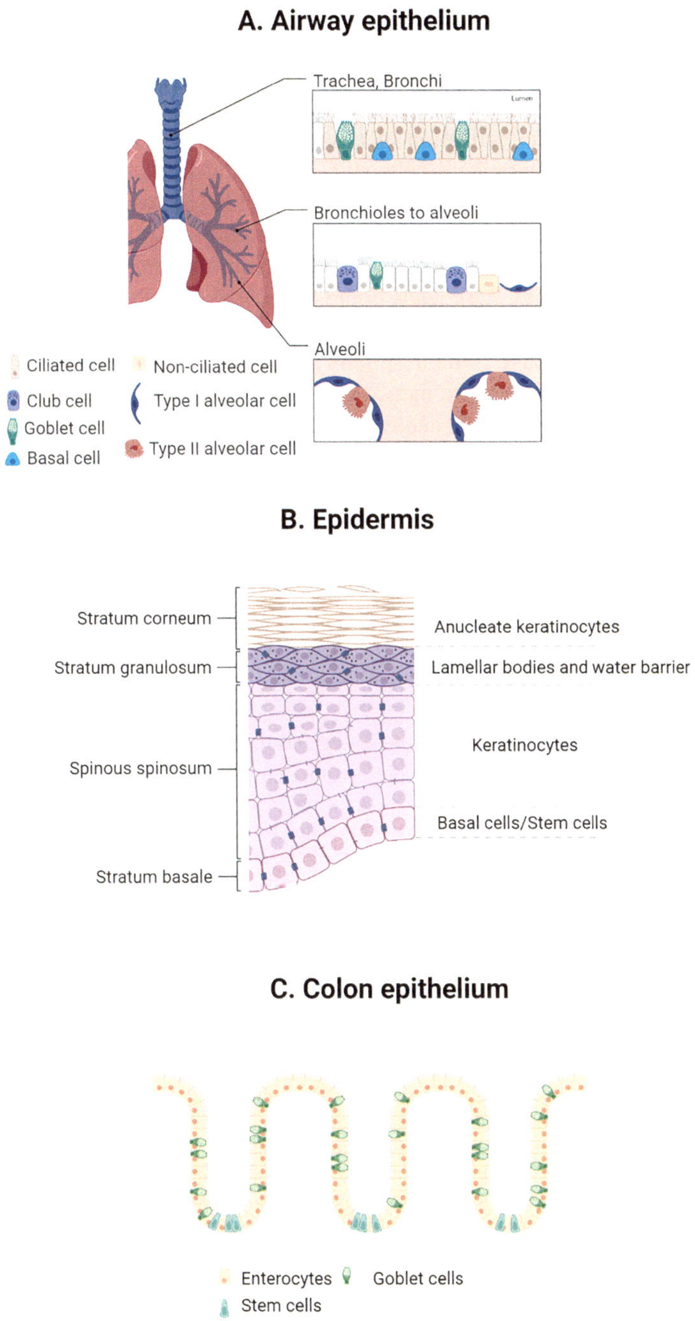

Fig. 2 The epithelial barrier in airway, skin, and gut. (**a**) The airway epithelium varies from the pseudostratified layer in the bronchi to the single squamous layer in the alveoli. It extends from the trachea and large bronchi to the smaller bronchioles and alveoli. The epithelium thus, forms a continuous layer that protects the underlying interstitial connective tissue from pathogens and pollutant-rich external air. In the trachea and large bronchi, the pseudostratified layers are composed

suboptimal epithelial barrier integrity, mainly as a result of direct oxidant damage and inflammation with loss of tight junction integrity [23–25].

In bronchial asthma, repeated injury to the airway mucosal barrier enhances mucosal permeability to pathogens and injurious chemicals. This epithelial barrier damage results from the activation of airway epithelial cells, dendritic cells, and innate group 2 innate lymphoid cells (ILC2), leading to the release of epithelial cytokines, such as thymic stromal lymphopoietin (TSLP), as well as interleukins IL-25, and IL-33 and to a Th2-biased inflammatory response. The associated infiltration and activation of inflammatory cells from the circulation, also reduced by azithromycin (see sect. 2.4), leads to the characteristic hallmarks of asthma [26] (Fig. 3).

Upon epithelial damage in the respiratory tract, basal, club, and type 2 alveolar cells are activated collectively to induce a recovery phase and healing of the barrier by generating new differentiated and functionally active cells. This recovery phase is activated very rapidly as epithelial barrier failure allows infectious agents and other materials from the external environment such as allergens or pollutant particles to enter the subepithelial stroma, triggering an inflammatory response and/or infection of submucosal tissues that may exacerbate further tissue damage. Thus, finding drugs that enhance the integrity of the epithelial barrier in the airways of people with underlying airway diseases such as COPD may reduce the risk of exacerbations, reduce symptoms and improve the quality of life.

Fig. 2 (continued) of mucociliary epithelium and basal cells which represent progenitor cells. In the bronchioles, club cells replace the basal cells as the progenitor cells. The distal part of the airway epithelium terminates in the alveoli where gas exchange takes place. The type II alveolar cells are responsible for surfactant production and also for the generation of new type I alveolar cells that are responsible for gas exchange. In vitro and in vivo work indicates that azithromycin may enhance the epithelial barrier via tight junction remodeling, enhancing epithelial cell growth, and differentiation, reducing epithelial-derived proinflammatory cytokines, and reducing mucus (see sect. 4) (**b**) The epidermis forms stratified squamous epithelium. The epidermis is composed of four layers of epithelial cells (keratinocytes). Stratum basale sits on top of the basement membrane, which separates the epidermis from the underlying dermis. Keratinocyte stem cells (basal cells) are located in the stratum basale. These stem cells give rise to keratinocytes which move up to the stratum spinosum. In the stratum spinosum, interconnections between cells are apparent, presumably through desmosomes. Keratinocytes differentiate further and move up to the stratum granulosum. This layer forms the water barrier. Keratinocytes are filled with lipids packed in lamellar bodies that make this layer highly hydrophobic and which may possibly be enhanced by barrier-protective macrolides (cf sect. 5.3). At the interface of the stratum granulosum and stratum corneum, keratinocytes undergo keratinization which is a specific form of apoptosis, losing their nuclei and other cellular organelles and accumulate to form the keratin- and lipid-rich stratum corneum. (**c**) The colon epithelium forms a columnar single-layer barrier. The colon epithelium is mainly composed of absorptive enterocytes, mucin-producing goblet cells, and stem cells located at the bottom of the crypt. The stem cells give rise to new enterocytes and goblet cells. Microfold (M) cells and enteroendocrine cells are also found within the colon epithelium (not shown in this figure), where they contribute to the immune and hormonal systems, respectively. Potential sites of action of barrier-protective macrolides in the gut have yet to be determined. Figures generated by BioRender.com

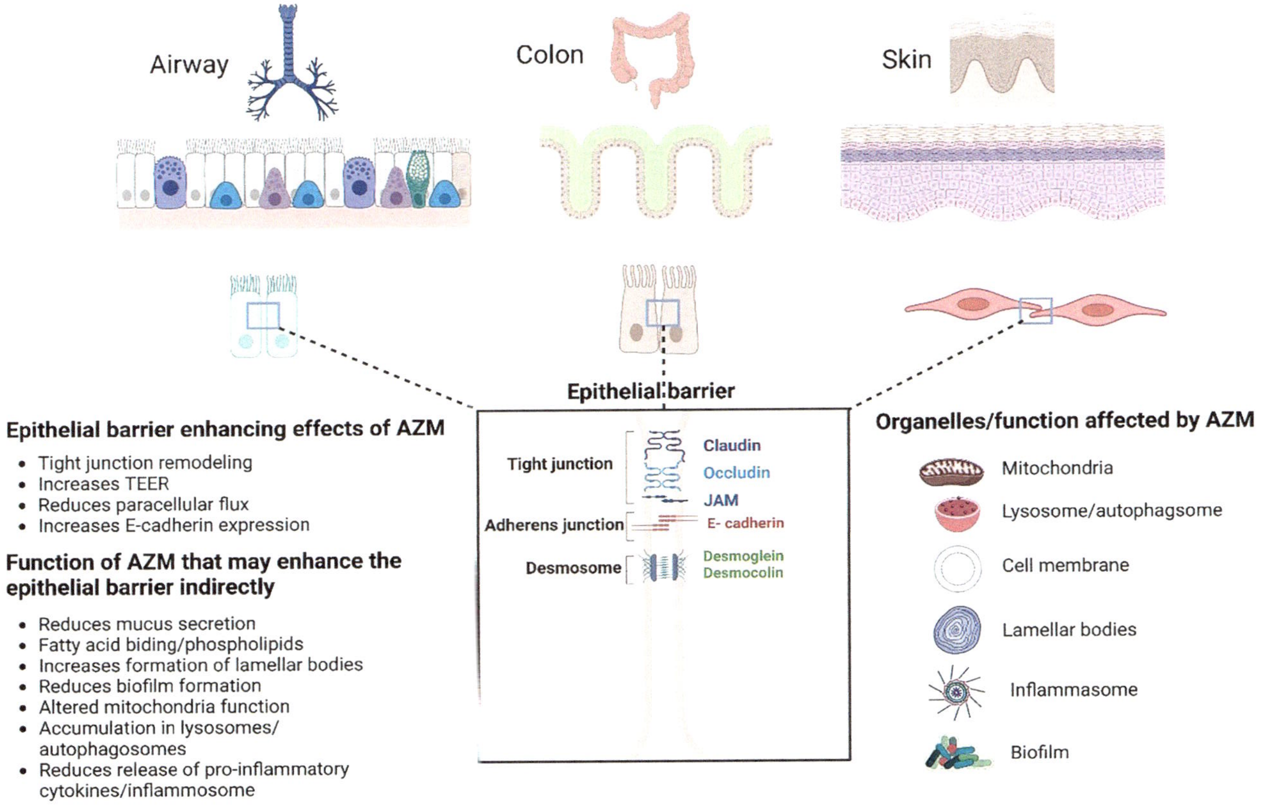

Fig. 3 Macrolides, especially azithromycin (AZM), interfere with a number of cellular organelles and signaling pathways to elicit their effects in epithelial and other cells. Binding to membrane phospholipids, probably by charge interactions, activates a series of signaling cascades resulting in altered gene regulation. As a result of intracellular macrolide accumulation, particularly in lysosomes, lipid accumulation occurs with lamellar body formation and alterations in

2.1.2 Epidermis

The cellular turnover in the stratified squamous epithelium, the epidermis, is fast and requires active stem or progenitor cells to generate new keratinocytes [27]. The keratinocyte stem cells sit on the basement membrane in the stratum basale [28] and give rise to keratinocytes which reach maximal differentiation in the stratum granulosum, forming the water barrier. The water barrier between the stratum granulosum and stratum corneum is composed of accumulated lipids (e.g., phospholipids, glucosylceramide, sphingomyelin, and cholesterol) that together with proteins form lamellar bodies (LBs) [28–31]. These stratified layers are of major importance for the barrier function of the skin and help prevent transepidermal water loss (TEWL).

Epidermal barrier failure and the accompanying inflammatory response are considered a primary component of skin diseases such as atopic dermatitis (AD), rosacea, and ichthyoses [32–35]. AD, a chronic, relapsing skin disease characterized by dry erythematous lesions and severe itching (pruritis), has a very high prevalence, affecting up to 3% of the worldwide population. Furthermore, the frequency of AD and other atopic diseases has increased by two- to threefold during the past decades in industrialized countries [36, 37]. Histological features of AD include intercellular edema (spongiosis) of the keratinocytes within the stratum spinosum, resulting from a lack of cell-cell binding [38]. Although the cause of AD is unknown, barrier failure and inflammatory responses are both key features of the disease [39]. A hallmark of AD is elevated serum concentrations of allergen-specific IgE antibodies against various inhaled, food, and environmental allergens, probably resulting from the epithelial barrier failure, leading to passage of allergens into the underlying connective tissues which initiate an inflammatory response triggered by cross-linking of allergens with IgE on mast cells [40].

Loss-of-function (LOF) studies on the gene *FLG*, which encodes for the precursor of the filament-associated protein filaggrin, have shown a strong association with AD [41]. LOF *FLG* mutations are also responsible for the onset of ichthyosis vulgaris, the most common skin disorder within ichthyoses (IC). IC are a heterogeneous group of skin diseases sharing the feature of barrier failure leading to water loss and compensatory hyperproliferation of keratinocytes [42]. Common phenotypes include dry skin (xerosis) and scaling, and IC patients are at increased risk for AD, asthma, and other allergic disorders, probably due to the disrupted skin barrier, subsequently allowing easier epidermal penetration of allergens and other external inflammatory stimuli [41]. As in IC and AD, rosacea is also characterized by

Fig. 3 (continued) mitochondrial oxygen consumption. As a consequence of these membrane and intracellular changes, release of cytokines and enzymes is modified. In airway epithelial cells, mucus secretion is decreased, and tight junction proteins are remodeled, resulting in an increase in transepithelial electrical resistance (TEER) with reduced paracellular flux. With time, epithelial growth and differentiation are enhanced, further facilitating the barrier function of the cells. Since junction proteins are crucial to skin and gut epithelium, it is likely that nonantibiotic macrolides will beneficially affect these molecules as well as other epithelial processes

increased TEWL with compromised tight junction proteins, while filaggrin remains unchanged [43, 44]. The pathophysiology of rosacea is still not understood but increased epithelial cell expression of cathelicidin (LL-37) and IL-33 play a key role, together with increased expression of vascular endothelial growth factor (VEGF) [45]. The epithelium of the skin, although multilayered compared to airway and gut, is susceptible to breaches of the barrier resulting in imbalance and subsequent inflammation.

2.1.3 Intestinal and Colon Epithelium

The intestine and colon epithelium are composed of multiple cell types. In the intestine, large folding of the epithelium generates villi and crypts. Cellular remodeling is undertaken in the crypts where stem cells deep in the crypts generate daughter cells that differentiate either downwards to become Paneth cells (intestine) or upwards to generate enterocytes, goblet cells and enteroendocrine cells [46]. The epithelial barrier in the gut is of great importance for maintaining homeostasis of the gastrointestinal tract, and barrier failure contributes to a variety of conditions such as leaky gut [47, 48], and inflammatory bowel diseases (IBD) such as Crohn's disease [49], ulcerative colitis [50] and celiac disease [51]. A common denominator of barrier failure in the gut is the aberrant regulation of tight junctions [51]. Recently, Parikh et al. used single-cell profiling to demonstrate the intestinal and colonic epithelial diversity in normal gut and epithelial cells derived from patients with IBD [52]. At the top of the crypts, they found a previously unknown absorptive cell, expressing the proton channel otopetrin 2 (OTOP2) and the satiety peptide uroguanylin, that senses pH and is dysregulated in inflammation. In IBD, they observed a positional remodeling of goblet cells that coincides with the downregulation of WFDC2-an antiprotease molecule that they found to be expressed by goblet cells and that preserves the integrity of tight junctions and prevents the invasion of bacteria and inflammation [52]. The expression patterns of various claudins, expressed both by gut epithelial and other mesodermal cells, have been investigated in both humans and in murine models of IBD and shown to reflect the interactions between the different cells involved in the disease [53].

It is apparent, therefore, that tight junctions play an important role in maintaining gut epithelial integrity. Others have shown that increased expression of claudin 2 increases paracellular flux [54], whilst the reduced function of occludin has been linked to increased barrier failure. IL-13 has been shown to increase claudin 2 expression resulting in increased paracellular flux, and TNF-alpha has been shown to induce the activity of myosin light chain kinase (MLCK) that further induces caveoli endocytosis of occludin resulting in increased leakiness of the gut [55]. Based on the importance of the epithelial barrier for healthy organs, drugs that maintain and/or increase the strength of the epithelial integrity may therefore be of great importance in a range of diseases of the airways, skin, and gastrointestinal tract and potentially open to therapy with barrier-protecting macrolides.

3 In Vitro Models to Study Epithelial Integrity and the Mechanism of Action of Macrolides

Advanced cell culture models are useful tools for studying epithelial biology both in health and disease. Since many epithelial tissues are exposed to hazardous environments, cell culture models have been useful in analyzing the effects of various toxicants and infectious agents on epithelial cells. Furthermore, these cell culture models now provide convenient assays for analyzing the efficacy of drugs as they can provide simple readout assays allowing for the reasonably rapid screening of large numbers of compounds. Testing cell viability in conventional monolayer culture is simple and fast. However, monolayer cultures have limitations, such as a lack of an in vivo-like environment, cellular phenotype plasticity, and association with the micro-environment [56]. For analysis of epithelial barrier integrity, culturing cells on transwell filters can provide a good option, either as liquid–liquid (LL) or air–liquid interface (ALI) cell culture. ALI cultures are suitable for analysis of the barrier integrity of the airway, gastrointestinal, and skin epithelium. ALI cultures are generated by initiating cell culture in liquid-liquid conditions on coated porous filters representing a basement membrane, and after a few days in culture, media is removed from the apical compartment, which allows for further differentiation into organotypic structures.

Regarding airway epithelium, culture of basal cells in ALI conditions results in pseudostratified-like histology. This is demonstrated by formation of apical-basolateral polarity, and formation of goblet and ciliated cells [57, 58]. Tight junctions are responsible for the apical to basolateral polarity of the cells and fencing, meaning they form the tight barrier between epithelial cells, which controls the paracellular flux between cells. A simple readout for barrier integrity in ALI cultures is to measure transepithelial electrical resistance (TEER) and paracellular flux (p-flux). Thus, increased TEER and reduced p-flux are good indicators of a functionally active barrier maintained by tight junctions and other adhesion molecules [59]. Additional readout assays include RNA sequencing, proteomic, ELISA, and metabolomic analysis. Mimicking the appropriate in vivo-like phenotype in vitro as closely as possible is of great importance as this allows for a better understanding of the communication between cells and histological appearance and allows investigation of the effect of external stimuli and drugs on the function of the epithelial barrier.

Reflecting in vivo pathological conditions in cell models using challenging assays can be a useful tool to either investigate the clinical condition in question or to study drugs or methods to ameliorate the clinical condition. It can be said that there are broadly three categories of challenging assays, biological, chemical, and mechanical. Biological assays include challenging the cell culture model with inflammatory cytokines and fibrosis-inducing agents such as TGFβ [60]. Chemical challenging can be performed using, for instance, EDTA, to bind calcium and subsequently impair cell-to-cell adhesion properties [61]. Mechanical challenging includes insults such as stretching cell models or increasing pressure in a way that deforms the cells, mimicking, for instance, what happens in ventilator-induced lung injury [62]. The challenge, however, needs to be adapted carefully to the cell type used, as bacterial lipopolysaccharide (LPS), for instance, does not exert the same response in different cell lines [63].

Using ALI cultures, it has been shown how azithromycin enhances the epithelial barrier by increasing TEER, an indicator of a strong barrier [64, 65], and in lung epithelial cells, it was shown that this drug also induces epidermal differentiation and the formation of lamellar bodies [66], which may be useful pharmacological properties to explain the effectiveness of macrolides in a number of diseases discussed below.

4 Macrolides and the Epithelial Barrier

Macrolide antibiotics as a class of drugs are known to have numerous additional non-antibacterial effects, such as immunomodulatory/antiinflammatory activity, targeted mainly at neutrophils and macrophages, together with the ability to enhance epithelial barrier function [6]. They inhibit adhesion, diapedesis, and activation of leukocytes, reducing inflammation, as well as reducing the epithelial-to-mesenchymal transition which occurs in fibrosis. In addition, they promote the formation of M2 macrophages – involved in active resolution of inflammation – and enhance the differentiation of epithelial cells, while regulating airway mucus hypersecretion [6]. Azithromycin, particularly, has been shown in bronchial epithelial cells to enhance processing of the tight junction proteins, claudin-1 and claudin-4, occludin, and junctional adhesion molecule-A, enhance intracellular lipid generation and to promote cell differentiation, all of which facilitate epithelial barrier function as observed by increased transepithelial resistance and decreased permeability [64, 66]. The actions of macrolides in modulating the production by airway epithelial cells of the neutrophil chemotactic and activating cytokine, interleukin-8 (IL-8) and inhibiting the secretion of mucus from airway secretory cells, in part by inhibition of MUC5AC, further contribute to protection of the epithelium from injury, including that to cigarette smoke [6, 67, 68]. Azithromycin has also been reported to inhibit, in human airway epithelial cells, the stimulation by the viral product polyinosinic-polycytidylic (poly (I:C)) acid of the T2-biasing cytokine TSLP, a response of potential therapeutic benefit in asthma [69]. Moreover, in a rat ovalbumin-induced asthma model, azithromycin promoted epithelial thickening and inhibited epithelial apoptosis [70].

It is of interest therefore, that recently, EpiEndo Pharmaceuticals has developed EP395, a macrolide with greatly reduced antimicrobial activity which has entered clinical development. This is the first macrolide analogue to have entered clinical trials for the treatment of nonbacterial airway diseases since solithromycin was tested for non-antibacterial efficacy in patients with COPD and terminated due to tolerability issues [71]. While solithromycin is a 14-membered fluoroketolide with good antibiotic potency, but a poor long-term safety profile, EP395 is an azithromycin-related, nitrogen-containing, 15-membered macrolactone that has been structurally and functionally optimized away from the antimicrobial class effects of macrolides, to minimize induction of host flora resistance [72, 73]. The compound has effects on epithelial barrier function, enhancing epithelial integrity, as well as possessing antiinflammatory actions that are shared by other 14- and 15-membered macrolides that have proven efficacy in patients with diffuse panbronchiolitis (DPB). Importantly, EP395 exhibits augmented barrier-modulating pharmacology in vitro compared to azithromycin, but similar effects have not been observed for erythromycin in the same assay [64, 73]. Moreover, inhibitory actions of EP395 on murine lung injury induced in vivo by cigarette smoke or SO_2 are commensurate with its epithelial barrier-protecting effect [72].

5 Macrolide-Sensitive Inflammatory Diseases

5.1 Distinctions between Macrolide Antibiotics

There has been an ongoing interest in clarifying the disease modifying pharmacology of macrolides ever since the late sixties and seventies when the dramatic antiinflammatory and even curative effect of erythromycin on DPB was recognized in Japan [74]. As DPB has an essentially unknown etiology and the exact pathophysiology is still not completely understood, it has remained unclear which of the multiple pharmacological properties of azithromycin, erythromycin, and other macrolides are responsible for this clinical benefit of a relatively rapid remission of inflammation and suppression of further disease progression [75–77].

However, it seems likely that the disease-modifying efficacy of macrolides on inflammatory responses lies within the 14-membered and 15-membered analogues, since the 16-membered compounds are not disease modifying in DPB or other macrolide-sensitive indications [78]. The potential efficacy of solithromycin, a 14-membered fluoroketolide, was investigated against non-bacterial airway diseases, but this drug was not well tolerated on long-term use and the trial was terminated due to safety issues when tested in patients with COPD [71].

In this regard, it is of interest therefore, that a patient with DPB who did not respond to erythromycin therapy did respond to clarithromycin [79], while in contrast the 16-membered josamycin, despite having prominent 14-membered like PMNC inhibitory effects, has been found to be clinically ineffective in treating DPB [78]. It is worth mentioning, in this context, that clarithromycin, in addition to its well-established antiinflammatory/immunomodulatory actions, also exerts beneficial effects on epithelial cell function [67]. Thus, it seems likely that both the 14-membered and 15-membered macrolide antibiotics share features essential for treating most cases with DPB, while those experimental antiinflammatory features shared by them with josamycin appear less important for therapeutic benefit in DPB [75, 78].

Nevertheless, beyond shared properties, each structure has distinct pharmacological characteristics differing from those of the others, depending on the assays and models of inflammation used. It is also unclear what specific pharmaceutical properties of macrolides are more relevant than others in macrolide-sensitive disease indications. Moreover, no statistically significant head-to-head studies exist to help in discerning whether one of the 14-membered or the 15-membered azalide structures is generally more effective than the others in any of the sensitive indications. Nevertheless, it is relevant in this context that clarithromycin is inactive in progressive CF lung disease, a condition repeatedly shown to be sensitive to azithromycin [80].

In view of the supportive data and despite the absence of direct head-to-head trial designs for any of the macrolide-sensitive indications, azithromycin seems to have become the go-to macrolide for off-label use, at least for some airway conditions, for example, GOLD (COPD) and GINA (asthma), [81, 82]. This is noteworthy as azithromycin was not introduced onto the market until 1988 and by then already much of the evidence for the 14-membered macrolides in DPB and CF had been established.

Consequently, the structural basis for most early documented attempts to develop non-antibiotic macrolides was the 14-membered ring. These compounds emulated the erythromycin-like effects on macrophages and neutrophils, their activation, chemotaxis, and reactive functions, while the 15-membered azithromycin-like structure has dominated more recent novel structural approaches. A summary of past attempts to develop non-antibiotic macrolides was given recently by Kricker et al. [6].

5.2 *Macrolide Antibiotics in COPD and Asthma*

Arising from the initial studies on DPB, there has been interest in the clinical utility of macrolides in the treatment of several respiratory diseases, including COPD, asthma, chronic allergic rhinosinusitis, non-CF bronchiectasis, CF, and cryptogenic organizing pneumonia (COP), previously termed bronchiolitis obliterans organizing pneumonia (BOOP) [83]. More detailed discussions of the use of macrolides in specific disorders are given in other chapters in this present volume. We focus here on the key clinical studies in patients with asthma and COPD, which are clearly associated with epithelial injury, and these are summarized below.

In asthma, small clinical trials have looked at the effects of macrolides on markers of inflammation. For example, it has been shown that 8 weeks of treatment with clarithromycin reduced IL-8 and neutrophilic inflammation in the sputum of patients with refractory asthma. The effect was most marked in those with refractory non-eosinophilic asthma [84]. In children on maintenance inhaled fluticasone propionate, 4 weeks treatment with clarithromycin reduced eosinophilic inflammation as assessed by blood levels of eosinophils and ECP [85]. In the AMAZES trial, 48 weeks of azithromycin reduced the number of combined moderate and severe exacerbations compared to placebo (1.07 versus 1.86 events/patient/year; incidence rate ratio 0.59 (95% CI 0.47–0.74) in patients with symptomatic asthma despite ICS/LABA therapy [2]. Subgroup analysis of the AMAZES trial indicated that azithromycin is effective at reducing exacerbations in both eosinophilic and non-eosinophilic asthma [86]. ERS/ATS guidelines suggest consideration of a trial macrolide treatment to reduce asthma exacerbations in adult asthma subjects on step 5 therapy that remain persistently symptomatic or uncontrolled. The potential benefit should be carefully considered against the risk of the emergence of antimicrobial resistance at both the individual patient and wider community levels. In the GINA treatment guidelines, in patients with no evidence of type 2 inflammation, a trial of low dose macrolide is a treatment option for consideration [82]. In this respect, it is worth noting the results of a study in mice sensitized to house dust mite (HDM), then exposed to poly(I:C), as a model of asthma complicated with viral infection. Four days oral treatment with 25 mg/kg of the non-antibiotic, 14-membered macrolide EM900 resulted in significant reduction of bronchial airway lavage fluid (BALF) of all cell counts, including the predominant eosinophils, and concentrations of the type 2 inflammatory cytokines IL-13, IL-5, RANTES, IL-17A, and MIP-2 [87]. These data indicate that the use of non-antibiotic macrolides is also likely to be of benefit in allergic airway inflammation.

In a small study ($n = 30$) in patients with COPD and neutrophilic bronchitis, patients were randomized to azithromycin 250 mg a day or placebo for 12 weeks. Azithromycin treatment resulted in a non-significant reduction in sputum neutrophils and IL-8 levels [88]. In a randomized, double-blind, placebo-controlled study in 109 COPD patients, 250 mg of erythromycin twice daily for 12 months reduced moderate to severe exacerbations compared to placebo [89]. Two studies have also been conducted looking at azithromycin on exacerbations in COPD patients. In the first such study performed, 1142 patients at risk of exacerbation were randomized to receive either 250 mg once a day or placebo for 1 year, in addition to their usual care. The median time to the first exacerbation was 266 days (95% confidence interval [CI], 227 to 313), among participants receiving azithromycin, as compared with 174 days (95% CI, 143 to 215) among participants receiving placebo ($P < 0.001$). The frequency of exacerbations was 1.48 exacerbations per patient-year in the azithromycin group, as compared with 1.83 per patient-year in the placebo group ($P = 0.01$) [1]. In a second study, COPD patients with 3 or more exacerbations in the previous year were randomized to azithromycin 500 mg three times a week ($n = 47$) or placebo ($n = 45$) for 12 months. Eighty-four exacerbations were recorded in the azithromycin group compared with 129 in the placebo group. Azithromycin resulted in a significant reduction in the exacerbation rate versus placebo (0·58, 95% CI 0·42–0·79; $p = 0{\cdot}001$) [4]. Interestingly, a sub-analysis of this study suggests that COPD patients with higher blood eosinophils (≥2%) derive greater benefit in terms of lower number of exacerbations and hospitalizations compared to those with blood eosinophils <2% [90]. Treatment recommendations suggest consideration of azithromycin in patients who continue to exacerbate despite LABA/LAMA treatment if blood eosinophil counts are <100 cells/μl (i.e., those who are unlikely to derive benefit from ICS) or those who continue to exacerbate despite LABA/LAMA/ICS, particularly if ex-smokers [81].

TSLP is a key epithelial cytokine released in response to multiple triggers, and blocking TSLP with tezepelumab is effective at reducing exacerbations in asthma [91]. The inhibition of TSLP generation from airway epithelium by azithromycin may contribute to its therapeutic benefit in asthma [69], in addition to the other beneficial effects of this drug on airway epithelium described previously.

Given the broad patient populations who derive clinical benefit from azithromycin in terms of exacerbation reduction, taken together with the data from HBEC and poly I:C stimulation, effects on the epithelium could at least in part explain the efficacy of macrolides in reducing exacerbations in asthma and COPD.

5.3 *Macrolides in Other Inflammatory Disorders*

Based on the foregoing discussion, it is likely that macrolide protective effects on the epithelial barrier may also contribute to the therapeutic benefit observed in the topical treatment of rosacea or atopic dermatitis with macrolide dermal formulations, or the oral macrolide therapy of psoriasis [92–94]. While these dermal disorders are also associated with barrier disruption, the effects of macrolides, up till now, have been associated with inhibition of inflammatory cell and mediator reduction and attributed exclusively to either antibacterial or antiinflammatory actions [92]. We have also recently suggested that oral macrolides without antibacterial activity and thus, without adverse effects on the gut microbiome, may also be of benefit in the treatment of epithelial damage in IBD [6]. A recent article connects gut and skin health, showing that fiber-derived short-chain fatty acids formed in the gut promote keratinocyte metabolism and differentiation in keratinocytes from the skin [95]. In this respect, it is worth noting that the beneficial effects of azithromycin on airway epithelial growth and differentiation are associated both with increased expression of a set of 51 genes also associated with epidermal differentiation and with increased deposition of intracellular fatty acids [66], suggesting a potential common mechanism in airway and skin and even intestinal epithelial protection.

In a recent review article from 2019 entitled "Azithromycin is the answer in pediatric respiratory medicine, but what was the question?" the author, Andrew Bush, is critical of the evolution of inappropriate over-prescription and widespread use of macrolides in chronic inflammatory diseases both in children and adults, as such "off-label" therapy leads to extensive resistance formation [76]. Furthermore, he urges the medical and scientific community to focus on better understanding the endotype of inflammatory conditions where the non-antibiotic effects of macrolides have proven to be beneficial beyond DPB and to develop new non-antibiotic macrolides to target strategically these identified endotypes of inflammation [76].

6 Concluding Remarks

The efficacy of macrolides in treating inflammatory disorders, particularly those of the respiratory tract, arose from the serendipitous observation of the dramatic benefit of erythromycin, given as an antibiotic to patients with DPB. In the succeeding years, this therapeutic benefit has been attributed to the antiinflammatory/immunomodulatory actions of erythromycin and of the next generation macrolides, particularly clarithromycin and azithromycin, subsequently developed as antibiotics. As a result, azithromycin has been used widely off-label in the treatment of COPD and asthma, this use supported by several randomized, double-blind, placebo-controlled clinical trials. Evidence, albeit associative, has suggested that such actions may play a role in the effects of macrolides in inflammatory skin disorders.

These findings on immunomodulatory actions of macrolide antibiotics have now been complemented by studies on the role of epithelial cell directed actions. In view of the increasing data on the importance of epithelial cell injury in the pathogenesis of inflammatory respiratory, intestinal and skin disorders, the recent data on the enhancing effects of azithromycin on epithelial barrier protection suggest that this may represent a therapeutically rewarding avenue for novel macrolide development. However, the almost inevitable occurrence of bacterial resistance in response to long-term macrolide antibiotic administration is a constant limitation to this approach. It is likely that the clinical testing of non-antibiotic macrolides, such as EP395, will facilitate the pursual of this possibility.

Conflict of Interest Statement FRG, JAK, MJP, and VN are all employees of EpiEndo Pharmaceuticals. CPP holds equity in Verona Pharma and MJP in Phialogics AG.

Ethical Compliance Statement All published studies reported here that were performed in the authors' laboratories complied with international guidelines.

References

1. Albert RK, Connett J, Bailey WC, Casaburi R, Cooper JA Jr, Criner GJ, et al. Azithromycin for prevention of exacerbations of COPD. N Engl J Med. 2011;365(8):689–98.
2. Gibson PG, Yang IA, Upham JW, Reynolds PN, Hodge S, James AL, et al. Effect of azithromycin on asthma exacerbations and quality of life in adults with persistent uncontrolled asthma (AMAZES): a randomised, double-blind, placebo-controlled trial. Lancet. 2017;390(10095):659–68.
3. Pomares X, Monton C, Espasa M, Casabon J, Monso E, Gallego M. Long-term azithromycin therapy in patients with severe COPD and repeated exacerbations. Int J Chron Obstruct Pulmon Dis. 2011;6:449–56.
4. Uzun S, Djamin RS, Kluytmans JA, Mulder PG, van't Veer NE, Ermens AA, et al. Azithromycin maintenance treatment in patients with frequent exacerbations of chronic obstructive pulmonary disease (COLUMBUS): a randomised, double-blind, placebo-controlled trial. Lancet. Respir Med. 2014;2(5):361–8.

5. Khoshnood S, Shirani M, Dalir A, Moradi M, Haddadi MH, Sadeghifard N, et al. Antiviral effects of azithromycin: a narrative review. Biomed Pharmacother. 2022;147:112682.
6. Kricker JA, Page CP, Gardarsson FR, Baldursson O, Gudjonsson T, Parnham MJ. Nonantimicrobial actions of macrolides: overview and perspectives for future development. Pharmacol Rev. 2021;73(4):233–62.
7. Oliver ME, Hinks TSC. Azithromycin in viral infections. Rev Med Virol. 2020;31:e2163.
8. Parrish AR. The impact of aging on epithelial barriers. Tissue Barriers. 2017;5(4):e1343172.
9. Akdis CA. Does the epithelial barrier hypothesis explain the increase in allergy, autoimmunity and other chronic conditions? Nat Rev Immunol. 2021;21(11):739–51.
10. Georas SN, Rezaee F. Epithelial barrier function: at the front line of asthma immunology and allergic airway inflammation. J Allergy Clin Immunol. 2014;134(3):509–20.
11. Rezaee F, Georas SN. Breaking barriers. New insights into airway epithelial barrier function in health and disease. Am J Respir Cell Mol Biol. 2014;50(5):857–69.
12. Graham WV, He W, Marchiando AM, Zha J, Singh G, Li HS, et al. Intracellular MLCK1 diversion reverses barrier loss to restore mucosal homeostasis. Nat Med. 2019;25(4):690–700.
13. Mann TS, Larcombe AN, Wang KCW, Shamsuddin D, Landwehr KR, Noble PB, et al. Azithromycin inhibits mucin secretion, mucous metaplasia, airway inflammation, and airways hyperresponsiveness in mice exposed to house dust mite extract. Am J Physiol Lung Cell Mol Physiol. 2022;322(5):L683–L98.
14. Shimizu T, Shimizu S. Azithromycin inhibits mucus hypersecretion from airway epithelial cells. Mediat Inflamm. 2012;2012:265714.
15. Parekh KR, Nawroth J, Pai A, Busch SM, Senger CN, Ryan AL. Stem cells and lung regeneration. Am J Physiol Cell Physiol. 2020;319(4):C675–C93.
16. Zuo WL, Shenoy SA, Li S, O'Beirne SL, Strulovici-Barel Y, Leopold PL, et al. Ontogeny and biology of human small airway epithelial Club cells. Am J Respir Crit Care Med. 2018;198(11): 1375–88.
17. Guillot L, Nathan N, Tabary O, Thouvenin G, Le Rouzic P, Corvol H, et al. Alveolar epithelial cells: master regulators of lung homeostasis. Int J Biochem Cell Biol. 2013;45(11):2568–73.
18. Cereijido M, Valdes J, Shoshani L, Contreras RG. Role of tight junctions in establishing and maintaining cell polarity. Annu Rev Physiol. 1998;60:161–77.
19. Kojima T, Go M, Takano K, Kurose M, Ohkuni T, Koizumi J, et al. Regulation of tight junctions in upper airway epithelium. Biomed Res Int. 2013;2013:947072.
20. Paradis T, Begue H, Basmaciyan L, Dalle F, Bon F. Tight junctions as a key for pathogens invasion in intestinal epithelial cells. Int J Mol Sci. 2021;22(5)
21. Bailey KL, Bonasera SJ, Wilderdyke M, Hanisch BW, Pavlik JA, DeVasure J, et al. Aging causes a slowing in ciliary beat frequency, mediated by PKCepsilon. Am J Physiol Lung Cell Mol Physiol. 2014;306(6):L584–9.
22. Angelidis I, Simon LM, Fernandez IE, Strunz M, Mayr CH, Greiffo FR, et al. An atlas of the aging lung mapped by single cell transcriptomics and deep tissue proteomics. Nat Commun. 2019;10(1):963.
23. Schamberger AC, Mise N, Jia J, Genoyer E, Yildirim AO, Meiners S, et al. Cigarette smoke-induced disruption of bronchial epithelial tight junctions is prevented by transforming growth factor-beta. Am J Respir Cell Mol Biol. 2014;50(6):1040–52.
24. Heijink IH, Brandenburg SM, Postma DS, van Oosterhout AJ. Cigarette smoke impairs airway epithelial barrier function and cell-cell contact recovery. Eur Respir J. 2012;39(2):419–28.
25. Strzelak A, Ratajczak A, Adamiec A, Feleszko W. Tobacco smoke induces and alters immune responses in the lung triggering inflammation, allergy, asthma and other lung diseases: a mechanistic review. Int J Environ Res Public Health. 2018;15(5)
26. Gon Y, Hashimoto S. Role of airway epithelial barrier dysfunction in pathogenesis of asthma. Allergol Int. 2018;67(1):12–7.
27. Fuchs E. Skin stem cells: rising to the surface. J Cell Biol. 2008;180(2):273–84.
28. Feingold KR. Lamellar bodies: the key to cutaneous barrier function. J Invest Dermatol. 2012;132(8):1951–3.

29. Braff MH, Di Nardo A, Gallo RL. Keratinocytes store the antimicrobial peptide cathelicidin in lamellar bodies. J Invest Dermatol. 2005;124(2):394–400.
30. Lundwall A, Brattsand M. Kallikrein-related peptidases. Cell Mol Life Sci. 2008;65(13): 2019–38.
31. Oren A, Ganz T, Liu L, Meerloo T. In human epidermis, beta-defensin 2 is packaged in lamellar bodies. Exp Mol Pathol. 2003;74(2):180–2.
32. Kezic S, Novak N, Jakasa I, Jungersted JM, Simon M, Brandner JM, et al. Skin barrier in atopic dermatitis. Front Biosci (Landmark Ed). 2014;19(3):542–56.
33. Natsuga K. Epidermal barriers. Cold Spring Harb Perspect Med. 2014;4(4):a018218.
34. Smith FJ, Irvine AD, Terron-Kwiatkowski A, Sandilands A, Campbell LE, Zhao Y, et al. Loss-of-function mutations in the gene encoding filaggrin cause ichthyosis vulgaris. Nat Genet. 2006;38(3):337–42.
35. Woo YR, Lim JH, Cho DH, Park HJ. Rosacea: molecular mechanisms and Management of a Chronic Cutaneous Inflammatory Condition. Int J Mol Sci. 2016;17(9)
36. Nutten S. Atopic dermatitis: global epidemiology and risk factors. Ann Nutr Metab. 2015;66 (Suppl 1):8–16.
37. Asher MI, Montefort S, Bjorksten B, Lai CK, Strachan DP, Weiland SK, et al. Worldwide time trends in the prevalence of symptoms of asthma, allergic rhinoconjunctivitis, and eczema in childhood: ISAAC phases one and three repeat multicountry cross-sectional surveys. Lancet. 2006;368(9537):733–43.
38. Weidinger S, Novak N. Atopic dermatitis. Lancet. 2016;387(10023):1109–22.
39. Kim J, Kim BE, Leung DYM. Pathophysiology of atopic dermatitis: clinical implications. Allergy Asthma Proc. 2019;40(2):84–92.
40. Suto H, Matsuda H, Mitsuishi K, Hira K, Uchida T, Unno T, et al. NC/Nga mice: a mouse model for atopic dermatitis. Int Arch Allergy Immunol. 1999;120(Suppl 1):70–5.
41. Weidinger S, Illig T, Baurecht H, Irvine AD, Rodriguez E, Diaz-Lacava A, et al. Loss-of-function variations within the filaggrin gene predispose for atopic dermatitis with allergic sensitizations. J Allergy Clin Immunol. 2006;118(1):214–9.
42. Irvine AD, McLean WH, Leung DY. Filaggrin mutations associated with skin and allergic diseases. N Engl J Med. 2011;365(14):1315–27.
43. Deng Z, Chen M, Xie H, Jian D, Xu S, Peng Q, et al. Claudin reduction may relate to an impaired skin barrier in rosacea. J Dermatol. 2019;46(4):314–21.
44. Dirschka T, Tronnier H, Folster-Holst R. Epithelial barrier function and atopic diathesis in rosacea and perioral dermatitis. Br J Dermatol. 2004;150(6):1136–41.
45. Suhng E, Kim BH, Choi YW, Choi HY, Cho H, Byun JY. Increased expression of IL-33 in rosacea skin and UVB-irradiated and LL-37-treated HaCaT cells. Exp Dermatol. 2018;27(9): 1023–9.
46. Umar S. Intestinal stem cells. Curr Gastroenterol Rep. 2010;12(5):340–8.
47. Ahmad R, Sorrell MF, Batra SK, Dhawan P, Singh AB. Gut permeability and mucosal inflammation: bad, good or context dependent. Mucosal Immunol. 2017;10(2):307–17.
48. Camilleri M. Leaky gut: mechanisms, measurement and clinical implications in humans. Gut. 2019;68(8):1516–26.
49. DeMeo MT, Mutlu EA, Keshavarzian A, Tobin MC. Intestinal permeation and gastrointestinal disease. J Clin Gastroenterol. 2002;34(4):385–96.
50. Martini E, Krug SM, Siegmund B, Neurath MF, Becker C. Mend your fences: the epithelial barrier and its relationship with mucosal immunity in inflammatory bowel disease. Cell Mol Gastroenterol Hepatol. 2017;4(1):33–46.
51. Odenwald MA, Turner JR. The intestinal epithelial barrier: a therapeutic target? Nat Rev Gastroenterol Hepatol. 2017;14(1):9–21.
52. Parikh K, Antanaviciute A, Fawkner-Corbett D, Jagielowicz M, Aulicino A, Lagerholm C, et al. Colonic epithelial cell diversity in health and inflammatory bowel disease. Nature. 2019;567 (7746):49–55.

53. Cuzic S, Antolic M, Ognjenovic A, Stupin-Polancec D, Petrinic Grba A, Hrvacic B, et al. Claudins: beyond tight junctions in human IBD and murine models. Front Pharmacol. 2021;12: 682614.
54. Obermuller B, Frisina N, Meischel M, Singer G, Stanzl-Tschegg S, Lichtenegger H, et al. Examination of intestinal ultrastructure, bowel wall apoptosis and tight junctions in the early phase of sepsis. Sci Rep. 2020;10(1):11507.
55. Heller F, Florian P, Bojarski C, Richter J, Christ M, Hillenbrand B, et al. Interleukin-13 is the key effector Th2 cytokine in ulcerative colitis that affects epithelial tight junctions, apoptosis, and cell restitution. Gastroenterology. 2005;129(2):550–64.
56. Edmondson R, Broglie JJ, Adcock AF, Yang L. Three-dimensional cell culture systems and their applications in drug discovery and cell-based biosensors. Assay Drug Dev Technol. 2014;12(4):207–18.
57. Arason AJ, Jonsdottir HR, Halldorsson S, Benediktsdottir BE, Bergthorsson JT, Ingthorsson S, et al. deltaNp63 has a role in maintaining epithelial integrity in airway epithelium. PLoS One. 2014;9(2):e88683.
58. Jiang D, Schaefer N, Chu HW. Air-liquid Interface culture of human and mouse airway epithelial cells. Methods Mol Biol. 2018;1809:91–109.
59. Srinivasan B, Kolli AR, Esch MB, Abaci HE, Shuler ML, Hickman JJ. TEER measurement techniques for in vitro barrier model systems. J Lab Autom. 2015;20(2):107–26.
60. Andrews C, McLean MH, Durum SK. Cytokine tuning of intestinal epithelial function. Front Immunol. 2018;9:1270.
61. Deli MA. Potential use of tight junction modulators to reversibly open membranous barriers and improve drug delivery. Biochim Biophys Acta. 2009;1788(4):892–910.
62. Cavanaugh KJ, Cohen TS, Margulies SS. Stretch increases alveolar epithelial permeability to uncharged micromolecules. Am J Physiol Cell Physiol. 2006;290(4):C1179–88.
63. Bisig C, Voss C, Petri-Fink A, Rothen-Rutishauser B. The crux of positive controls–pro-inflammatory responses in lung cell models. Toxicol In Vitro. 2019;54:189–93.
64. Asgrimsson V, Gudjonsson T, Gudmundsson GH, Baldursson O. Novel effects of azithromycin on tight junction proteins in human airway epithelia. Antimicrob Agents Chemother. 2006;50 (5):1805–12.
65. Slater M, Torr E, Harrison T, Forrester D, Knox A, Shaw D, et al. The differential effects of azithromycin on the airway epithelium in vitro and in vivo. Physiol Rep. 2016;4(18):e12960.
66. Arason AJ, Joelsson JP, Valdimarsdottir B, Sigurdsson S, Gudjonsson A, Halldorsson S, et al. Azithromycin induces epidermal differentiation and multivesicular bodies in airway epithelia. Respir Res. 2019;20(1):129.
67. Kanoh S, Rubin BK. Mechanisms of action and clinical application of macrolides as immunomodulatory medications. Clin Microbiol Rev. 2010;23(3):590–615.
68. Chen M, Yang T, Meng X, Sun T. Azithromycin attenuates cigarette smoke extract-induced oxidative stress injury in human alveolar epithelial cells. Mol Med Rep. 2015;11(5):3414–22.
69. Zhu C, Lei W, Huang J. Azithromycin inhibits double-stranded RNA-induced thymic stromal lymphopoietin release from human airway epithelial cells. Pharmazie. 2013;68(11):899–903.
70. Liu Y, Pu Y, Li D, Zhou L, Wan L. Azithromycin ameliorates airway remodeling via inhibiting airway epithelium apoptosis. Life Sci. 2017;170:1–8.
71. London IC, Melinta TI. A study to evaluate the anti-inflammatory effects of solithromycin in chronic obstructive pulmonary disease. https://ClinicalTrials.gov/show/NCT02628769; 2015.
72. Kricker JA, Ingthorsson S, Valdimarsdottir B, Joelsson JP, Sigurdsson S, Gardarsson FR, et al. Targeting the lung epithelial barrier to inhibit neutrophilic inflammation. 15th world congress on inflammation; 5–8 June 2022; Rome, Italy: Pharmadvances, SIF; 2022.
73. Kricker JA, Valdimarsdottir B, Joelsson JP, Ingthorsson S, Parnham MJ, Sigurdsson S, et al. Barriolides: non-antibacterial compounds with epithelial barrier enhancing properties and anti-inflammatory effects in vitro. 15th world congress on inflammation; 5–8 June 2022; Rome, Italy: Pharmadvances, SIF; 2022.
74. Azuma A, Kudoh S. Diffuse panbronchiolitis in East Asia. Respirology. 2006;11(3):249–61.

75. Feldman C, Anderson R. The cytoprotective interactions of antibiotics with human ciliated airway epithelium. 2005. In: Antibiotics as anti-inflammatory and immunomodulatory agents [internet]. Basel: Birkhäuser Basel; 2005. p. 1. Progress in Inflammation Research; [49-63].
76. Bush A. Azithromycin is the answer in paediatric respiratory medicine, but what was the question? Paediatr Respir Rev. 2020;34:67–74.
77. Reijnders TDY, Saris A, Schultz MJ, van der Poll T. Immunomodulation by macrolides: therapeutic potential for critical care. Lancet Respir Med. 2020;8(6):619–30.
78. Rubin BK. Immunomodulatory properties of macrolides: overview and historical perspective. Am J Med. 2004;117(Suppl 9A):2S–4S.
79. Mikasa K, Sawaki M, Kita E, Konishi M, Maeda K, Hamada K, et al. Long-term chemotherapy using erythromycin (EM) for chronic lower airway infection: effectiveness of clarithromycin in EM ineffective cases–the fourth report. Kansenshogaku Zasshi. 1992;66(8):1097–104.
80. Robinson P, Schechter MS, Sly PD, Winfield K, Smith J, Brennan S, et al. Clarithromycin therapy for patients with cystic fibrosis: a randomized controlled trial. Pediatr Pulmonol. 2012;47(6):551–7.
81. GOLD. Global strategy for prevention, diagnosis and management of COPD: 2022 report. www.goldcopd.org: Global initiative for chronic obstructive lung disease, Inc.; 2022.
82. GINA. Global Strategy for Asthma Management and Prevention. https://ginasthma.org/; 2022.
83. Crosbie PA, Woodhead MA. Long-term macrolide therapy in chronic inflammatory airway diseases. Eur Respir J. 2009;33(1):171–81.
84. Simpson JL, Powell H, Boyle MJ, Scott RJ, Gibson PG. Clarithromycin targets neutrophilic airway inflammation in refractory asthma. Am J Respir Crit Care Med. 2008;177(2):148–55.
85. Wan KS, Liu YC, Huang CS, Su YM. Effects of low-dose clarithromycin added to fluticasone on inflammatory markers and pulmonary function among children with asthma: a randomized clinical trial. Allergy Rhinol (Providence). 2016;7(3):131–4.
86. Gibson PG, Yang IA, Upham JW, Reynolds PN, Hodge S, James AL, et al. Efficacy of azithromycin in severe asthma from the AMAZES randomised trial. ERJ Open Res. 2019;5 (4):00056.
87. Sadamatsu H, Takahashi K, Tashiro H, Kato G, Noguchi Y, Kurata K, et al. The non-antibiotic macrolide EM900 attenuates HDM and poly(I:C)-induced airway inflammation with inhibition of macrophages in a mouse model. Inflamm Res. 2020;69(1):139–51.
88. Simpson JL, Powell H, Baines KJ, Milne D, Coxson HO, Hansbro PM, et al. The effect of azithromycin in adults with stable neutrophilic COPD: a double blind randomised, placebo controlled trial. PLoS One. 2014;9(8):e105609.
89. Seemungal TA, Wilkinson TM, Hurst JR, Perera WR, Sapsford RJ, Wedzicha JA. Long-term erythromycin therapy is associated with decreased chronic obstructive pulmonary disease exacerbations. Am J Respir Crit Care Med. 2008;178(11):1139–47.
90. Djamin RS, Bafadhel M, Uzun S, Russell REK, Ermens AAM, Kerstens R, et al. Blood eosinophil count and GOLD stage predict response to maintenance azithromycin treatment in COPD patients with frequent exacerbations. Respir Med. 2019;154:27–33.
91. Corren J, Pham TH, Garcia Gil E, Salapa K, Ren P, Parnes JR, et al. Baseline type 2 biomarker levels and response to tezepelumab in severe asthma. Allergy. 2022;77(6):1786–96.
92. Alzolibani AA, Zedan K. Macrolides in chronic inflammatory skin disorders. Mediat Inflamm. 2012;2012:159354.
93. Bakar O, Demircay Z, Yuksel M, Haklar G, Sanisoglu Y. The effect of azithromycin on reactive oxygen species in rosacea. Clin Exp Dermatol. 2007;32(2):197–200.
94. Huang SW, Chen YJ, Wang ST, Ho LW, Kao JK, Narita M, et al. Azithromycin impairs TLR7 signaling in dendritic cells and improves the severity of imiquimod-induced psoriasis-like skin inflammation in mice. J Dermatol Sci. 2016;84(1):59–70.

95. Trompette A, Pernot J, Perdijk O, Alqahtani RAA, Domingo JS, Camacho-Munoz D, et al. Gut-derived short-chain fatty acids modulate skin barrier integrity by promoting keratinocyte metabolism and differentiation. Mucosal Immunol. 2022;15(5):908–26.
96. Takeyama K. Macrolides and mucus production. 2005. In: Antibiotics as anti-inflammatory and immunomodulatory agents [internet]. Basel: Birkhäuser Basel; 2005. p. 1. Progress in Inflammation Research; [123-32].

Macrolides and Inflammatory Cells, Signaling, and Mediators

Mitsuko Kondo

Abstract Low-dose long-term macrolide therapy had a remarkable effect on the prognosis of diffuse panbronchiolitis and suppression of airway secretion and neutrophilic inflammation in this disease. Macrolides inhibit airway water secretion, mucin secretion, and mucus production. Macrolides also suppress neutrophilic infiltration through suppression of proinflammatory cytokines, chemokines, and adhesion molecules. However, macrolides do not appear to be immunosuppressive but rather immunomodulatory, to reset and normalize inflammation. In order to elucidate the mechanism of action of macrolides, the intracellular signal transduction mechanism has been investigated using animal models and cell lines, and in these models, it is important to inhibit mitogen-activated protein kinases and transcription factors such as NFκB. However, the effects of macrolides are widespread and diverse, as are their target proteins and receptors. Since macrolides affect lysosome, autophagy, and apoptosis, their affinity with the membranes that constitute the cell membrane and intracellular organelles attracts attention. This can explain many of the actions of macrolides, intracellular accumulation, and temporal transition of actions.

Keywords Airway secretion · Mucin · Neutrophil · Proinflammatory cytokine · Mitogen-activated protein kinase · NFκB · Apoptosis · Cell membrane

1 Introduction

Low-dose long-term therapy with erythromycin (EM) brought about a breakthrough improvement in the prognosis of diffuse panbronchiolitis (DPB) [1]. The principal mechanisms of action for macrolide therapy are thought to be suppressing airway hypersecretion and neutrophil inflammation. Macrolides improve mucociliary clearance by directly suppressing excessive water and mucin secretion [2–4]. Macrolides

M. Kondo (✉)
Department of Respiratory Medicine, Tokyo Women's Medical University School of Medicine, Tokyo, Japan
e-mail: kondo.mitsuko@twmu.ac.jp

B. K. Rubin, M. Shinkai (eds.), *Macrolides as Immunomodulatory Agents*, Progress in Inflammation Research 92, https://doi.org/10.1007/978-3-031-42859-3_2

also suppress neutrophil activation and accumulation in the airway, which acts indirectly on airway epithelial cells to suppress hypersecretion [5]. The characteristic features of macrolide therapy are as follows. (1) Macrolides are effective at low-dose and long-term administration, (2) Macrolides are effective even in *Pseudomonas aeruginosa*-infected pathologies that are resistant to macrolides, (3) 14-membered macrolides [EM, clarithromycin (CAM), roxithromycin (RXM)] and 15-membered macrolide/azilide azithromycin (AZM) are more effective than 16-membered macrolides [2]. Macrolide concentrations are at least tenfold higher in the epithelial lung fluid than serum [2]. Currently, macrolides are widely used for chronic airway inflammatory diseases with neutrophil inflammation such as chronic sinusitis, bronchiectasis, cystic fibrosis (CF), and COPD. In addition, the usefulness of macrolides has been established in some cases of intractable and noneosinophilic asthma and is being studied for the therapy of pulmonary fibrosis. In this chapter, we introduce the effects of macrolides on airway secretion and inflammatory cells/cytokines and describe the broad effects of macrolides on intracellular signaling mechanisms.

2 Regulation of Airway Secretion and Inflammatory Cells/Cytokines and Chemokines by Macrolides

1. Regulation of water secretion

Over 90% of airway surface fluid is water, and water secretion is regulated by active Cl ion transport in airway epithelial cells. EM suppresses Cl ion transport in airway epithelial cells, when the short-circuit current, an indicator of active ion transport, is measured by Ussing chamber [3]. Using the patch clamp technique with nasal gland cells, RXM suppresses activation of Cl ion channels induced by acetylcholine [6]. That is, 14-membered macrolides cause a decrease in water secretion associated with inhibition of Cl ion channels. The main Cl ion channels in the airway are cAMP-dependent CFTR and Ca-activated Cl ion channels (CaCC). CaCC is a transmembrane protein 16A (TMEM16A) [7]. We found that TMEM16A-dependent Cl ion transport in IL-13-treated airway epithelial cells was suppressed by pretreatment with CAM [8]. EM also suppresses intracellular Ca^{2+} elevation induced by ATP stimulation through Ca^{2+} influx from extracellular spaces and Ca^{2+} oscillations [9]. Cl ion transport suppression by macrolides may also be due to inhibiting the increase in intracellular Ca^{2+}. However, macrolides appear to have no effect on Cl ion transport in CFTR-knockout mouse and patients with CF [10].

CAM, amoxicillin, and cefaclor were administered for 1 week to patients with chronic bronchitis and bronchiectasis, and changes in the sputum volume were measured, and a decrease in sputum volume of 30% or more was observed in the CAM group. In the sputum, the proportion of solid components increased, and the Cl ion concentration decreased [11], suggesting that the decrease in sputum content was due to a decrease in water content, perhaps due to inhibiting Cl ion transport. When CAM was administered to patients with COPD for 8 weeks, the volume of sputum was reduced by half, and an increase in sputum elasticity was measured while viscosity was unchanged [4].

2. Suppression of mucin secretion

Mucin accounts for more than 30% of the solid components of airway mucus. Mucin is a large glycoprotein, and its core protein is composed of repeating serine and threonine peptides decorated with sugar chains linked by O-glycosidic bonds. There are secretory and membrane-bound mucins in the respiratory tract, the former being gel-forming and a component of mucus. Secretory mucin-producing cells in the airway are goblet cells, mucous cells, and serous cells in the submucosal glands. MUC5AC and MUC5B are produced from goblet cells, and MUC5B is abundantly produced from mucous cells of the submucosal gland [12]. When secretory stimulants are administered to goblet cells, degranulation from the secretory granules occurs rapidly. Airway mucus hypersecretion results from degranulation from secretory cells and from increased mucin production. Stimulation of the autonomic nervous system and mediators such as elastase and histamine causes degranulation. In animal experiments, administration of CAM and EM once a day for 1 week suppresses degranulation caused by lipopolysaccharide (LPS) stimulation, but not with ampicillin or cefaclor [13].

3. Suppression of mucin production

The epithelial growth factor receptor (EGFR) plays an important role in mucin production [14]. There are many EGFR ligands such as epidermal growth factor (EGF), TGFα, HB-EGF, amphiregulin and tobaccos smoke, and when EGFR is stimulated by these ligands, its phosphorylation occurs and the ERK1/2 pathway is activated via Ras, Raf, and MEK [14, 15]. Transcription factors such as NFκB then enter the nucleus to promote gene expression and mucin. Macrolides suppress TGFα- and LPS-stimulated mucin production in NCI-H292 cells, perhaps at the transcriptional level of NFκB [16]. EGFR can be phosphorylated when stimulated with TNFα or H_2O_2 is added to NCI-H292 cells [17]. Because the antioxidant, N-acetyl cysteine, suppresses this reaction, it is thought that this is due to reactive oxygen species (ROS) derived from neutrophils phosphorylating EGFR [17]. The addition of neutrophil elastase to NCI-H292 cells also causes phosphorylation of EGFR and enhances mucin production [18]. Macrolides suppress the infiltration and activation of neutrophils, resulting in suppression of ROS and elastase production, suppression of EGFR activation, and reduction in mucin production. The culture supernatant of *Pseudomonas aeruginosa* stimulates EGFR and enhances mucin production [19]; therefore, macrolides can decrease mucin gene expression by decreasing EGFR activation.

4. Regulation of inflammatory cells/cytokines

Neutrophils release chemokines including IL-8/CXCL8, leukotrienes, proteases, and ROS. Low-dose long-term macrolide therapy decreases neutrophil numbers, IL-8/CXCL8, and IL-1β in bronchoalveolar lavage fluid of subjects with DPB or bronchiolitis [20]. Administration of LPS to rats enhances airway neutrophil accumulation, IL-8/CXCL8, TNFα, and MUC5AC production, and these can be decreased by macrolides [21]. The expression of neutrophil adhesion molecules Mac1 (CD11b/CD18) and L-selection is also suppressed by macrolides [22, 23]. EM administered to cultured human airway epithelial cells decreases the production of IL-6 and IL-8/CXCL8 and the expression of ICAM-1. Macrolides also reduce VCAM-1 expression and leukocyte migration in a murine bleomycin-induced lung fibrosis model [24]. EM inhibits leukocyte recruitment in the lung through downregulation of adhesion molecules in vivo study using LPS stimulation [25]. That is, macrolides can suppress neutrophil infiltration through suppression of proinflammatory cytokines, chemokines, and adhesion molecules.

Macrolides have also been shown to be effective against eosinophil inflammation. EM suppresses the secretion of the eosinophil chemotactic chemokine, RANTES, and eotaxin from IL-1β and TNFα-stimulated fibroblasts [26]. Roxithromycin decreases the production of IL-5 from T cells [27]. In a murine asthma model induced by human dust mite antigen, AZM decreased the number of eosinophils and neutrophils in BAL, with a decrease in IL-4, 5, 6, 10, 12, 13, RANTES, and goblet cells. AZM also decreased goblet cell metaplasia and mucus secretion [28].

5. Application of macrolides to hypersecretion in COPD and asthma

Long-term macrolide therapy with EM or azithromycin (AZM) has been shown to decrease COPD exacerbations [29, 30]. Macrolides can suppress the expression of the adhesion molecule, ICAM-1, needed for the invasion of viruses and decrease inflammatory cytokines released from airway epithelial cells [31]. As airway defenses are impaired by smoking or oxidants, persistent infection can occur, leading to chronic neutrophil accumulation and hypersecretion. Macrolides suppress chronic airway inflammation in COPD by inhibiting virus infection, biofilm formation, infiltration of inflammatory cells, and hypersecretion [32].

IL-8/CXCL8 and neutrophils are involved in non-T2 asthma, and in these patients, macrolide therapy inhibits neutrophilic inflammation and improves quality of life [33]. Airway obstruction due to mucus leads to decreased respiratory function and contributes to fatal asthma [12]. MUC5AC is abundant in the sputum of persons with asthma, and MUC5AC, but not MUC5B, is tethered to the cell surface after being secreted from goblet cells, increasing sputum viscosity and tenacity. IL-13, a T2 cytokine is abundant in the asthma airway; IL-13 causes goblet cell metaplasia and increased MUC5AC in airway epithelial cells in vivo and in vitro. IL-13-induced goblet cell metaplasia is decreased by macrolides but not by corticosteroids [34, 35]. CAM inhibits the IL-13 receptor-JAK-STAT6 pathway and EGFR-MAP kinase pathway and inactivates NFκB transcriptional activity [35]. IL-13 induces secretion of CLCA1 from airway epithelial cells, and this is associated with goblet cell metaplasia. CAM also decreases CLCA1 expression [36]. CLCA1 is also a regulator of TMEM16A and is involved in the stabilization of TMEM16A in the cell membrane [37]. Expression of TMEM16A is also strongly associated with goblet cell metaplasia, and CAM suppresses IL-13-induced TMEM16A expression [8] (Fig. 1). Macrolides also enhance the barrier function of the airway epithelium by differentiation of epithelial cells into ciliated cells and enhancing epithelial repair

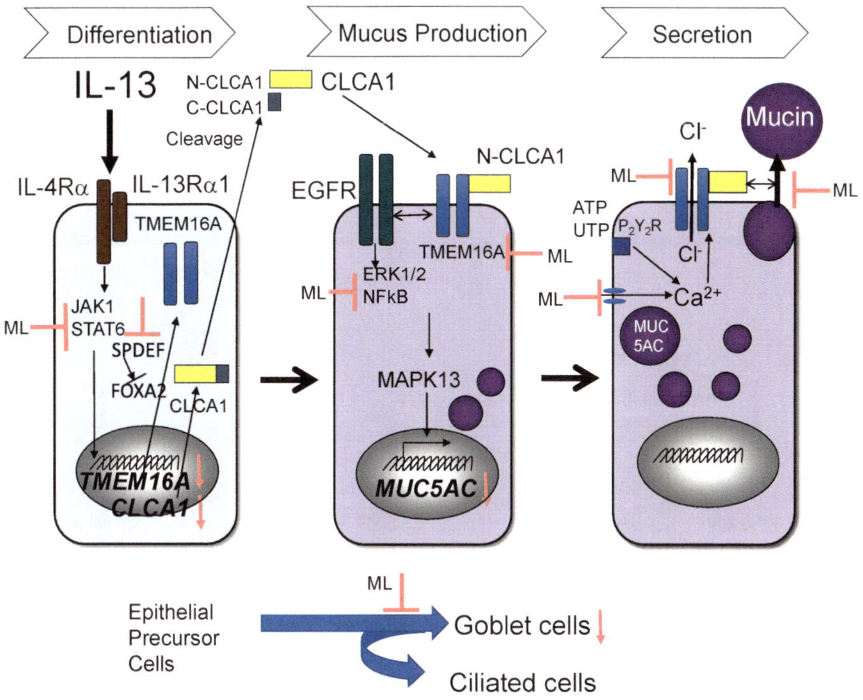

Fig. 1 The hypothesis from goblet cell metaplasia to the secretion of airway epithelial cells induced by IL-13 and the reported points of action of macrolides Stimulation of IL-13 induces TMEM16A via JAK1 and STAT6, after which TMEM16A migrates to the cell membrane. Similarly, CLCA1 is also produced and secreted extracellularly by stimulation with IL-13. CLCA1 is autolyzed, and N-CLCA1 acts on TMEM16A, contributing to the stabilization of TMEM16A on the cell membrane. In addition, TMEM16A interacts with EGFR, MUC5AC is induced via activation of ERK1/2, NFκB, and MAPK13-dependent pathway, mucin granules are formed, and goblet cell formation is completed. IL-13 stimulation suppresses FOXA2 through activation of SPDEF and suppresses differentiation into ciliated cells. In goblet cells, secretory stimuli such as ATP and UTP increase intracellular Ca^{2+} via P2Y2 receptors and induce extracellular Ca^{2+} influx. As a result, TMEM16A shows CaCC activity and causes Cl ion transport and mucin granule secretory reaction. In this hypothesis, the blocking marks are reported as the points of action of macrolides (ML). Created with reference to References 8, 9, 34–36

[2, 8]. Macrolide therapy is expected to be effective for neutrophil-dominant asthma, which is steroid-resistant, and severe asthma with mucus hypersecretion. It is reported that AZM therapy for refractory asthma can decrease exacerbations and improve quality of life [38].

6. Time course of macrolide action on inflammatory cells

After the first administration of macrolides, the effects of macrolides on neutrophil inflammation are known to be biphasic, nonlinear, and time-dependent [2, 39]. In a very acute phase, neutrophil degranulation, phagocytosis, and the formation of neutrophil extracellular traps (NETS) are enhanced [40, 41], and the

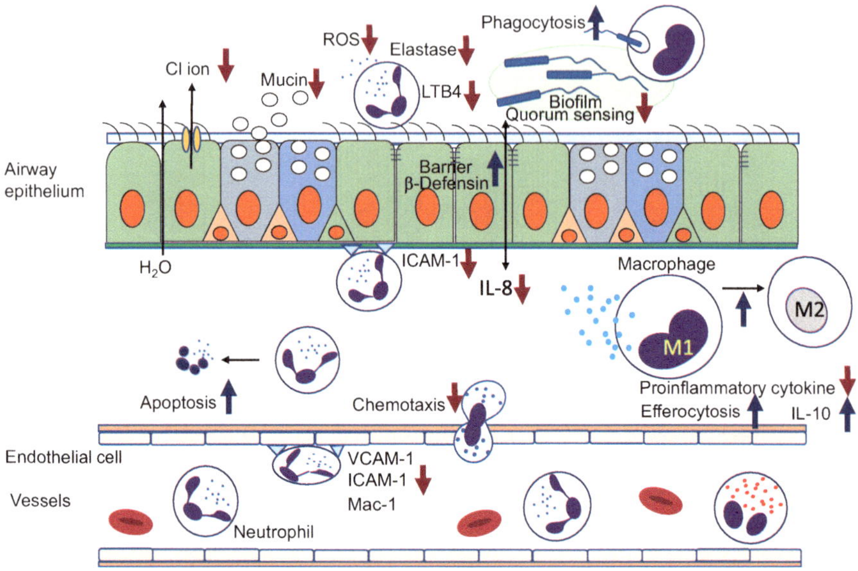

Fig. 2 Effect of macrolides on chronic inflammatory airways. In the chronic inflammatory airway, barrier dysfunction of the airway epithelium, infiltration of inflammatory cells, goblet cell metaplasia, hypersecretion, impairment of mucociliary clearance, and recurrent airway infection are observed. Macrolides have antiinflammatory effects such as suppression of proinflammatory cytokine productions, adhesion molecules, chemical mediators release, reactive oxygen species (ROS) production, and induction of apoptosis of neutrophils. For airway epithelium, macrolides suppress secretory responses, enhance barrier function, and suppress proinflammatory cytokines and adhesion molecules. For bacteria, macrolides suppress biofilm and quorum-sensing function. Downward-facing arrows, inhibition by macrolides; upward-facing arrows, enhancement by macrolides

antibacterial effect and host defense are stimulated. However, after 24 h, macrolides decrease IL-8, proteases, and ROS and promote resolution from inflammation. Apoptosis of neutrophils is also involved in this process such that neutrophil necrosis decreases and the release of inflammatory mediators mitigates. Macrolides also suppress the release of proinflammatory cytokines and inducible nitric oxide synthase (iNOS) from monocytes and alveolar macrophages and convert M1 to M2 macrophages after 2–3 days. M2 macrophages release the antiinflammatory cytokine, IL-10 [42]. Macrophages enhance phagocytosis and efferocytosis of apoptotic neutrophils in the presence of macrolides [43]. The effect of macrolides on the resolution of inflammation lasts for weeks to months [44]. Macrolides also reduce the expression of Toll-like receptors and the expression of IL-12 in dendritic cells [45]. This causes macrolides to suppress differentiation into Th1 cells and, as a result, to reduce IFNγ released from Th1 cells. Macrolides induce immune-tolerant dendritic cells and suppress the expression of co-stimulatory molecules [45–47].

In summary, the effects of macrolides on the airway are shown in Fig. 2 and Table 1.

Table 1 Antiinflammatory and immunomodulatory effects of macrolides on airway epithelial cells, inflammatory cells, and other cells

Airway epithelial cells	Neutrophils	Macrophages/Monocytes	Lymphocytes	Fibroblasts	Endothelial cells
Inhibition of cytokine etc.					
IL-8	TNFα	IL-1β	IL-4, IL-5, IL-13	VEGF	VCAM-1
TNFα	LTB4	TNFα	TNFα	RANTES	VEGF
GM-CSF	IL-1β	IL-6	IL-2	Eotaxin	
Eotaxin	Mac1	IL-8	IL-17	IL-8	
IL-6		(G)M-CSF	IFNγ	MMP	
ICAM-1		IL-12	IL-10		
		IFNγ			
Inhibition of function					
Cl ion transport	Elastase	Inducible NO production	T cell skewing Th1	Proliferation	Angiogenesis
Mucin secretion	Myeloperoxidase	Phagosomal acidification	Perforin	Migration	
MUC5AC Production	ROS	Co-stimularoty molecules	CD69		
Goblet cell metaplasia	NETS	TLR2,4,6,9	Granzyme B		
	Chemotaxis	MHC class II	CD8		
		M1 macrophage			
Stimulation of function					
Mucociliary clearance	Apoptosis	Efferocytosis	IgA		
Tight junction		Phagocytosis	Apoptosis		
β-Defensin		Differentiation to M2	Treg		

It is classified into inhibition of cytokine etc., inhibition or stimulation of function by macrolides. *ROS* reactive oxygen species; *NETS* neutrophil extracellular traps

3 Intracellular Signaling Mechanisms

Macrolides are concentrated in tissues and cells, and their concentration is reported to reach 10–100 times that of serum [48], suggesting a role of macrolides in intracellular signaling. However, the target proteins and receptors are still unknown. Intracellular signaling pathways affected by macrolides are shown in Fig. 3.

1. Intracellular calcium

Intracellular Ca^{2+} plays an important role in intracellular signal transduction. In airway epithelial cells and A549 cells, EM suppresses intracellular Ca^{2+} level and Ca^{2+} influx from the extracellular space caused by purinergic receptor stimulation [49]. EM and AZM can decrease mucus secretion from the submucosal glands of the airways, in part, by inhibiting calcium influx [50]. In mast cells, roxithromycin also decreases the activation by β-defensin 2 via the Ca^{2+} signaling pathway [51]. In neutrophils, EM suppresses FMLP-stimulated superoxide production and Ca^{2+} influx [52]. In addition, since intracellular Ca^{2+} is also involved in the activation of mitogen-activated protein kinases (MAPKs) and NFκB, it is speculated that macrolides may affect a wide range of cell functions through the regulation of intracellular Ca^{2+} [2].

2. Mitogen-activated protein kinases (MAPKs)

MAPKs form a network responding to both internal and external stimuli for signal transduction and play an important role in controlling inflammatory gene expression, cell proliferation, cell differentiation, and apoptosis [53]. There are three main classes of MAPKs: extracellular signal-regulated kinase (ERK), c-Jun N-terminal kinase (JNK), and p38 MAPK. MAPKs induce IL-8/CXCL8 expression by both an NFκB-dependent and independent pathway. Shinkai et al. investigated the effect of macrolides on MAPK and IL-8/CXCL8 expression using airway epithelial cells. CAM suppressed ERK phosphorylation in the initial 30–90 min, the level was increased at 2 h to 3 days, and it normalized to the unstimulated level by 5 days. As a result, IL-8/CXCL8 was maximal at 24 h, and then gradually decreased [54]. The action of macrolides is not to suppress inflammation in one direction but to reset and normalize it and thus is immunomodulatory with long-term therapy. Macrolides also protect cells by moving the cell cycle to G_1/G_0, and they decrease the phosphorylation of ERK in airway epithelial cells [55]. Furthermore, the inhibitory effect of CAM and AZM on MUC5AC production from airway epithelial cells and neutrophil infiltration during *Pseudomonas aeruginosa* infection is also mediated by the inhibition of the ERK activity [56–58]. It has been reported that EM restored steroid sensitivity by suppressing the activation of the JNK/c-JUN pathway induced by tobacco smoke [59].

3. Transcription factors; NFκB and AP-1

Macrolides decrease cytokine production by suppressing the transcription factors NFκB and AP-1 in airway epithelial cells and monocytes [60–62]. NFκB is inactive

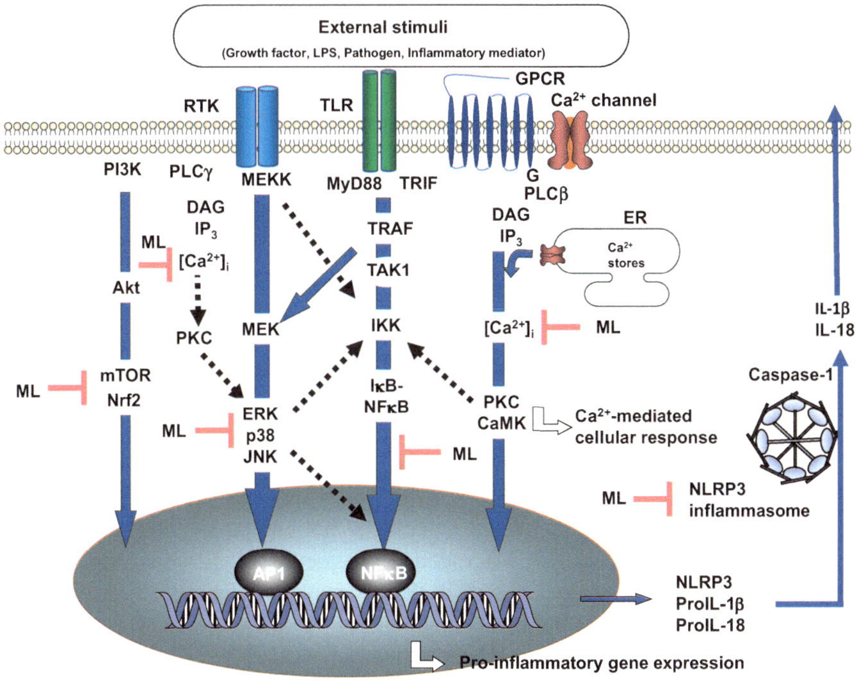

Fig. 3 Intracellular signaling transduction pathways and the related sites of macrolide immunomodulation. Receptor tyrosine kinases (RTKs) are receptors for many growth factors and cytokines. For example, epithelial growth factor receptor (EGFR) activates MEKK, MEK, and ERK1/2. Toll-like receptors (TLRs) activated by pathogens and LPS stimulate the IκB kinase (IKK) complex and the MAPK pathway. IKK complex activates NFκB through the digestion of IκB, and then NFκB is translocated. The MAPK pathway leads to AP-1 induction. Macrolides inhibit these pathways and then inhibit proinflammatory gene expression. NLRP3, ProIL-1β, and ProIL-18 gene expression form NLRP3 inflammasome, leading to IL-β and IL-18 release decomposed by Caspase-1. G-protein-coupled receptor (GPCR) or RTK-mediated activation of phospholipase C (PLC) produces inositol triphosphate (IP3) and diacylglycerol (DAG). IP3 increases intracellular Ca from endoplasmic reticulum Ca stores, and DAG activates protein kinase C (PKC). RTK- or GPCR-stimulation also induces activation of PI3K/Akt pathway. Macrolides inhibit these pathways and as a result, modulate various cell functions. Blue arrows are major pathways influenced by macrolides. Dashed arrows are cross-talk pathways. Red lines indicate the sites of macrolide's inhibition. Modified from Reference 2. Abbreviations: *Akt* AKT8 virus oncogene cellular homolog; *AP-1* activator protein 1; *CaMK* calmodulin kinase; *ER* endoplasmic reticulum; *ERK* extracellular signal-regulated kinase; *GFR* cytokine receptor/growth factor receptor; *IKK* IκB kinase; *IP_3R* inositol triphosphate receptor; *JNK* c-Jun N-terminal kinase; *MEK* MAPK/ERK kinase; *MEKK* MAPK/ERK kinase kinase; *mTOR* serine/threonine kinase mammalian target of rapamycin; *MyD88* myeloid differentiation factor 88; *PI3K* phosphoinositide 3-kinase; *PKC* protein kinase C; *TAK1* transforming growth factor-activated protein kinase 1; *TRAF* TNF receptor-associated factor; *TRIF* TIR-domain-containing adaptor-inducing interferon-β; *TLR* Toll-like receptor; *Nrf2* Nuclear factor-erythroid 2-related factor 2

in the cytoplasm when bound to IκB. When IκB is phosphorylated via IκB kinase (IKK), the bond with NFκB is dissociated; NFκB then becomes free and translocates into the nucleus, initiating transcription. Macrolides suppress IKK and IκB phosphorylation and inhibit IκB degradation [63]. AZM decreases IL-8/CXCL8 production by suppressing the transcriptional activity of NFκB and AP-1 in CF airway epithelial cells [64]. AZM also inhibits MAC5AC production in airway epithelial cells via the c-Jun/AP-1 pathway [65]. AZM can decrease AP-1-mediated IL-1β production from macrophages in a model of LPS-stimulated neutrophil inflammation in the lung [66].

4. PI3K/Akt/mTOR pathway

Rapamycin, very large macrolide with antiproliferative and immunosuppressive effects, inhibits the serine/threonine kinase mammalian target of rapamycin (mTOR), forming a complex with FK506 binding protein 12 (FK-BP12) attenuating T-cell responses [67, 68]. In an asthma model, AZM also inhibits remodeling by suppressing hypoxia-inducible factor (HIF)-α and VEGF via the phosphoinositide 3-kinase (PI3K)/AKT8 virus oncogene cellular homolog (Akt)/mTOR pathway [69]. The enhancement of SLE macrophage phagocytosis and conversion to M2 macrophages by AZM is mediated by PI3K/Akt phosphorylation [70]. Macrolides may suppress inflammation induced by smoking, in part, via the PI3K/Akt-Nuclear factor-erythroid 2-related factor 2 (Nrf2) pathway [71].

5. Inflammasome

The inflammasome is a multiprotein complex formed in the cytoplasm by exposure to pathogen-associated molecular pattern (PAMP) or danger-associated molecular pattern (DAMP). The best-characterized inflammasome is the NOD-like receptor thermal protein domain associated protein 3 (NLRP3) inflammasome complex. The NLRP3 inflammasome is activated in a two-step process. First, NF-κB signaling is induced by PAMP or DAMP-mediated activation of TLR4 or TNFR and enhances the expression of NLRP3, pro-IL-1β, and pro-IL-18 (priming step, Signal 1). Next, diverse signals (whole pathogens, PAMP/DAMP, potassium efflux, environment factors such as silica, endogenous factors such as amyloid-β, and mitochondrial damage) can indirectly activate NLRP3, resulting in complex formation and activation of caspase-1 (Signal 2). Activated caspase-1 induces the secretion of the proinflammatory cytokines IL-1β and IL-18, as well as the expression of metabolic enzymes, phagosome maturation, vasodilation, and pyrotosis or inflammatory programmed cell death [72]. The inflammasome is observed in many cells, but its role has been clarified especially in monocytes, macrophages, and neutrophils. AZM suppresses the inflammasome complex after LPS stimulation and suppresses IL-1β production in monocytes [73]. In addition, NLRP3 inflammasome is involved in neutrophilic asthma. It is reported that macrolides inhibit IL-I-β-induced IL-8/CXCL8 production and mucin production [74, 75], which may be inflammasome mediated.

Aged cells produce proinflammatory cytokines called senescence-associated secretory phenotype (SASP), which can cause chronic inflammation and tissue damage. SASP and inflammasome are closely related, as SASP is regulated by IL-1 signaling via the inflammasome [76]. AZM appears to selectively eliminate aged fibroblasts by glycolysis and autophagy, acting as a senolytic drug [77]. In idiopathic pulmonary fibrosis (IPF), SASP induces myofibroblast induction and collagen production enhancement via Wnt/β-catenin signaling [78]. Along with autophagy, AZM can also enhance mitophagy, a mechanism for the elimination of injured mitochondria [79].

6. Lysosomes, autophagy, apoptosis

The lysosome is an organelle containing digestive enzymes that decomposes and recycles intracellular and extracellular components [80]. Since macrolides have amphiphilic properties, they accumulate in lysosomes, and the hydrophilic amino group of macrolides affects the function of lysosomes [81]. Autophagy is a mechanism that takes in damaged intracellular components and pathogens into autophagosomes, transports them to lysosomes, fuses them, forms autolysosomes, decomposes the components, and reuses them [82, 83]. There are reports that AZM enhances smooth muscle autophagy [84] and, conversely reduces fibroblast and macrophage autophagy [85]. In a pulmonary fibrosis model, it has been reported that AZM suppresses NADPH oxidase 4 by suppressing autophagy and the differentiation of fibroblasts into myofibroblasts [86]. Autophagy of cancer cells is advantageous to cancer growth, so macrolides have been used to suppress autophagy during cancer therapy [87]. However, inhibition of autophagy appears to depend on the intracellular concentration of the macrolide and the cell type involved. Apoptosis causes cell death by cell shrinkage, nuclear chromatin condensation, and nuclear fragmentation, forming extracellular vesicles that preserve the cell membrane and are phagocytosed and eliminated by macrophages. Autophagy and apoptosis have common proteins such as Atg5 and Beclin-1 [88]. In smooth muscle, macrolides initially cause autophagy, which, when prolonged, leads to apoptosis [84]. Apoptosis in neutrophils is related to high concentrations of AZM [89]. Neutrophil apoptosis contributes to the resolution of inflammation [44, 90]. However, in macrophages, accumulation of macrolides does not cause apoptosis but induces efferocytosis that phagocytoses apoptotic cells in COPD.

7. Interaction with membranes

Azithromycin has amphiphilic properties, like surfactants, that are both hydrophobic and hydrophilic, so the cell membrane takes it up and acts on the cell membrane and organelles in various ways [44, 91]. The hydrophobic group enters through fatty acid constituents, and the hydrophilic cyclic lactone enters via phosphoric acid. Because the cyclic lactone is positively charged, it neutralizes the negatively charged site inside the cell membrane. This increases the rigidity of the cell membrane and inhibits the release of arachidonic acid. Lipid remodeling modifies intracellular signaling, especially MAPK systems, suppressing transcription factor activation, particularly when the cells are activated. Membrane remodeling affects cell surface molecule recycling and phagocytosis. Molecules affected by negative charges are also affected, affecting lysosomal uptake and autophagy. Apoptosis is induced by inhibition of Bcl at high concentrations of AZM, suggesting that macrolides accumulate in lysosomes and alter their function, leading to increased phagocytosis and efferocytosis, modified autophagy, and increased apoptosis. Changes in the cell membrane also affect intracellular signal transduction, resulting in the inhibition of cytokines, mucins, and inflammation-related genes. The intracellular target of josamycin was comprehensively examined by a genome-wide shRNA screen. It was found that josamycin is associated with mitochondrial transcription and protein, anaerobic metabolism, and MAP kinase kinase kinase 4 (MAP 3 K4) and is able to suppress oxidative phosphorylation and shift to glycolysis [92].

4 Conclusion

Low-dose long-term macrolide therapy has progressed from the discovery of remarkable clinical effects in DPB to basic research and further to clinical application in other airway diseases. Macrolides suppress mucus hypersecretion and neutrophilic infiltration through the suppression of proinflammatory cytokines, chemokines, and adhesion molecules. Macrolide antibiotics are immunomodulatory, meaning that they reset and normalize the immune response. In order to elucidate the mechanism of action of macrolides, the intracellular signal transduction mechanism has been studied, and the importance of MAPK pathways and transcription factors such as NFκB has been clarified. However, the target proteins and receptors for macrolides are still unclear. The affinity with the membranes that constitute the cell membrane and intracellular organelles suggests effects on cellular integrity and cell death.

Compliance with ethical standards This article does not contain any studies with human participants or animals performed by the author.

Conflict of Interest The author has no conflict of interest.

References

1. Kudoh S, Azuma A, Yamamoto M, Izumi T, Ando M. Improvement of survival in patients with diffuse panbronchiolitis treated with low-dose erythromycin. Am J Respir Crit Care Med. 1998;157(6 Pt 1):1829–32.
2. Kanoh S, Rubin BK. Mechanisms of action and clinical application of macrolides as immunomodulatory medications. Clin Microbiol Rev. 2010;23(3):590–615.
3. Tamaoki J, Isono K, Sakai N, Kanemura T, Konno K. Erythromycin inhibits cl secretion across canine tracheal epithelial cells. Eur Respir J. 1992;5(2):234–8.
4. Tamaoki J, Takeyama K, Tagaya E, Konno K. Effect of clarithromycin on sputum production and its rheological properties in chronic respiratory tract infections. Antimicrob Agents Chemother. 1995;39(8):1688–90.
5. Tamaoki J. The effects of macrolides on inflammaotry cells. Chest. 2004;125(2 Suppl):41S–50S.

6. Ikeda K, Wu D, Takasaka T. Inhibition of acetylcholine-evoked cl- currents by 14-membered macrolide antibiotics in isolated acinar cells of the Guinea pig nasal gland. Am J Respir Cell Mol Biol. 1995;13(4):449–54.
7. Caputo A, Caci E, Ferrera L, Pedemonte N, Barsanti C, Sondo E, et al. TMEM16A, a membrane protein associated with calcium-dependent chloride channel activity. Science. 2008;322(5901): 590–4.
8. Hara K, Kondo M, Tsuji M, Takeyama K, Tamaoki J. Clarithromycin suppresses IL-13-induced goblet cell metaplasia via the TMEM16A-dependent pathway in Guinea pig airway epithelial cells. Respir Investig. 2019;57(1):79–88.
9. Kondo M, Kanoh S, Tamaoki J, Shirakawa H, Miyazaki S, Nagai A. Erythromycin inhibits ATP-induced intracellular calcium responses in bovine tracheal epithelial cells. Am J Respir Cell Mol Biol. 1998;19(5):799–804.
10. Barker PM, Gillie DJ, Schechter MS, Rubin BK. Effect of macrolides on in vivo ion transport across cystic fibrosis nasal epithelium. Am J Respir Crit Care Med. 2005;171(8):868–71.
11. Tagaya E, Tamaoki J, Kondo M, Nagai A. Effect of a short course of clarithromycin therapy on sputum production in patients with chronic airway hypersecretion. Chest. 2002;122(1):213–8.
12. Fahy JV, Dickey BF. Airway mucus function and dysfunction. N Engl J Med. 2010;363(23): 2233–47.
13. Tamaoki J, Takeyama K, Yamawaki I, Kondo M, Konno K. Lipopolysaccharide-induced goblet cell hypersecretion in the Guinea pig trachea: inhibition by macrolides. Am J Physiol. 1997;272 (1 Pt 1):L15–9.
14. Takeyama K, Dabbagh K, Lee HM, Agustí C, Lausier JA, Ueki IF, et al. Epidermal growth factor system regulates mucin production in airways. Proc Natl Acad Sci U S A. 1999;96(6): 3081–6.
15. Perrais M, Pigny P, Copin MC, Aubert JP, Van Seuningen I. Induction od MUC2 and MUC5AC mucins by factors of the epidermal growth factor (EGF)nfamily is mediated by EGF receptor/Ras/Raf/extracellular signal-regulated kinase cascase and Sp1. J Biol Chem. 2002;277:32258–67.
16. Takeyama K, Tamaoki J, Kondo M, Aoshiba K, Nakata J, Isono K, et al. Effect of macrolide antibiotics on MUC5AC production on human bronchial epithelial cells. Jpn J Antibiot. 2001;54:52–4.
17. Takeyama K, Dabbagh K, Jeong Shim J, Dao-Pick T, Ueki IF, Nadel JA. Oxidative stress causes mucin synthesis via transactivation of epidermal growth factor receptor: role of neutrophils. J Immunol. 2000;164(3):1546–52.
18. Kohri K, Ueki IF, Nadel JA. Neutrophil elastase induces mucin production by ligand-dependent epidermal growth factor receptor activation. Am J Physiol Lung Cell Mol Physiol. 2002;283(3): L531–40.
19. Kohri K, Ueki IF, Shim JJ, Burgel PR, Oh YM, Tam DC, et al. Pseudomonas aeruginosa induces MUC5AC production via epidermal growth factor receptor. Eur Respir J. 2002;20(5): 1263–70.
20. Sakito O, Kadota J, Kohno S, Abe K, Shirai R, Hara K. Interleukin 1 beta, tumor necrosis factor alpha, and interleukin 8 in bronchoalveolar lavage fluid of patients with diffuse panbronchiolitis: a potential mechanism of macrolide therapy. Respiration. 1996;63(1):42–8.
21. Ou XM, Feng YL, Wen FQ, Wang K, Yang J, Deng ZP, et al. Macrolides attenuate mucus hypersecretion in rat airways through inactivation of NF-kappaB. Respirology. 2008;13(1): 63–72.
22. Lin HC, Wang CH, Liu CY, Yu CT, Kuo HP. Erythromycin inhibits beta2-integrins (CD11b/ CD18) expression, interleukin-8 release and intracellular oxidative metabolism in neutrophils. Respir Med. 2000;94(7):654–60.
23. Enomoto F, Andou I, Nagaoka I, Ichikawa G. Effect of new macrolides on the expression of adhesion molecules on neutrophils in chronic sinusitis. Auris Nasus Larynx. 2002;29(3):267–9.
24. Li Y, Azuma A, Takahashi S, Usuki J, Matsuda K, Aoyama A, et al. Fourteen-membered ring macrolides inhibit vascular cell adhesion molecule 1 messenger RNA induction and leukocyte

migration: role in preventing lung injury and fibrosis in bleomycin-challenged mice. Chest. 2002;122(6):2137–45.
25. Sanz MJ, Nabah YN, Cerdá-Nicolás M, O'Connor JE, Issekutz AC, Cortijo J, et al. Erythromycin exerts in vivo anti-inflammatory activity downregulating cell adhesion molecule expression. Br J Pharmacol. 2005;144(2):190–201.
26. Sato E, Nelson DK, Koyama S, Hoyt JC, Robbins RA. Erythromycin modulates eosinophil chemotactic cytokine production by human lung fibroblasts in vitro. Antimicrob Agents Chemother. 2001;45(2):401–6.
27. Konno S, Adachi M, Asano K, Okamoto K, Takahashi T. Anti-allergic activity of roxithromycin: inhibition of interleukin-5 production from mouse T lymphocytes. Life Sci. 1993;52(4):PL25–30.
28. Mann TS, Larcombe AN, Wang KCW, Shamsuddin D, Landwehr KR, Noble PB, et al. Azithromycin inhibits mucin secretion, mucous metaplasia, airway inflammation, and airways hyperresponsiveness in mice exposed to house dust mite extract. Am J Physiol Lung Cell Mol Physiol. 2022;322(5):L683–98.
29. Seemungal TA, Wilkinson TM, Hurst JR, Perera WR, Sapsford RJ, Wedzicha JA. Long-term erythromycin therapy is associated with decreased chronic obstructive pulmonary disease exacerbations. Am J Respir Crit Care Med. 2008;178(11):1139–47.
30. Uzun S, Djamin RS, Kluytmans JA, Mulder PG, van't Veer NE, Ermens AA, et al. Azithromycin maintenance treatment in patients with frequent exacerbations of chronic obstructive pulmonary disease (COLUMBUS): a randomised, double-blind, placebo-controlled trial. Lancet. Respir Med. 2014;2(5):361–8.
31. Suzuki T, Yamaya M, Sekizawa K, Hosoda M, Yamada N, Ishizuka S, et al. Erythromycin inhibits rhinovirus infection in cultured human tracheal epithelial cells. Am J Respir Crit Care Med. 2002;165(8):1113–8.
32. Yamaya M, Azuma A, Takizawa H, Kadota J, Tamaoki J, Kudoh S. Macrolide effects on the prevention of COPD exacerbations. Eur Respir J. 2012;40(2):485–94.
33. Simpson JL, Powell H, Boyle MJ, Scott RJ, Gibson PG. Clarithromycin targets neutrophilic airway inflammation in refractory asthma. Am J Respir Crit Care Med. 2008;177(2):148–55.
34. Kanoh S, Tanabe T, Rubin BK. IL-13-induced MUC5AC production and goblet cell differentiation is steroid resistant in human airway cells. Clin Exp Allergy. 2011;41(12):1747–56.
35. Tanabe T, Kanoh S, Tsushima K, Yamazaki Y, Kubo K, Rubin BK. Clarithromycin inhibits interleukin-13-induced goblet cell hyperplasia in human airway cells. Am J Respir Cell Mol Biol. 2011;45(5):1075–83.
36. Nagashima A, Shinkai M, Shinoda M, Shimokawaji T, Kimura Y, Mishina K, et al. Clarithromycin suppresses Chloride Channel accessory 1 and inhibits Interleukin-13-induced goblet cell hyperplasia in human bronchial epithelial cells. Antimicrob Agents Chemother. 2016;60(11):6585–90.
37. Sala-Rabanal M, Yurtsever Z, Nichols CG, Brett TJ. Secreted CLCA1 modulates TMEM16A to activate ca(2+)-dependent chloride currents in human cells. elife. 2015;4:4.
38. Gibson PG, Yang IA, Upham JW, Reynolds PN, Hodge S, James AL, et al. Effect of azithromycin on asthma exacerbations and quality of life in adults with persistent uncontrolled asthma (AMAZES): a randomised, double-blind, placebo-controlled trial. Lancet. 2017;390 (10095):659–68.
39. Shinkai M, Henke MO, Rubin BK. Macrolide antibiotics as immunomodulatory medications: proposed mechanisms of action. Pharmacol Ther. 2008;117(3):393–405.
40. Porto BN, Stein RT. Neutrophil extracellular traps in pulmonary diseases: too much of a good thing? Front Immunol. 2016;7:311.
41. Zhang H, Qiu SL, Tang QY, Zhou X, Zhang JQ, He ZY, et al. Erythromycin suppresses neutrophil extracellular traps in smoking-related chronic pulmonary inflammation. Cell Death Dis. 2019;10(9):678.
42. Murphy BS, Sundareshan V, Cory TJ, Hayes D, Anstead MI, Feola DJ. Azithromycin alters macrophage phenotype. J Antimicrob Chemother. 2008;61(3):554–60.

43. Aderem A, Underhill DM. Mechanisms of phagocytosis in macrophages. Annu Rev Immunol. 1999;17:593–623.
44. Parnham MJ, Erakovic Haber V, Giamarellos-Bourboulis EJ, Perletti G, Verleden GM, Vos R. Azithromycin: mechanisms of action and their relevance for clinical applications. Pharmacol Ther. 2014;143(2):225–45.
45. Iwamoto S, Kumamoto T, Azuma E, Hirayama M, Ito M, Amano K, et al. The effect of azithromycin on the maturation and function of murine bone marrow-derived dendritic cells. Clin Exp Immunol. 2011;166(3):385–92.
46. Pollock J, Chalmers JD. The immunomodulatory effects of macrolide antibiotics in respiratory disease. Pulm Pharmacol Ther. 2021;71:102095.
47. Sugiyama K, Shirai R, Mukae H, Ishimoto H, Nagata T, Sakamoto N, et al. Differing effects of clarithromycin and azithromycin on cytokine production by murine dendritic cells. Clin Exp Immunol. 2007;147(3):540–6.
48. Foulds G, Shepard RM, Johnson RB. The pharmacokinetics of azithromycin in human serum and tissues. J Antimicrob Chemother. 1990;25(Suppl A):73–82.
49. Zhao DM, Xue HH, Chida K, Suda T, Oki Y, Kanai M, et al. Effect of erythromycin on ATP-induced intracellular calcium response in A549 cells. Am J Physiol Lung Cell Mol Physiol. 2000;278(4):L726–36.
50. Lu S, Liu H, Farley JM. Macrolide antibiotics inhibit mucus secretion and calcium entry in swine airway submucosal mucous gland cells. J Pharmacol Exp Ther. 2011;336(1):178–87.
51. Kase K, Hua J, Yokoi H, Ikeda K, Nagaoka I. Inhibitory action of roxithromycin on histamine release and prostaglandin D2 production from beta-defensin 2-stimulated mast cells. Int J Mol Med. 2009;23(3):337–40.
52. Mitsuyama T, Hidaka K, Furuno T, Hara N. Neutrophil-induced endothelial cell damage: inhibition by a 14-membered ring macrolide through the action of nitric oxide. Int Arch Allergy Immunol. 1997;114(2):111–5.
53. Johnson GL, Lapadat R. Mitogen-activated protein kinase pathways mediated by ERK, JNK, and p38 protein kinases. Science. 2002;298(5600):1911–2.
54. Shinkai M, Foster GH, Rubin BK. Macrolide antibiotics modulate ERK phosphorylation and IL-8 and GM-CSF production by human bronchial epithelial cells. Am J Physiol Lung Cell Mol Physiol. 2006;290(1):L75–85.
55. Shinkai M, Tamaoki J, Kobayashi H, Kanoh S, Motoyoshi K, Kute T, et al. Clarithromycin delays progression of bronchial epithelial cells from G1 phase to S phase and delays cell growth via extracellular signal-regulated protein kinase suppression. Antimicrob Agents Chemother. 2006;50(5):1738–44.
56. Imamura Y, Yanagihara K, Mizuta Y, Seki M, Ohno H, Higashiyama Y, et al. Azithromycin inhibits MUC5AC production induced by the Pseudomonas aeruginosa autoinducer N-(3-Oxododecanoyl) homoserine lactone in NCI-H292 cells. Antimicrob Agents Chemother. 2004;48(9):3457–61.
57. Tsai WC, Rodriguez ML, Young KS, Deng JC, Thannickal VJ, Tateda K, et al. Azithromycin blocks neutrophil recruitment in pseudomonas endobronchial infection. Am J Respir Crit Care Med. 2004;170(12):1331–9.
58. Kaneko Y, Yanagihara K, Seki M, Kuroki M, Miyazaki Y, Hirakata Y, et al. Clarithromycin inhibits overproduction of muc5ac core protein in murine model of diffuse panbronchiolitis. Am J Physiol Lung Cell Mol Physiol. 2003;285(4):L847–53.
59. Bin YF, Ma N, Lu YX, Sun XJ, Liang Y, Bai J, et al. Erythromycin reverses cigarette smoke extract-induced corticosteroid insensitivity by inhibition of the JNK/c-Jun pathway. Free Radic Biol Med. 2020;152:494–503.
60. Desaki M, Takizawa H, Ohtoshi T, Kasama T, Kobayashi K, Sunazuka T, et al. Erythromycin suppresses nuclear factor-kappaB and activator protein-1 activation in human bronchial epithelial cells. Biochem Biophys Res Commun. 2000;267(1):124–8.

61. Ichiyama T, Nishikawa M, Yoshitomi T, Hasegawa S, Matsubara T, Hayashi T, et al. Clarithromycin inhibits NF-kappaB activation in human peripheral blood mononuclear cells and pulmonary epithelial cells. Antimicrob Agents Chemother. 2001;45(1):44–7.
62. Kikuchi T, Hagiwara K, Honda Y, Gomi K, Kobayashi T, Takahashi H, et al. Clarithromycin suppresses lipopolysaccharide-induced interleukin-8 production by human monocytes through AP-1 and NF-kappa B transcription factors. J Antimicrob Chemother. 2002;49(5):745–55.
63. Aghai ZH, Kode A, Saslow JG, Nakhla T, Farhath S, Stahl GE, et al. Azithromycin suppresses activation of nuclear factor-kappa B and synthesis of pro-inflammatory cytokines in tracheal aspirate cells from premature infants. Pediatr Res. 2007;62(4):483–8.
64. Cigana C, Nicolis E, Pasetto M, Assael BM, Melotti P. Anti-inflammatory effects of azithromycin in cystic fibrosis airway epithelial cells. Biochem Biophys Res Commun. 2006;350(4):977–82.
65. Araki N, Yanagihara K, Morinaga Y, Yamada K, Nakamura S, Yamada Y, et al. Azithromycin inhibits nontypeable *Haemophilus influenzae*-induced MUC5AC expression and secretion via inhibition of activator protein-1 in human airway epithelial cells. Eur J Pharmacol. 2010;644 (1–3):209–14.
66. Bosnar M, Čužić S, Bošnjak B, Nujić K, Ergović G, Marjanović N, et al. Azithromycin inhibits macrophage interleukin-1β production through inhibition of activator protein-1 in lipopolysaccharide-induced murine pulmonary neutrophilia. Int Immunopharmacol. 2011;11 (4):424–34.
67. Weng D, Wu Q, Chen XQ, Du YK, Chen T, Li H, et al. Azithromycin treats diffuse panbronchiolitis by targeting T cells via inhibition of mTOR pathway. Biomed Pharmacother. 2019;110:440–8.
68. Ratzinger F, Haslacher H, Poeppl W, Hoermann G, Kovarik JJ, Jutz S, et al. Azithromycin suppresses CD4(+) T-cell activation by direct modulation of mTOR activity. Sci Rep. 2014;4: 7438.
69. Zhao X, Yu FQ, Huang XJ, Xu BY, Li YL, Zhao XY, et al. Azithromycin influences airway remodeling in asthma via the PI3K/Akt/MTOR/HIF-1α/VEGF pathway. J Biol Regul Homeost Agents. 2018;32(5):1079–88.
70. Wang J, Xie L, Wang S, Lin J, Liang J, Xu J. Azithromycin promotes alternatively activated macrophage phenotype in systematic lupus erythematosus via PI3K/Akt signaling pathway. Cell Death Dis. 2018;9(11):1080.
71. Sun X, Chen L, He Z. PI3K/Akt-Nrf2 and anti-inflammation effect of macrolides in chronic obstructive pulmonary disease. Curr Drug Metab. 2019;20(4):301–4.
72. Broz P, Dixit VM. Inflammasomes: mechanism of assembly, regulation and signalling. Nat Rev Immunol. 2016;16(7):407–20.
73. Gualdoni GA, Lingscheid T, Schmetterer KG, Hennig A, Steinberger P, Zlabinger GJ. Azithromycin inhibits IL-1 secretion and non-canonical inflammasome activation. Sci Rep. 2015;5:12016.
74. Seys SF, Lokwani R, Simpson JL, Bullens DMA. New insights in neutrophilic asthma. Curr Opin Pulm Med. 2019;25(1):113–20.
75. Otsu K, Ishinaga H, Suzuki S, Sugawara A, Sunazuka T, Omura S, et al. Effects of a novel nonantibiotic macrolide, EM900, on cytokine and mucin gene expression in a human airway epithelial cell line. Pharmacology. 2011;88(5–6):327–32.
76. Acosta JC, Banito A, Wuestefeld T, Georgilis A, Janich P, Morton JP, et al. A complex secretory program orchestrated by the inflammasome controls paracrine senescence. Nat Cell Biol. 2013;15(8):978–90.
77. Ozsvari B, Nuttall JR, Sotgia F, Lisanti MP. Azithromycin and Roxithromycin define a new family of "senolytic" drugs that target senescent human fibroblasts. Aging (Albany NY). 2018;10(11):3294–307.
78. Chen X, Xu H, Hou J, Wang H, Zheng Y, Li H, et al. Epithelial cell senescence induces pulmonary fibrosis through Nanog-mediated fibroblast activation. Aging (Albany NY). 2019;12 (1):242–59.

79. Fiorillo M, Tóth F, Sotgia F, Lisanti MP. Doxycycline, azithromycin and vitamin C (DAV): a potent combination therapy for targeting mitochondria and eradicating cancer stem cells (CSCs). Aging (Albany NY). 2019;11(8):2202–16.
80. Ballabio A, Bonifacino JS. Lysosomes as dynamic regulators of cell and organismal homeostasis. Nat Rev Mol Cell Biol. 2020;21(2):101–18.
81. Breiden B, Sandhoff K. Emerging mechanisms of drug-induced phospholipidosis. Biol Chem. 2019;401(1):31–46.
82. Randow F, Münz C. Autophagy in the regulation of pathogen replication and adaptive immunity. Trends Immunol. 2012;33(10):475–87.
83. Klionsky DJ. Autophagy participates in, well, just about everything. Cell Death Differ. 2020;27(3):831–2.
84. Stamatiou R, Paraskeva E, Boukas K, Gourgoulianis KI, Molyvdas PA, Hatziefthimiou AA. Azithromycin has an antiproliferative and autophagic effect on airway smooth muscle cells. Eur Respir J. 2009;34(3):721–30.
85. Renna M, Schaffner C, Brown K, Shang S, Tamayo MH, Hegyi K, et al. Azithromycin blocks autophagy and may predispose cystic fibrosis patients to mycobacterial infection. J Clin Invest. 2011;121(9):3554–63.
86. Tsubouchi K, Araya J, Minagawa S, Hara H, Ichikawa A, Saito N, et al. Azithromycin attenuates myofibroblast differentiation and lung fibrosis development through proteasomal degradation of NOX4. Autophagy. 2017;13(8):1420–34.
87. Moriya S, Che XF, Komatsu S, Abe A, Kawaguchi T, Gotoh A, et al. Macrolide antibiotics block autophagy flux and sensitize to bortezomib via endoplasmic reticulum stress-mediated CHOP induction in myeloma cells. Int J Oncol. 2013;42(5):1541–50.
88. Fimia GM, Piacentini M. Regulation of autophagy in mammals and its interplay with apoptosis. Cell Mol Life Sci. 2010;67(10):1581–8.
89. Koch CC, Esteban DJ, Chin AC, Olson ME, Read RR, Ceri H, et al. Apoptosis, oxidative metabolism and interleukin-8 production in human neutrophils exposed to azithromycin: effects of Streptococcus pneumoniae. J Antimicrob Chemother. 2000;46(1):19–26.
90. Reijnders TDY, Saris A, Schultz MJ, van der Poll T. Immunomodulation by macrolides: therapeutic potential for critical care. Lancet Respir Med. 2020;8(6):619–30.
91. Kricker JA, Page CP, Gardarsson FR, Baldursson O, Gudjonsson T, Parnham MJ. Nonantimicrobial actions of macrolides: overview and perspectives for future development. Pharmacol Rev. 2021;73(4):233–62.
92. Gupta A, Ökesli-Armlovich A, Morgens D, Bassik MC. Khosla C A genome-wide analysis of targets of macrolide antibiotics in mammalian cells. J Biol Chem. 2020;295(7):2057–67.

Part II
Clinical Use for Airway Disease

Macrolides as Immunomodulatory Agents

Namiko Taniuchi and Arata Azuma

Abstract Diffuse panbronchiolitis (DPB) is a disease characterized by diffuse bilateral centrilobular lesions consisting of peribronchial infiltration of inflammatory cells. More than 50 years after its first being reported in Japan, DPB is recognized as a disease that predominantly affects East Asians and disease susceptibility genes have been proposed. Kudo et al. found that low-dose long-term erythromycin (EM) therapy can be an effective treatment for DPB, resulting in a marked improvement in prognosis. The beneficial effect of EM therapy led to progress in understanding the pathogenesis of chronic inflammatory airway diseases and to new developments in the field of research on actions other than the antimicrobial activity of 14- and 15-membered ring macrolides. Macrolide therapy is most effective in the early stage of the disease and should be initiated as soon as possible. In case of exacerbation, infection with *Haemophilus influenzae*, *Streptococcus pneumoniae*, *Moraxella catarrhalis*, and *Pseudomonas aeruginosa* should be considered, and effective antimicrobial agents should be administered. In recent years, the number of cases complicated by pulmonary nontuberculous mycobacterial infections has been increasing. In particular, the induction of clarithromycin resistance by *Mycobacterium avium* complex has become a problem. Macrolide-resistant DPB is also becoming a clinical problem.

Keywords Diffuse panbronchiolitis (DPB) · Erythromycin (EM) · Clarithromycin (CAM) · 14- and 15-membered ring macrolides · Macrolide therapy

1 Introduction

In 1969, Homma, Yamanaka, and coworkers first reported diffuse panbronchiolitis (DPB) as a new clinicopathologic entity characterized by chronic recurrent bronchiolitis and peribronchiolitis with lymphocyte and plasma cell infiltration, often

N. Taniuchi (✉) · A. Azuma
Department of Pulmonary Medicine, Nippon Medical School Musashikosugi Hospital, Kanagawa, Japan
e-mail: taniuchi@nms.ac.jp; a-azuma@nms.ac.jp

B. K. Rubin, M. Shinkai (eds.), *Macrolides as Immunomodulatory Agents*, Progress in Inflammation Research 92, https://doi.org/10.1007/978-3-031-42859-3_3

causing small airway obstruction through the formation of lymph follicles, granulomas, and scars [1, 2]. After more than a decade of research in Japan, the first comprehensive report on DPB was published in Western countries in 1983 [3]. Today, more than 50 years later, DPB is widely recognized internationally as an airway disease predominantly affecting East Asians, and disease susceptibility genes have been identified [4].

For the first 10 years after DPB was reported, DPB had a poor prognosis when treatment with antibiotics and supportive therapy was used [5]. However, in 1984, Kudo et al. found that low-dose long-term erythromycin (EM) therapy could be an effective treatment for DPB, resulting in a marked improvement in prognosis [6–9] (Fig. 1). The beneficial effect of EM therapy led to progress in understanding the pathogenesis of chronic inflammatory airway diseases [9] and to new developments in the field of research on actions beyond the antimicrobial activity [9] of 14- and 15-membered ring macrolide antibiotics.

2 Epidemiology

In Japan, the male-to-female ratio of DPB is 1.4–2:1 [25], and consequently, no remarkable sex predominance is observed. Two-thirds of patients are nonsmokers, and patients have no specific history of inhalation of toxic fumes. Disease onset is most common in people in their 40 s and 50 s. DPB is a form of sinobronchial syndrome (SBS), with 70%–90% of patients with chronic sinusitis history [2, 10, 11]. Before the advent of low-dose EM therapy in the 1980s, DPB was a disease of high frequency and poor prognosis; DPB prevalence in Japan was reported to be 13.8/100,000 persons, with a 5-year survival rate of 50–70% [8, 12]. However, long-term treatment with EM has increased the 10-year survival rate to >90% [8]. In recent years, DPB prevalence has decreased, and DPB has become a nonfatal disease. This is partly due to the frequent use of macrolides for upper and lower respiratory infections in primary care [12].

3 HLA Antigens

DPB is predominantly seen in East Asia, and human leukocyte antigen (HLA) analysis of Japanese DPB patients reported that 63.2% of them were found to carry human leukocyte antigen (HLA) B54 [13], which is almost exclusively seen in East Asians. DPB has also been reported to run in families [14]. HLA typing reported the association between HLA-B*5401 and HLA-B*5404 in Japanese and HLA-A11 in Korean [15]. In addition, a significant increase of Bw54 and slight increases of Cw1 and MC1 were observed in HLA class I and class II antigens in Japanese. These increases might be explained by the fact that these two antigens, Cw1 and MC1, formed a haplotype with Bw54, which suggests that one or some of

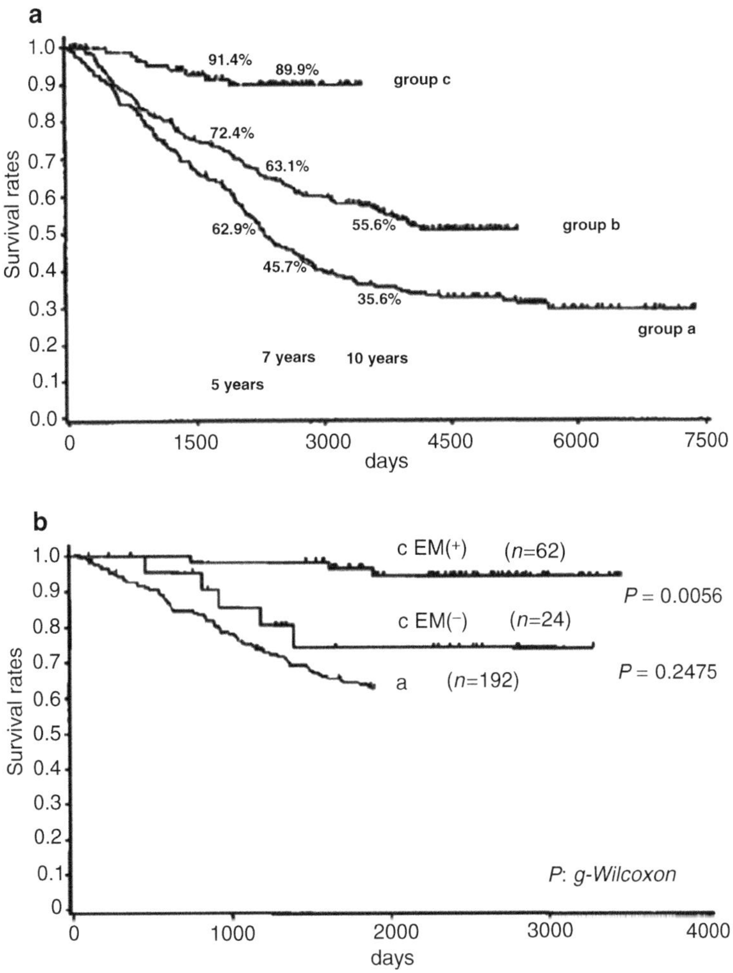

Fig. 1 (**a**) Survival curves according to the year of first medical examination for patients with diffuse panbronchiolitis (group a: 1970–1979, group b: 1980–1984, group c: 1985–1990). (**b**) Contribution of treatment with erythromycin (EM) on the survival of patients with diffuse panbronchiolitis. In patients in group c treated with EM ($n = 62$), the survival ratio was significantly higher than in simultaneous patients without EM treatment ($n = 24$) ($p = 0.0056$). In contrast, survival curves of patients in group a ($n = 192$) who were not treated with EM before 1985 were not significantly different from those of non-EM treated patients in group c ($p = 0.2475$)

the genes controlling the susceptibility and/or immune responsiveness of DPB might be located near HLA loci [13]. The presence of the haplotype B54-Cw1-A11, which is common to both Japanese and Koreans, has raised the hypothesis that one of the genes responsible for DPB is located between chromosome 6 HLA gene loci A and B and that genetic recombination may have occurred during ethnic division or integration [16].

However, cases of rheumatoid arthritis (RA) complicating DPB have been reported. HLA-DR4 has been reported to be associated with RA in various racial groups [17, 18], and of the eight cases of DPB and RA combined in Japanese, the three patients in whom both HLA-B54 and HLA-DR4 were measured were all positive. Because HLA-B54 and HLA-DR4 constitute a haplotype among Japanese, these diseases possibly occur together [19].

4 Pathophysiology

Chronic sinusitis is a frequent complication of chronic respiratory bronchiolitis, which is associated with impaired airway clearance and chronic infection [11, 20]. Due to the release of proteolytic enzymes and reactive oxygen species, the excessive mucin secretion from goblet cells and the recruitment of neutrophils increases the production of airway mucus and tissue damage, further impairing mucus transport. Histopathological findings show an accumulation of lymphocytes and foamy macrophages in the interstitium, consistent with chronic inflammation mainly by CD8+ lymphocytes and macrophages [21].

In macrolide-refractory and some advanced cases, the patient may expectorate up to 200–300 mL of sputum daily as well as changes in airway pathogens, eventually leading to chronic respiratory infections with *Pseudomonas aeruginosa* [22].

5 Diagnosis

In 1988, a working group of the Ministry of Health and Welfare in Japan proposed diagnostic criteria, shown in Table 1 [23, 24].

More than 80% of the patients have a history of or suffer from chronic paranasal sinusitis [25, 26]; even those who appear to be asymptomatic. Chronic cough with copious purulent sputum is usually present as well as exertional dyspnea. Auscultation can show crackles, wheezes, or both. In a review of 81 histologically proven cases, 44% had *Haemophilus influenzae* in their sputum at presentation and 22% had *Pseudomonas aeruginosa*. After 4 years, the detection rate of *P. aeruginosa* increased to 60% [25, 26]. Laboratory findings suggest the presence of immunological abnormalities and chronic nonspecific inflammation. The titer of cold hemagglutinin is raised in most patients [27].

Pulmonary function testing shows airflow limitation and a relative lack of bronchodilator reversibility. Decreased FEV_1/FVC (forced expiratory volume in 1 second/forced vital capacity) of less than 70%, decreased VC (vital capacity) of less than 80% predicted, and increased residual volume, greater than 150% predicted, are common. Hypoxia with PaO_2 (arterial oxygen tension) less than 80 torr subsequently develops [9, 25, 26].

Table 1 Diagnostic criteria for diffuse panbronchiolitis

Noninvasive (clinical manifestations)
1. Persistent cough, sputum, and exertional dyspnea.
2. History or current symptoms of chronic sinusitis.
3. Chest X-ray: Bilateral, diffuse, small nodular shadows. Chest CT (HRCT): Bilateral, diffuse, centrilobular micronodules
4. Coarse crackles.
5. FEV_1/FVC less than 70% and PaO_2 less than 80 mmHg (10.64 kPa).
6. Titer of cold agglutinins of 64 or greater.
Diagnosis
Cases definitely established should fulfill criteria 1, 2, and 3, along with at least two of criteria 4, 5, and 6.
Lung biopsy
Lung biopsy showing inflammation centered on the respiratory bronchioles with a transmural infiltrate composed of lymphocytes, plasma cells, and distinctive lipid-laden "foamy" macrophages, also known as foam cells[a]

FEV_1 forced expiratory volume in 1 second; *FVC* forced vital capacity; *PaO_2* arterial oxygen tension; *HRCT* high-resolution computed tomography
[a]In regions where diffuse panbronchiolitis is endemic (e.g., East Asia), a lung biopsy is not needed if the patient fulfills the first three criteria and at least two of the second three

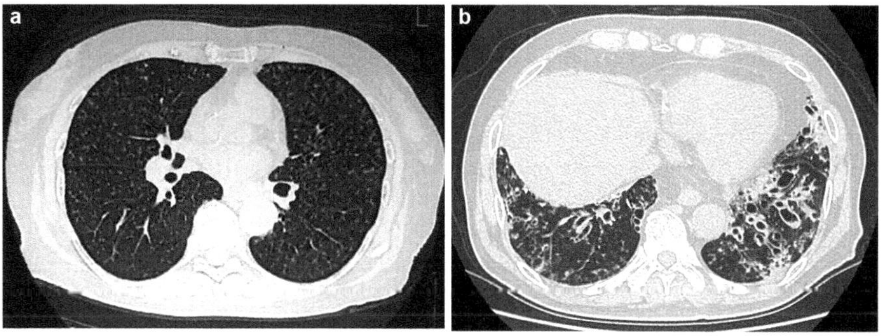

Fig. 2 (**a**) Chest HRCT in a typical DPB case. Diffusely distributed 1–2 mm sized centrilobular granular shadows, as well as linear and dendritic shadows associated with the granular shadows, are seen. Bronchiectasis with bronchial wall thickening is also seen. (**b**) Chest HRCT in an advanced DPB case. Marked bronchiectasis and bronchial wall thickening are seen in the basal and central bronchus. Granular and dendritic shadows are also shown in the typical DPB

Chest CT is useful for detecting the characteristic pulmonary lesions of DPB [9, 28, 29]. Nodular shadows are distributed in a centrilobular fashion, often extending to small, branching linear areas of attenuation in a "tree-in-bud" pattern. Peripheral air trapping is usually confirmed in expiratory films. There is dilatation of airways and bronchial wall thickening characteristic of bronchiectasis. In advanced disease, multiple cystic lesions predominate in the lower lung fields accompanied by dilated proximal bronchi showing extensive bronchiectasis (Fig. 2).

6 Treatment

Table 2 shows the treatment summary for DPB. In 2000, clinical guidelines on macrolide therapy for DPB were proposed by the Diffuse Lung Disease Committee members of the Ministry of the Health and Welfare in Japan, based mainly on evidence from the historical study [8], observational studies, and expert opinion [30]. Macrolide therapy is effective in the early stages of disease, so treatment should be initiated as soon as possible after diagnosis. Beneficial effect is usually observed within 2–3 months. If symptoms and laboratory findings improve, treatment is usually completed after 2 years.

Low-dose long-term macrolide therapy for DPB was first demonstrated using EM [6] and established through a large retrospective study [8] and a small randomized controlled trial [31]. Similar clinical efficacy was observed using CAM and RXM, 14-membered ring macrolides as is EM [32, 33]. There are historical changes in macrolide therapy for DPB. First, there was a period of investigation based on case experience in which complete cure was achieved with EM [8]. Later, AZM, a 15-membered macrolide, was introduced and proved to be effective in DPB. Although it has been reported that AZM was effective in 73% of patients in whom 14-membered macrolides were ineffective [34], a direct comparison between 14-membered macrolides and AZM has never been evaluated. In the modern era,

Table 2 Clinical guidelines for diffuse panbronchiolitis therapy

Macrolides
First choice: Erythromycin 400 or 600 mg oral/daily
Second choice: Clarithromycin 200 or 400 mg orally or roxithromycin 150 or 300 mg orally
Third choice: Azithromycin 250 mg orally, three times a week
Assessment of response and duration of treatment
Although clinical response is usually obtained within 2 or 3 months, treatment should be continued for at least 6 months, and then the overall response should be evaluated
Treatment can be completed after 2 years when clinical manifestations, radiological findings, and pulmonary function evaluations are improved or stable without significant loss of daily activity
Treatment should be restarted if symptoms reoccur after cessation
When it is effective in advanced cases with extensive bronchiectasis or respiratory failure, treatment should be continued for more than 2 years
Treatments other than macrolides
Use expectorants as adjunctive therapy, as appropriate
If nontuberculous mycobacteria (NTM) infection is present, treatment of NTM should also be considered
When exacerbation occurs, search for causative organisms by sputum culture. Additional antimicrobial agents should be administered to cover *Haemophilus influenzae*, *Streptococcus pneumoniae*, *Moraxella catarrhalis*, and *Pseudomonas aeruginosa*
Rehabilitation and airway clearance are helpful in advanced cases. Home oxygen therapy should be introduced in cases of respiratory failure
Improvement of nutritional status and vaccination are important to prevent exacerbations
Lung transplantation should be considered in patients with refractory progression of disease

one reason for first-line EM is that CAM, RXM, and AZM can induce resistance to nontuberculous mycobacteria (NTM). About 20% of DPB patients have comorbid NTM [35]. The differences between macrolide drugs, in terms of tissue translocation [36], inhibition of toxins in *P. aeruginosa*, and in the production of proinflammatory cytokines in dendritic cells [37], have been reported but these differences have not been directly associated with different clinical outcomes of therapy.

There are several randomized trials on the effect of expectorants in treating bronchiectasis in more severe DPB [38]. Bromhexine and cysteine-type expectorants have been reported to improve sputum, dyspnea, and FEV1 [39, 40].

In advanced cases with extensive bronchiectasis or respiratory failure, macrolides can be continued for a longer period. No criteria exist for macrolide discontinuation when macrolides are ineffective. In practice, there is often no next step, and macrolides are often continued indefinitely along with supportive care. In case of exacerbation, antimicrobial agents should be administered based on the susceptibility of the organisms, considering infections such as *Haemophilus influenzae*, *Streptococcus pneumoniae*, *Moraxella catarrhalis*, and *P. aeruginosa* [41, 42].

The mechanisms of action of macrolides in treating DPB cannot be attributed entirely to their antimicrobial effect. DPB can improve without eliminating the bacteria and improvement is seen even in patients with resistant *P. aeruginosa* infection [9]. As noted in other chapters, many studies have been conducted on the effects of macrolides on DPB. A summary of the actions of macrolides found in studies related to DPB is shown in Table 3; (i) inhibition of hypersecretion, (ii) inhibition of neutrophil activity, (iii) effects on lymphocytes, macrophages, and epithelial cells, (iv) Inhibition of chloride channels, (v) effects of cytokine/chemokine expression, and (vi) modulation of bacterial function. A schematic of the relationships among cytokines, chemokines, adhesion molecules, and lipid mediators involved in DPB inflammation in the airway epithelium is shown in Fig. 3 [43, 44].

Proposed actions of EM in the treatment of airway inflammation are summarized in the schematic diagram in Fig. 4 [9]. First, EM suppresses hypersecretion by the inhibition of mucus and water secretion from epithelial cells. Second, EM inhibits neutrophil accumulation at sites of inflammation by the inhibition of adhesion and migration of neutrophils into inflamed regions from capillary vessels, secretion of interleukin-8 and leukotriene B4 from the epithelial cells and from neutrophils [45]. These effects subsequently reduce the levels of injurious substances, such as elastase and superoxide anion [46], and clearly play important roles in the improvement of airway inflammation, although controversies exist concerning the effects of EM on neutrophil activity itself [47–50] and on lymphocytes and macrophages.

DPB is one of the indications for lung transplantation in Japan. The conditions for transplantation are as follows: the disease is refractory to treatment and there is no effective treatment other than lung transplantation, the patient is in imminent danger of death (2-year chance of survival is less than 50%), and the patient must be under 60 years of age. In Japan, 835 lung transplants were performed between 1998 and 2020, including 16 cases of DPB [51]. In a report summarizing five lung transplants for patients with DPB, all patients had successful transplants with no DPB

Table 3 Actions of macrolides found in studies related to diffuse panbronchiolitis

(i) Inhibition of hypersecretion
A large amount of sputum is a characteristic manifestation of DPB [43]. The reduction of sputum volume is the most sensitive parameter [59]. EM inhibits ion transport in epithelial cells in a dose-dependent fashion, and this inhibition depends on the blockade of chloride channels, resulting in reduced water secretion [60].
(ii) Inhibition of neutrophil activity
Many neutrophils are found in bronchoalveolar lavage fluid (BALF), frequently reaching 70 to 80% [43]. After EM treatment, the percentage of neutrophils in BALF markedly decreases and this is associated with attenuated neutrophil chemotaxis [61, 62]. Neutrophil elastase in sputum [63] and in BALF [61] is also decreased.
(iii) Effects on lymphocytes, macrophages, and epithelial cells
In the peribronchiolar areas, chronic inflammation with lymphocytes, plasma cells, and foamy macrophages is the characteristic pathological feature of DPB [43]. These resolve after EM treatment [43]. Memory T cells and activation of CD8+ cells, mainly cytotoxic cells, significantly increase in DPB but decrease after EM treatment [64]. EM has a suppressive effect on the proliferative response of human lymphocytes stimulated with mitogens and antigens. It has been suggested that EM may suppress T cell proliferation at a late stage in the activation process by impairing their response to IL-2 [65]. EM accelerates both the differentiation and proliferation of the monocyte-macrophage system [66].
(iv) Inhibition of chloride channel
In previous in vitro and in vivo studies, EM and other 14-membered ring macrolides can inhibit cl secretion across the airway epithelial cl channel [43]. The inhibition of cl secretion may decrease water secretion across the airway mucosa toward the lumen [1].
(v) Effects of cytokine/chemokine expression
Airway epithelial cells express and release cytokines/chemokines, adhesion molecules, and lipid mediators, and thereby participate in the regulation of inflammatory responses in the airways (Fig. 3) [43, 44]. Inflammatory cytokines such as CXCL-8, IL-1β, and TNF-α are increased in BALF from patients with DPB [32]. Treatment with a 14-membered ring macrolide decreases neutrophil number and these inflammatory cytokines and chemokines [32]. EM attenuates airway inflammatory responses by decreasing the local cytokine/chemokine levels and thus decreasing the recruitment of inflammatory cells such as neutrophils [43].
(vi) Modulation of bacterial function
Even sub-MIC macrolide concentrations can reduce the infectibility of bacteria, which includes virulence factor production and bacterial activity itself. Sub-MIC (minimum inhibitory concentration) of 14-membered ring macrolides exhibits inhibitory effects on biofilm formation and the expression of virulence factors of *P. aeruginosa* [9]. Subinhibitory levels of EM, CAM, and AZM enhance the susceptibility of P. aeruginosa to serum bactericidal activity by altering the cell membrane structure [67]. EM also modulates the effect of pyocianin indirectly. EM prevents the lesion infected with *P. aeruginosa* from tissue injury caused by pyocianin in both direct and indirect manners [68].

recurrence in the transplanted lungs [52]. On the other hand, there was a report of DPB developing after lung transplantation [53].

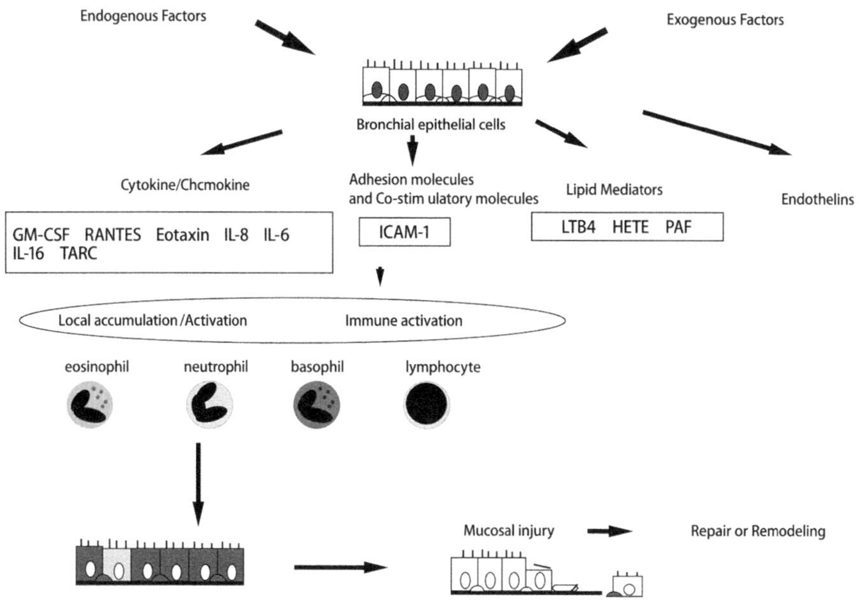

Fig. 3 Airway epithelial cells as sources of cytokines and chemokines in the airways. Airway epithelial cells express and release a variety of cytokines/chemokines, adhesion molecules, and lipid mediators, and thereby participate in the regulation of inflammatory responses in the airways

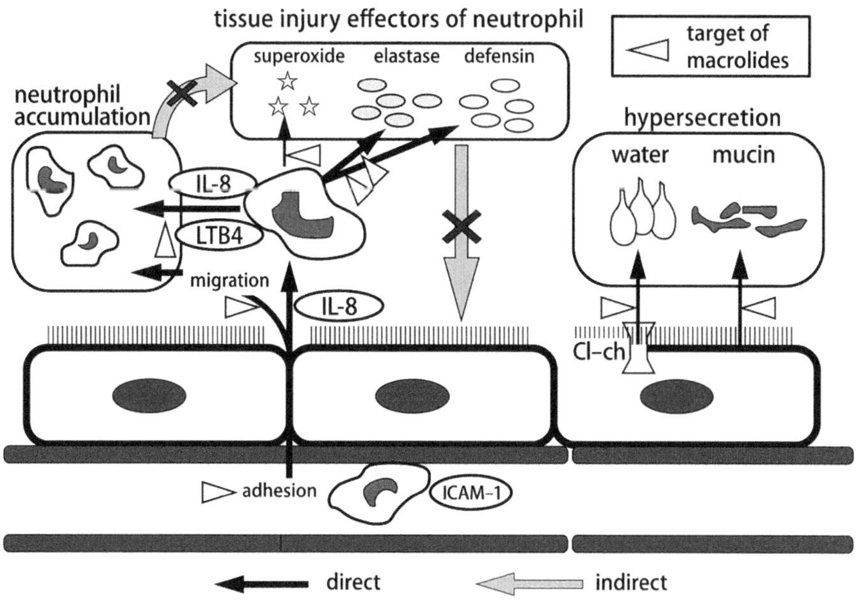

Fig. 4 Schematic diagram of airway inflammation and proposed mechanisms of action of erythromycin. *ICAM-1* intercellular adhesion molecule-1; *LTB4* leukotriene B4

7 Macrolide-Resistant DPB

In clinical practice, 20% of DPB cases are refractory to treatment [16]. EM therapy is considered to be ineffective in patients with long disease duration, persistent *P. aeruginosa* positive, severe bronchiectasis, and difficult to control infection [7] [54–56]. The reason for this may be an organizing progress from peripheral bronchioles to central bronchi due to long-term persistent inflammation leading to irreversible airway disease, which is different from the pathogenesis of DPB in the early stage when EM is effective [57]. It has also been reported that EM is not effective in DPB with severe emphysema. The following mechanisms have been postulated for the development of emphysematous change in DPB: first, alveolar destruction due to inflammation extending not only to respiratory bronchioles but also to alveoli; second, check valve mechanism due to stenosis of respiratory bronchioles; and third, age-related effects [58].

8 Conclusion

The first case of DPB was identified in Japan over 50 years ago. Since then, considerable research has focused on the disease etiology, and genetic associations unique to East Asian populations has been suggested. The advent of EM therapy has changed the prognosis and clinical outcome of the disease to a remarkable extent. DPB is now regarded as a disease with a good prognosis that can be cured by early diagnosis and macrolide therapy. In contrast, the cases complicated by NTM infections, the macrolide-resistant DPB, and the association and differentiation of DPB from other diseases with similar pathophysiology have become clinical problems.

The etiology of DPB is that it is a complex disease, and no single factor is clearly responsible. The beneficial effect of EM therapy led to progress in understanding the pathogenesis of chronic inflammatory airway diseases and to new developments in the field of research on the immunomodulatory activity of 14- and 15-membered ring macrolides.

Conflict of Interest The authors have no conflicts of interest directly relevant to the content of this chapter.

References

1. Yamanaka A, Saiki S, Tamura S, Saito K. Problems in chronic obstructive baronial diseases, with special reference to diffuse panbronchiolitis. Naika. 1969;23:442–51. (in Japanese)
2. Homma H. Diffuse panbronchiolitis. Nihon Kyobu Shikkan Gakkai Zasshi. 1975;13:383–95. (in Japanese)
3. Homma H, Yamanaka A, Tanimoto S, Tamura M, Chijimatsu Y, Kira S, Izumi T. Diffuse panbronchiolitis. A disease of the transitional zone of the lung. Chest. 1983;83:63–9.

4. Keicho N, Ohashi J, Tamiya G, et al. Fine localization of a major disease-susceptibility locus for diffuse panbronchiolitis. Am J Hum Genet. 2000;66:501–7.
5. Kudoh S, Kimua H, Uetake M, et al. Abstract of annual meeting. Nihon Kyobu Shikkan Gakkai Zasshi. 1984;22:254. (in Japanese)
6. Kudoh S, Kimura H. Clinical effect of low-dose long-term administration of macrolides on diffuse panbronchiolitis. Nihon Kyobu Shikkan Gakkai Zasshi. 1984;22:254. (in Japanese)
7. Kudoh S, Uetake T, Hagiawra K, Hirayama M, Hus LH, Kimura H, Sugiyama Y. Clinical effects of low-dose long-term erythromycin chemotherapy on diffuse panbronchiolitis. Nihon Kyobu Shikkan Gakkai Zasshi. 1987;25:632–42. (in Japanese)
8. Kudoh S, Azuma A, Yamamoto M, Izumi T, Ando M. Improvement of survival in patients with diffuse panbronchiolitis treated with low-dose erythromycin. Am J Respir Crit Care Med. 1998;157:1829–32.
9. Azuma A, Kudoh S. Diffuse panbronchiolitis in East Asia. Respirology. 2006;11:249–61.
10. Sugiyama Y. Diffuse panbronchiolitis. Clin Chest Med. 1993;14:765–72.
11. Greenberg SD, Ainsworth JZ. Comparative morphology of chronic bronchitis and chronic sinusitis, with discussion of "Sinobronchial" syndrome. South Med J. 1966;59:64–74.
12. Kono C, Yamaguchi T, Yamada Y, Uchiyama H, Kono M, Takeuchi M, Sugiyamas Y, Azuma A, Kudoh S, Sakurai T, Tatsumi K. Historical changes in epidemiology of diffuse panbronchiolitis. Sarcoidosis Vasc Diffuse Lung Dis. 2012;29:19–25.
13. Sugiyama Y, Kudoh S, Maeda H, Suzaki H, Takaku F. Analysis of HLA antigens in patients with diffuse panbronchiolitis. Am Rev Respir Dis. 1990;141:1459–62.
14. Kudoh S, Keicho N. Racial dependency of diffuse panbronchiolitis and search for disease-susceptibility gene. J Nippon Med Sch. 1999;66(5):336–9. (in Japanese)
15. Keicho N, Hijikata M. Genetic predisposition to diffuse panbronchiolitis. Respirology. 2011;16:581–8.
16. Azuma A, Kudoh S. Diffuse panbronchiolitis. Nihon Rinsho. 2002;60(Suppl 1):32–45. (in Japanese)
17. Maeda H, Juji T, Mitsui H, Sonozaki H, Okitsu K. HLA DR4 and rheumatoid arthritis in Japanese people. Ann Rheum Dis. 1981;40:299–302.
18. Gran JT, Husby G, Thorsby E. The association between rheumatoid arthritis and the HLA antigen DR4. Ann Rheum Dis. 1983;42:292–6.
19. Sugiyama Y, Ohno S, Kano S, Maeda H, Kitamura S. Diffuse panbronchiolitis and rheumatoid arthritis: a possible correlation with HLA-B54. Intern Med. 1994;33:612–4.
20. Committee for the Japanese respiratory society guidelines for management of cough, Kohno S, Ishida T, et al. The Japanese respiratory society guidelines for management of cough. Respirology. 2006;11(Suppl 4):S135–86.
21. Matsumoto T, Fujita M. Practical treatment of diffuse panbronchiolitis. Jpn J Clin Exp Med. 1989;96(12):1469–73. (in Japanese)
22. Kamio K. Obstructive lung disease–Other chronic airway inflammation. Review of respiratory medicine 2022–23; section II-14. 2021:89–94. Sogo Igaku Sha. (in Japanese).
23. Nakata K. Revision of clinical guidelines for diffuse panbronchiolitis. Annual report on the study of diffuse lung disease in 1998. Grant-in aid from the Ministry of Health and Welfare of Japan, Tokyo. 1999:109-111.
24. Kudoh S, Keicho N. Diffuse panbronchiolitis. Clin Chest Med. 2012;33:297–305.
25. Izumi T, Doi O, Nobechi A, Homma Y, Kino N, Nakata K, Inatomi K, Homma H. Annual report on the study of interstitial lung disease in 1982. In: Grant-in aid from the Ministry of Health and Welfare on Japan. Tokyo, Japan; 1983. p. 3–41. (in Japanese).
26. Homma H. Diffuse panbronchiolitis. Jpn J Med. 1986;25:329–34.
27. Homma S, Sakamoto S, Kawabata M, et al. Comparative clinicopathology of obliterative bronchiolitis and diffuse panbronchiolitis. Respiration. 2006;73:481–7.
28. Akira M, Kitatani F, Lee YS, Kita N, Yamamoto S, Higashihara T, Morimoto S, Ikezoe J, Kozuka T. Diffuse panbronchiolitis: evaluation with high-resolution CT. Radiology. 1988;168 (2):433–8.

29. Nishimura K, Kitaichi M, Izumi T, Itoh H. Diffuse panbronchiolitis: correlation of high-resolution CT and pathologic findings. Radiology 184(3):779–85, 1992. (Hansell DM. Small airways diseases: detection and insights with computed tomography). Eur Respir J. 2001;17(6): 1294–313.
30. Nakata K, Taguchi Y, Kudoh S. [Therapeutic Guidelines for DPB (Author's Translation)]. Annual Report on the study of diffuse lung disease in 1999. Grant-in aid from the Ministry of Health and Welfare of Japan, Tokyo, Japan. 2000:111. (in Japanese).
31. Akira M, Higashihara T, Sakatani M, et al. Diffuse panbronchiolitis: follow-up CT examination. Radiology. 1993;189:559–62.
32. Sakito O, Kadota J, Khono S, et al. Interleukin 1 beta, tumor necrosis factor alpha, and interleukin 8 in bronchoalveolar lavage fluid of patients with diffuse panbronchiolitis: a potential mechanism of macrolide therapy. Respiration. 1996;63:42–8.
33. Kadota J, Mukae H, Ishii H, et al. Long-term efficacy and safety of clarithromycin treatment in patients with diffuse panbronchiolitis. Respir Med. 2003;97:844–50.
34. Kobayasi H, Takeda H, Sakayori T, et al. Clinical study of azithromycin in the treatment of diffuse panbronchiolitis. Kansenshogaku Zasshi. 1995;69:711–21. (in Japanese)
35. Tsuji T, Tanaka E, Yasuda I, Nakatsuka Y, Kaji Y, Yasuda T, Hashimoto S, Hwang MH, Hajiro T, Taguchi Y. Nontuberculous mycobacteria in diffuse panbronchiolitis. Respirology. 2015;20(1):80–6.
36. Rodvold KA, Gotfried MH, Danziger LH, et al. Intrapulmonary steady-state concentration of clarithromycin and azithromycin in healthy adult volunteers. Antimicrob Agents Chemother. 1997;41:1399–402.
37. Sugiyama K, Shirai R, Mukae H, et al. Differing effects of clarithromycin and azithromycin on cytokine production by murine dendritic cells. Clin Exp Immunol. 2007;147:540–6.
38. Wilkinson M, Sugumar K, Milan SJ, et al. Mucolytics for bronchiectasis. Cochrane Database Syst Rev. 2014;5:CD001289.
39. Olivieri D, Ciaccia A, Marangio E, et al. Role of bromhexine in exacerbations of bronchiectasis. Double-blind randmised multicenter study versus placebo. Respiration. 1991;58:117–21.
40. Crisafulli E, Coletti O, Costi S, et al. Effectiveness of erdosteine in elderly patients with bronchiectasis and hypersecretion: a 15-day, prospective, parallel, open-label, pilot study. Clin Ther. 2007;29:2001–9.
41. Wallace RJ Jr, Brown BA, Griffith DE, Girard WM, Murphy DT, Onyi GO, Steingrube VA, Mazurek GH. Initial clarithromycin monotherapy for Mycobacterium avium-intracellulare complex lung disease. Am J Respir Crit Care Med. 1994;149(5):1335–41.
42. Griffith DE, Brown-Elliott BA, Langsjoen B, Zhang Y, Pan X, Girard W, Nelson K, Caccitolo J, Alvarez J, Shepherd S, Wilson R, Graviss EA, Wallace RJ Jr. Clinical and molecular analysis of macrolide resistance in Mycobacterium avium complex lung disease. Am J Respir Crit Care Med. 2006;174(8):928–34.
43. Kudoh S, Azuma A, Tamaoki J, Nakata K, Takizawa H, Goto H. Novel activity of erythromycin and its derivatives. Macrolide antibiotics (Second Edition) Chemistry, biology, and practice--Chapter 12. 2003:533–569.
44. Takizawa H. Airway epithelial cells as regulators of airway inflammation. Int J Mol Med. 1998;1:367–78.
45. Sakito O, Kadota J, Kohno S, Abe K, Shirai R, Hara K. Interleukin 1 beta, tumor necrosis factor alpha, and interleukin 8 in bronchoalveolar lavage fluid of patients with diffuse panbronchiolitis: a potential mechanism of macrolide therapy. Respiration. 1996;63:42–8.
46. Umeki S. Anti-inflammatory action of erythromycin. Its inhibitory effect on neutrophil NADPH oxidase activity. Chest. 1993;104:1191–3.
47. Nelson S, Summer WR, Terry PB, Warr GA, Jakab GJ. Erythromycin induced suppression of pulmonary antibacterial defenses. Am Rev Respir Dis. 1987;136:1207–12.
48. Hirata T, Matsunobe S, Matsui Y, Kado M, Mikiya K, Oshima S. Effect of erythromycin on the generation of neutrophil chemiluminescence in vitro. Nippon Kyoubu Shikkan Gakkai Zasshi. 1990;28:1066–71. (in Japanese)

49. Oda H, Kadota JI, Kohno S, Hara K. Erythromycin inhibits neutrophil chemotaxis in bronchoalveoli of diffuse panbronchiolitis. Chest. 1994;106:1116–23.
50. Hojo M, Fujita I, Hamasaki Y, Miyazaki M, Miyazaki S. Erythromycin does not directly affect neutrophil functions. Chest. 1994;105:520–3.
51. The Japanese Society of Lung and Heart-Lung Transplantation. Registry report of Japanese lung transplantation –2021. Ishoku. 2021;56(3):245–51. (in Japanese)
52. Sugimoto S, Miyoshi K, Yamane M, Oto T. Lung transplantation for diffuse panbronchiolitis: 5 cases from a single Centre. Interact Cardiovasc Thorac Surg. 2016;22(5):679–81.
53. Beyoglu MA, Sahin MF, Turkkan S, et al. Diffuse Panbronchiolitis after lung transplantation: first case in the literature. Transplant Proc. 2021;53(8):2622–5.
54. Yamaguchi T, Goto H, Okamura T, et al. Clinical study of long-term administration of clarithromycin on DPB. Report of the Diffuse lung disease investigative research group. 1992:263-5 (in Japanese).
55. Taguchi Y, Taneda K, Kori Y, et al. Guidelines for erythromycin therapy for diffuse panbronchiolitis. Report of the Diffuse lung disease investigative research group. 1996:77-79. (in Japanese).
56. Yamaguchi T, Onozaki I, Kuriyama T, et al. Efficacy of erythromycin therapy in DPB patients with P. aeruginosa infection. Nihon Kyobu Shikkan Gakkai Zasshi. 1989;27:473–8. (in Japanese)
57. Ohashi Y, Motojima S, Ogata E, et al. Study of the usefulness of erythromycin in diffuse panbronchiolitis. Dokkyo Med J. 1991;7:9–15. (in Japanese)
58. Kamoshida T. Pathological study of diffuse panbronchiolitis–relationship between the duration of disease and respiratory bronchial lesions. Nihon Kyobu Shikkan Gakkai Zasshi. 1993;31: 169–79. (in Japanese)
59. Yamamoto M, Kudoh S, Ina Y, Tamura A. Clinical efficacy of erythromycin for patients with diffuse panbronchiolitis–A double blind study. Saishin Igaku. 1990;45:103–8. (in Japanese)
60. Tamaoki J, Isono K, Sasaki N, Kanemura T, Konno K. Erythromycin inhibits cl secretion across canine tracheal epithelial cells. Eur Respir J. 1992;5:234–8.
61. Ichikawa Y, Ninomiya H, Koga H, Tanaka M, Kinoshita M, Tokunaga N, Yano T, Oizumi K. Erythromycin reduces neutrophils and neutrophil-derived elastolytic-like activity in the lower respiratory tract of bronchiolitis patients. Am Rev Respir Dis. 1992;146(1):196–203.
62. Kadota J, Sakito O, Khono S, Sawa H, Mukae H, Oda H, Kawakami K, Fukushima K, Hiratani K, Hara K. A mechanism of erythromycin treatment in patients with diffuse panbronchiolitis. Am Rev Respir Dis. 1993;147(1):153–9.
63. Mikami M. Clinical and pathophysiological significance of neutrophil elastase in sputum and the effect of erythromycin in chronic respiratory diseases. Nippon Kyoubu Shikkan Gakkai Zasshi. 1992;29:72–83. (in Japanese)
64. Kawakami K, Kadota J, Iida K, Fujii T, Shirai R, Matsubara Y, Kohno S. Phenotypic characterization of T cells in bronchoalveolar lavage fluid (BALF) and peripheral blood of patients with diffuse panbronchiolitis; the importance of cytotoxic T cells. Clin Exp Immunol. 1997;107 (2):410–6.
65. Keicho N, Kudoh S, Yotsumoto H, Akagawa KS. Anti-lymphocytic activity of erythromycin distinct from that of FK506 or cyclosporin a. J Antibiot. 1993;46:1406–13.
66. Keicho N, Kudoh S, Yotsumoto H, Akagawa KS. Erythromycin promotes monocyte to macrophage differentiation. J Antibiot. 1994;47:80–9.
67. Tateda K, Hirakata Y, Furuya N, Ohno A, Yamaguchi K. Effects of sub-MICs of erythromycin and other macrolide antibiotics on serum sensitivity of pseudomonas aeruginosa. Antimicrob Agents Chemother. 1993;37:675–80.
68. Denning GM, Wollenweber LA, Railsback MA, Cox CD, Stoll LL, Britigan BE. Pseudomonas pyocyanine increases interleukin-8 expression by human airway epithelial cells. Infect Immun. 1998;66:5777–84.

Macrolides and Cystic Fibrosis

Rishi Pabary, Adam Jaffe, and Andrew Bush

Abstract Macrolide antibiotics attracted interest as a potential therapy in cystic fibrosis (CF) due to remarkable similarities in pathogenic features with diffuse panbronchiolitis (DPB), as described in the chapter by Azuma and Taniuchi. Azithromycin in particular is widely used for acute pulmonary exacerbations in CF, both for its direct antimicrobial and indirect immunomodulatory properties. A number of randomised clinical trials also support the long-term use of macrolides in CF, predominantly in patients chronically infected with *Pseudomonas aeruginosa*, which is surprising given that they have little inherent antibacterial activity against this ubiquitous CF pathogen. In this chapter, we recapitulate the pathophysiology of CF, discuss the purported mechanisms of action of macrolides and summarise the key evidence for their use in this multisystem disease.

Keywords Azithromycin · Cystic fibrosis · *Pseudomonas aeruginosa* · Neutrophil · Airway inflammation · Rhinovirus · Pulmonary exacerbation

---

R. Pabary (✉)
Paediatric Respiratory and Sleep Medicine, Royal Brompton Hospital, London, UK

Imperial College, London, UK
e-mail: r.pabary@rbht.nhs.uk

A. Jaffe
Discipline of Paediatrics and Child Health, School of Clinical Medicine, UNSW, Sydney, Australia

Sydney Children's Hospital, Randwick, Sydney, Australia

A. Bush
National Heart and Lung Institute, and Imperial Centre for Paediatrics and Child Health, Imperial College London, London, UK

B. K. Rubin, M. Shinkai (eds.), *Macrolides as Immunomodulatory Agents*, Progress in Inflammation Research 92, https://doi.org/10.1007/978-3-031-42859-3_4

1 Introduction

Cystic fibrosis (CF) is a multisystem disorder primarily affecting the respiratory and gastrointestinal systems. Whilst life expectancy has increased since it was first described by Dorothy Andersen in 1938 [1], CF remains a life-limiting illness; current median survival is between 44 and 53 years [2], with death usually due to respiratory failure. It is anticipated that the new disease modulators will dramatically improve this.

2 Pathophysiology

CF is the commonest autosomal recessive disease in the Northern European population; between 1/28 and 1/40 [3] are carriers of an abnormal variant of the gene, which is localised to the long arm of chromosome 7 [4]. This gene encodes cystic fibrosis transmembrane conductance regulator (CFTR), a cAMP-regulated anion channel that regulates chloride transport across the apical membrane of epithelial cells [5]. CFTR also influences bicarbonate transport, both directly and indirectly [6, 7] and other conductance pathways within the cell membrane including the epithelial sodium channel (EnAC) and outwardly rectifying chloride channels [8, 9]. Over 2000 different *CFTR* mutations, categorised into six classes, of which approximately 400 are known to be disease-causing, have been identified [10], and it is therefore unsurprising that the clinical phenotype is variable. Furthermore, there are significant inconsistencies between CF genotype and phenotype [11], even in patients that have identical mutations and from the same family kindred, suggesting that environment, polymorphisms or modifier genes also influence CFTR function. It is therefore unsurprising that precisely how defective CFTR results in disease is still not completely understood, with several pathways and mechanisms being postulated, many of which are thought to cause an increase in inflammation.

2.1 *Low Volume Hypothesis*

A combination of sodium reabsorption and chloride secretion maintains the periciliary fluid layer (PCL) that separates mucus from the cilia in the lung [12]. Absorption of airway surface liquid (ASL) in CF is increased, depleting the PCL and allowing mucus to interfere with ciliary function, leading to impaired mucociliary clearance and airway plugging [13]. This predisposes to infection, which can induce a persistent inflammatory response and ultimately lead to the destruction of surrounding lung tissue [14].

2.2 Primary Inflammation Hypothesis

Elimination of viral pathogens is impaired in CF airway epithelia, allowing increased replication and airway inflammatory changes that predispose to earlier acquisition of bacterial infections such as *Pseudomonas aeruginosa* [15]. Resolution of the inflammatory response is necessary to prevent collateral damage to normal tissue, and several pathways responsible for this process appear impaired in CF [16]. Macrophages express CFTR and, in CF, appear unable to switch from the M1 to the M2 phenotype, a process required for the resolution of inflammatory response; in the CF pig, it has been demonstrated that this impacts the response to pathogens including *Pseudomonas aeruginosa* [17, 18]. Whether or not inflammation precedes infection in CF remains unclear and is reviewed in detail elsewhere [19, 20], but neutrophils have been detected in bronchoalveolar lavage fluid (BAL) in babies as young as 4 weeks without evidence of infection [21]. Following exposure to microorganisms, neutrophils certainly become predominant in the CF airway [22], a finding that persists even in clinically stable patients with mild lung disease [23]. The antimicrobial capacity of neutrophils through mechanisms such as phagocytosis is impaired in CF [24]. Neutrophils lacking *CFTR* have less intrinsic apoptotic potential [24], which leads to increased formation of neutrophil extracellular traps (NETs) [25], which in turn drive inflammation and lung destruction. Neutrophils also produce elastase; this digests proteins, including elastin, in the airway wall, contributing to bronchiectasis [26] and driving mucus secretion [27], worsening airways obstruction and promoting the generation of CXCL8 (also known as IL-8) and LTB_4, both potent chemoattractants that recruit more neutrophils [28], perpetuating the cycle of inflammation and lung destruction. It is, therefore, unsurprising that anti-inflammatory therapies, in particular neutrophil modulation, are of interest in CF. However, the paradigm that reduced inflammation equates to better outcomes is oversimplistic; the BIIL 284 BS (an LTB_4 receptor antagonist) trial provides a cautionary lesson as early cessation of the study was mandated due to an excess of infection-related adverse events, likely secondary to suppression of the inflammatory response [29] to subnormal levels [30].

2.3 Aberrant Mucin Secretion Hypothesis

Mucus is a protective coating secreted by healthy airways. Mucin glycoproteins are the major constitution of the mucus gel, which is responsible for the rheological properties of mucus [31], and are encoded by *MUC* genes, 23 of which have been identified [32]. It is speculated that defective CFTR leads to dehydration of mucosal surfaces and changes in mucin properties. MUC5AC and MUC5B are the predominant gel-forming mucins secreted in the airway; it is suggested that overexpression of these contributes to increased mucin secretion into the lumen of the respiratory tract with the resulting formation of mucus plaques, infection and inflammation

[32, 33]. In a study of expectorated sputum in patients with CF, however, DNA was shown to play a more prominent role than mucins, with a decrease in MUC5AC and MUC5B observed, compared to normal non-CF mucus [34]. This suggests that there may be a relative increase in other components of CF sputum or a primary defect of mucin secretion in CF.

2.4 Cell Receptor Hypothesis

Adherence of *Pseudomonas* to airway epithelial cells is critical for establishing infection. The exact mechanism for this remains unclear. Abnormally low pH of the ASL related to defective CFTR-mediated bicarbonate transport is thought to predispose to innate host defence abnormalities in CF [35] including increased expression of the asialylated glycoprotein (asialoGM1) receptor on the surface of CF epithelial cells [36–38]. *Pseudomonas aeruginosa* binds to asialoGM1 and induces CXCL8 secretion via the nuclear factor kappa B (NF-κB) signalling pathway [39]. CFTR itself has been shown to be a receptor for *Pseudomonas aeruginosa*; in cultured human airway epithelial cells expressing the commonest CFTR variant phe508del, uptake of *Pseudomonas aeruginosa* is defective [40, 41], limiting phagocytosis and leading to increased bacterial load in a murine model of pulmonary infection [40]. These findings might help explain the preferential infection of CF airways by *Pseudomonas aeruginosa*. At later stages of infection however, these bacteria form hypoxic macrocolonies in the airway and are not in direct contact with the epithelial cells [42–44]. This suggests that chronic infection is a process in which initial adherence is just one important step and that factors initiating infection are probably different from those perpetuating chronic infection.

3 Clinical Features in CF

Most patients with CF die from lung disease perpetuated by the inflammatory response to recurrent and persistent infections with pathogens including *Staphylococcus aureus, Aspergillus fumigatus,* non-tuberculous mycobacteria and, ultimately, chronic infection with *Pseudomonas aeruginosa* in 60-70% of adult patients [45]. This is similar to DPB, where various different bacterial species may initially infect the airway, but *Pseudomonas aeruginosa* ultimately causes chronic infection with biofilm formation [46]. Interest in macrolides in DPB followed a case report suggesting a benefit from long-term erythromycin use, which was subsequently demonstrated even in patients chronically infected with *Pseudomonas aeruginosa,* which is typically resistant to this class of antibiotics [46]. In patients treated with macrolides, DPB 10-year survival increased from 12% to over 90% [47, 48] and, given the similarities between the phenotype of lung disease in DPB and CF, this raised the question of whether macrolides might be of similar benefit in

CF. Whilst the clinical phenotype of DPB and CF are similar, pathophysiologic mechanisms are likely to differ. phe508del [49] and rarer CFTR mutations have not been described [50] in patients with DPB, although some of the proposed mechanisms of macrolide benefit may be applicable to both conditions.

4 Proposed Mechanisms for Action of Macrolides in CF

Whilst macrolides have direct antimicrobial properties against a number of pathogens commonly detected in patients with CF (such as *Haemophilus influenzae* and *Staphylococcus aureus*), and there are data suggesting that azithromycin may prevent acquisition of new CF pathogens [51], it is the immunomodulatory properties and indirect actions on other organisms such as *Pseudomonas aeruginosa* that are of greater interest. However, there is a need to balance these possible benefits of long-term use against the potential for selection of macrolide-resistant strains of organisms such as *Staphylococcus aureus* [52, 53].

4.1 Signalling Pathways and Chemokine Release

An early step in the inflammatory cascade is the signalling to effector cells via proinflammatory molecules of various cytokines and chemokine families. As discussed previously, neutrophils predominate in the airways of patients with CF and activation of the neutrophil response results in parenchymal lung damage through the production of elastase. Work in animal models [54] and in patients with DPB [55] demonstrates reduction in neutrophil influx into the airways following treatment with erythromycin. Rather than having a direct modulating effect on the neutrophil itself, macrolides are likely to influence neutrophil chemotactic activity indirectly by modulating the production of specific cytokines such as IL-1β, IL-6 and, in particular, the potent neutrophil chemoattractants CXCL8 [56–61], TNF-α [62, 63], and GM-CSF [59]. It is likely that NF-κB, a protein transcription factor considered a master regulator of biochemical cascades in innate immunity [64, 65] is required for transcription of all these cytokines.

In children with CF, CXCL8 release from blood and airway neutrophils is higher than in controls and not further enhanced by the presence of lipopolysaccharide (LPS) [66]. CXCL8 production is greater in airway neutrophils compared to blood and, whilst able to partially suppress production by blood neutrophils, dexamethasone is not effective at reducing CXCL8 production by airway neutrophils in CF [66]. This is relevant to potential benefits of macrolides in CF, as it has been shown that these antibiotics are able to modulate CXCL8 secretion. In a small open study in CF patients, a 1-month course of erythromycin significantly reduced sputum CXCL8 in four out of six patients [67] and CXCL8 reduction was also seen in BAL from adults with DPB, asthma and bronchiectasis following macrolide therapy

[60]. Macrolides are likely to exert a direct effect on the airway epithelial cell; in cultured cells exposed to physiological levels of erythromycin or clarithromycin, there is a reduction in CXCL8 mRNA and protein in both healthy subjects and those with chronic airway inflammation [60]. Erythromycin has also been shown to reduce IL-6 and CXCL8 secretion from human bronchial epithelia stimulated by endotoxin [58] and IL-6 and TNF-α in human blood stimulated with *Streptococcus pneumonia* [68]. In a murine model of *Pseudomonas* infection, azithromycin reduced TNF-α levels and inhibited neutrophil recruitment to the lung [69], and clarithromycin has been shown to be as effective as prednisolone in reducing IL-5, CXCL8 and GM-CSF in nasal tissue cultures from patients with chronic rhinosinusitis [70]. *In vitro* evidence suggests that macrolides may reduce CXCL8 gene expression by suppression of ERK1/2 and thus both activator protein-1 (AP-1) binding sites and the transcription factor NF-κB [71–73]. This could be of particular relevance as human airway epithelial cells derived from CF patients demonstrate elevated NF-κB activation compared to control cells, both at baseline and following *Pseudomonas aeruginosa* stimulation, with CXCL8 mRNA levels remaining elevated for longer in CF cells [74]. In healthy bronchial epithelial cells stimulated with LPS, clarithromycin initially decreases CXCL8 production but then potentiates it over twofold before returning to normal level [61]; this highlights that suppression of proinflammatory cytokines is not purely time-dependent and that macrolides are in fact immunomodulatory rather than simply immunosuppressive [75] and why longer-term use might be key in reducing exacerbations and inflammation in patients with chronic respiratory disease [76].

4.2 *Direct Neutrophil Effect*

In addition to the indirect effects of macrolides on neutrophil pathways discussed above, there is evidence macrolides also affect neutrophil function directly via a number of different mechanisms.

4.2.1 Endothelial and Airway Adhesion

Neutrophils and other inflammatory cells require adhesion molecules to migrate into the airway in response to inflammation. Intercellular adhesion molecule (ICAM)-1 plays an important role in the adhesion of neutrophils to airway epithelium [77] and is overexpressed in CF airway epithelium [78–80], a process that may be regulated by NF-κB. Any treatment that reduces neutrophil adherence to either epithelial or endothelial cells may therefore downregulate the inflammatory cascade. Studies on cultures of human bronchial epithelial cells stimulated with *Haemophilus influenzae* endotoxin have shown that erythromycin causes a reduction in IL-6, CXCL8, soluble ICAM-1 and decreased neutrophil migration and adhesion to epithelial cells [58], a finding replicated in a study using roxithromycin [59]. ICAM-1 and

CXCL8 expression may also be reduced by inhibition of neutrophil elastase (NE); erythromycin is an alternate substrate inhibitor of NE, and flurythromycin inactivates it *in vitro* [81].

Integrin CD11b/CD18 (Mac-1) expression on peripheral neutrophils in patients with DPB is higher than in controls [82] and is significantly reduced by roxithromycin, correlating with a reduction in neutrophils in BAL. Macrolides also reduce Mac-1 expression in neutrophils stimulated by LPS and inhibit their oxidative burst [83], with a significant reduction in CD-11b/CD18 demonstrated on the surface of whole blood cells following erythromycin treatment [84]. In a model using cultured fibroblasts, clarithromycin decreased the expression of several adhesion molecules including ICAM-1, vascular cell adhesion molecule (VCAM)-1 and lymphocyte function-associated antigen-3 (LFA-3), whilst in a murine model of lung fibrosis, erythromycin inhibited VCAM-1 mRNA and neutrophil airway infiltration, suggesting a role in both resolution of inflammation and prevention of fibrosis [85].

4.2.2 Migration

As previously discussed, an increased presence of neutrophils in the CF airway predisposes to lung damage [22]. When compared to controls, CF neutrophils demonstrate higher migratory responsiveness to CXCL8, which in addition is detected at higher concentrations in CF serum, sputum and BAL compared to controls [86], suggesting that CF neutrophils are primed to CXCL8 [87]. In a small study in CF patients, erythromycin did not reduce neutrophil chemotaxis over a 4-week period [87] and, in fact, macrolide doses required to inhibit *in vitro* chemotaxis of blood neutrophils from healthy volunteers are far greater than that used therapeutically [88]. These findings suggest that erythromycin does not directly modulate neutrophil function [89] and that reduced neutrophil migration demonstrated in animal models of lung injury [47, 69] is mediated via the signalling and adhesion pathways outlined above.

4.2.3 Reactive Oxygen Species (ROS)

A key component of innate immunity is the generation of ROS by neutrophil NADPH oxidase [90]. However, ROS can also damage surrounding tissues, causing a cascade of inflammation; inherent antioxidant mechanisms are crucial to protect cells from injury [91]. Given the degree of neutrophilic inflammation in CF, findings such as an increase in ROS in the BAL fluid of children with CF are unsurprising [92], but it is likely that there is also an intrinsic defect in antioxidant defence due to lack of CFTR that exacerbates this [93–95]. In a zebrafish model, loss of CFTR function leads to an exaggerated neutrophil response and excessive ROS generation from epithelia, irrespective of whether typical CF pathogens are present [96]. Different classes of macrolides are able to inhibit ROS production by neutrophils, both *in vitro* and *in vivo* [75, 97–103], and may therefore attenuate this response. The mechanism remains uncertain but may be due in part to stabilisation of the cell membrane [104]. As with the effect on CXCL8 production, this is not a time-dependent effect, the semicolon afterwards alludes to a trial that shows enhancement of he burst followed by down regulation of the oxidative burst and increased neutrophil apoptosis up to 28 days later [102]. This suggests that macrolides initially stimulate neutrophil antimicrobial activity before later dampening down deleterious inflammation.

4.2.4 Apoptosis

It has been demonstrated in CF piglets and patients with CF that neutrophils survive longer due to delayed apoptosis, allowing the formation of NETs and increasing inflammation [25]. Erythromycin increases cyclic AMP (cAMP) levels in neutrophils *in vitro*, leading to accelerated apoptosis at 24 h in a dose-dependent manner [105]. This has also been seen in healthy controls up to 28 days after a short course of azithromycin [102]. *In vitro*, in the presence of *Streptococcus pneumoniae* the pro-apoptotic effect of azithromycin is impaired [106] indicating that this proposed mechanism of action might not be as relevant in CF, given the almost ubiquitous presence of microbial pathogens in the airway from a young age.

4.3 *Effect on* Pseudomonas aeruginosa

Clinical improvement in patients with DPB treated with macrolides is independent of whether they are chronically infected with *Pseudomonas aeruginosa* [46]. Since this is seen below the minimum inhibitory concentration (MIC) for *Pseudomonas aeruginosa*, and in fact there are no published breakpoints [107], it is suggested that the effects of macrolides on *Pseudomonas* in DPB are anti-inflammatory rather than antibacterial [57, 108, 109]. There are a number of purported mechanisms by which macrolides indirectly counteract inflammation secondary to *Pseudomonas* infection, which is of relevance when considering their use in CF.

4.3.1 Adherence

In CF, increased binding of *Pseudomonas aeruginosa* to respiratory epithelial cells, likely due to overexpression of receptors and mutant CFTR [36, 37], has been demonstrated. In 11 children with CF treated with azithromycin for 3 months, a 70% decrease in adherence of *Pseudomonas aeruginosa* to buccal epithelial cells was observed [110], but this was not reproduced in seven adult CF patients who underwent nasal brushing after 2 weeks of oral azithromycin [111]. It is difficult, therefore, to be certain whether *in vitro* studies showing that macrolides decrease

Pseudomonas adherence to silicon filters [112], mouse tracheal epithelium [113] and human type IV basement collagen [114] translate to clinical efficacy in CF via this mechanism.

4.3.2 Suppression of Bacterial Exoproducts and Mucus Secretion

Pseudomonas aeruginosa produces extracellular toxins and exopolysaccharide that contribute to pathogenesis by stimulating inflammation and tissue destruction in the host [115, 116]. *In vitro,* it has been shown that erythromycin attenuates nasal epithelial damage caused by neutrophils in the presence of *Pseudomonas aeruginosa,* with no effect seen where neutrophils were incubated with erythromycin alone, suggesting that macrolides attenuate production of virulence factors that damage epithelia [117]. Chronic infections in CF develop a mucoid phenotype due to hypersecretion of alginate, creating a biofilm that coats airway surfaces [118] and protects bacteria within the biofilm from antimicrobials and host immune defences [44, 119, 120], making eradication difficult. Biofilms also act as an antigen and induce an antigen-antibody reaction on the surface of the airway [121], resulting in immune complex deposition and neutrophilia. Sub-MIC concentrations of macrolides inhibit production of alginate and the formation and stability of biofilms [122, 123]; with an increase in biofilm permeability, penetration of bactericidal antibiotics may be facilitated, a mechanism that could explain why a combination of azithromycin and ciprofloxacin leads to increased killing of biofilm *Pseudomonas aeruginosa* compared to ciprofloxacin alone [121].

Sub-MIC macrolide concentrations also reduce mucus secretion by airway epithelial cells, both *in vitro* and *in vivo* [124, 125]. An 80% reduction in viscosity of sputa from 29 CF patients infected with *Pseudomonas aeruginosa* has been demonstrated *in vitro* with the addition of roxithromycin [126] and twice weekly treatment with azithromycin for 3 months reduced sputum viscosity in 9/10 adolescents with CF who were chronically infected with *Pseudomonas aeruginosa* [127]. The effect on mucus secretion occurs via MUC5AC gene expression [125]; this is upregulated in a murine model of DPB and *Pseudomonas aeruginosa* infection and reduces after macrolide treatment via modulation of intracellular signal transduction, including phosphorylation of extracellular signal-regulated kinase 1/2 [128]. Clinically in CF patients, this mechanism might attenuate the inflammatory response by facilitating the clearance of secretions.

Erythromycin suppresses the production of elastase and protease in *Pseudomonas aeruginosa* cultures without affecting bacterial growth over a 24hr period [129]. Macrolides appear to differ in their abilities to suppress *Pseudomonas aeruginosa* virulence factors, with azithromycin appearing more efficacious, particularly in terms of pyocyanin [130, 131], exotoxin A, exoenzyme and phospholipase C [132] production. The mechanisms by which sub-MIC concentrations of macrolides are able to suppress virulence factors are not entirely clear; direct inhibition of ribosomal translation seems unlikely as this would be expected to also suppress bacterial growth although inhibition of protein synthesis, leading to decreased expression of heat shock proteins and loss of viability of *Pseudomonas aeruginosa* has been demonstrated [133]. Interaction of azithromycin with the 50s ribosomal subunit selectively inhibits expression of quorum sensing genes such as *rhlR* at both transcriptional and post-transcriptional levels [107, 134], leading to a reduction in virulence factors, oxidative stress and motility of *Pseudomonas aeruginosa* [135]. Loss of motility is mediated by inhibition of flagellin production [130, 136] and effects on the assembly of type IV pili [137] by macrolides at sub-MIC concentrations, making phagocytosis of bacteria by alveolar macrophages easier.

4.3.3 Non-inflammatory Effects

Whilst most data indicate that macrolides exert effects via immunomodulatory and anti-virulence mechanisms, it is also suggested that *Pseudomonas aeruginosa* accumulates azithromycin over a period of chronic exposure, directly affecting viability and protein synthesis [138]. This effect was seen at 48hrs, but not at earlier time points, in agar cultures of PAO-1 and 13/14 clinical isolates of *Pseudomonas aeruginosa,* with protein synthesis decreasing in a time-dependent manner. This suggests that macrolides may in fact be directly bactericidal in circumstances where bacteria are exposed for longer periods due to intracellular accumulation of the antibiotic.

4.4 Antiviral Effects

In human CF bronchial epithelial cells infected with rhinovirus, a sevenfold reduction in viral replication is seen in cells that are treated with azithromycin compared to controls [139]. The likely mechanism for this is via amplification of the antiviral response mediated by interferon pathways, as evidenced by upregulated expression of interferon-stimulated genes [139, 140]. This is of particular relevance as rhinoviruses frequently trigger pulmonary exacerbations [141], and the innate immune response to them is impaired in CF; CF bronchial epithelial cells express up to 1000 times less interferon type I (β) and type III (λ) mRNA compared with controls in response to rhinovirus with a resulting increase in rhinovirus RNA and virus release [142]. It is also thought that coinfection with *Pseudomonas aeruginosa* also suppresses interferon responses to rhinovirus in CF bronchial epithelial cells compared with control cells [143]; if macrolides upregulate interferon pathways, this provides a plausible biological mechanism to explain the reduction in CF pulmonary exacerbations that has been reported in a number of clinical trials.

4.5 Effects on Ion Transport

It is suggested that one mechanism by which azithromycin may exert an effect on CF is via the modulation of alternate chloride channels. This theory followed a case report in which a CF patient had improved lung function after receiving chemotherapy for fibrosarcoma [157]. An increase in multidrug resistance (MDR) protein mRNA in nasal epithelial cells was demonstrated, which was not seen in a CF patient not exposed to chemotherapy; it is thought that long-term upregulation of genes encoding proteins promoting MDR may complement CFTR function that is lacking in CF [158]. CFTR and MDR, a P-glycoprotein, both belong to the ATP-binding cassette (ABC) family of chloride channels and share sequence homology [159]. The ABC transporter family are a group of proteins whose function is the transport of a wide variety of substrates. It is known that erythromycin can upregulate P-glycoprotein expression [160]. However, despite potentially upregulating chloride-secreting channels, some data suggest that macrolides inhibit chloride secretion rather than accentuate it [161, 162], which would be detrimental in CF, where chloride secretion is reduced. One potential pathway by which this might occur is by an effect on endothelin-1 (ET-1), a potent vaso- and bronchoconstrictor produced by endothelial cells [163]. Macrolides reduce ET-1 gene expression and release in human bronchial epithelial cells [164] and, as ET-1 is a chloride secretagogue in the airways [165], this could potentially explain a reduction in chloride secretion.

In another study, nasal chloride secretion improved in 6/10 CF patients treated with azithromycin for 1 month [166], subsequently suggested to be secondary to MDR overexpression [167]. These findings were not replicated in other studies of nasal PD measurements in CF mice and patients [111, 168]. In human bronchial epithelial cells, a significant dose-dependent increase of chloride efflux is seen in CF (but not in non-CF) cells after azithromycin treatment, in the absence of increased expression of either MDR or CFTR [169], suggesting that another mechanism rather than upregulation of these proteins is responsible. In Ussing chamber studies of healthy murine colon tissue, there is an increase in anion secretion with azithromycin, which is also seen in sheep trachea treated with erythromycin [162]. From these data, it appears that macrolides have a role in modulating ion transport, but whether this is a mechanism by which they may be efficacious in CF remains unclear.

4.6 Nitric Oxide (NO)

NO is a gaseous free radical produced from the amino acid L-arginine by NO synthase (NOS). NO is involved in a number of important physiological processes within the lung including inflammation and bacterial killing. Given the degree of inflammation in the lower airway, exhaled NO is surprisingly low in CF [170] for reasons that are not entirely clear but may include reduced inducible NOS expression (iNOS) in the bronchial epithelium [171] or increased degradation by NO reductase by *Pseudomonas aeruginosa* in the lower airways [172]. Macrolide antibiotics inhibit immune complex-induced lung injury in rats; it is thought that this is through modulation of cytokine release that downregulates type II iNOS gene expression, and thereby reduces NO production by alveolar macrophages [173, 174]. Conversely, erythromycin has also been shown to stimulate endogenous NO production by a protein kinase A-dependent mechanism [175] and release of NO from non-adrenergic, non-cholinergic neurones, a system that is thought to modulate airway inflammation [176]. It is not entirely clear how macrolides effect NO production in the CF airway but, low NO is thought to enhance adherence of *Pseudomonas aeruginosa* to human bronchial epithelial cells [177] and increase susceptibility to bacterial and viral infections [178, 179], and there is a focus on possible therapeutic benefits of exogenous NO in CF [180].

4.7 Airway Remodelling

Airway changes such as dilatation, fibrosis and neovascularisation that are observed with disease progression in CF [181] may be modulated by macrolides. 14-member macrolides appear to reduce tumour angiogenesis by an unknown mechanism [182], and it is therefore possible that bronchial neovascularisation in CF could be reduced. Roxithromycin inhibits TNF-α induced vascular endothelial growth factor (VEGF) production [183], and macrolides may have indirect effects on angiogenesis via CXCL8, which is angiogenic as well as proinflammatory [184]. An analogue of rapamycin (a macrolide immunosuppressant) inhibited epidermal growth factor-induced proliferation [185] and attenuated fibrotic pathways induced by transforming growth factor-α [186] in murine models of lung inflammation and remodelling. If these effects were recapitulated in the human lower airway, this could have profound implications for prevention of remodelling that has been demonstrated in children with CF [187].

4.8 Bioactive Phospholipids

Cell injury causes the release of cell membrane phospholipid-derived arachidonic acid and is converted into platelet-activating factor (PAF), leukotrienes, prostaglandins and thromboxane A [188]. Many of these membrane-derived phospholipids modulate direct and leucocyte-mediated damaging effects on the airway epithelium [75]. PAF, in particular, is implicated, with elevated levels in seen in many conditions where inflammation and cell damage are a feature of pathogenesis [189]. Macrolides attenuate the adverse effects of bioactive phospholipids on the human respiratory epithelium *in vitro* [190], potentially through inhibition of the

PAF/PAF-receptor and/or thrombin-protease-activated receptor-1 systems [191]. Ketolides, a relatively new class of macrolides designed to combat respiratory infections that have acquired resistance to conventional macrolides [192], have been shown to be cytoprotective against the effects of bioactive phospholipids, lysophosphatidylcholine, PAF and lyso-PAF on nasal epithelial strips from healthy volunteers [193]. However, the extent to which macrolides protect airway epithelium in CF remains unclear; this is further discussed in the chapter authored by Clive Page.

4.9 Antibacterial Effects in CF

Macrolides are potentially beneficial in CF for their broad-spectrum antibacterial properties, particularly against organisms such as *Staphylococcus aureus*, *Haemophilus influenzae* and non-tuberculous mycobacteria (NTM) and are widely used for acute exacerbations. Interestingly, no clinical trial in CF has yet demonstrated a clinically significant long-term effect on microbiology, despite evidence for clinical improvement [194]. A cautionary tale again the long-term use of macrolides is that some studies do report an increased risk of acquisition of macrolide-resistant organisms [194]; this is discussed in further detail below.

4.10 Summary

Despite a plethora of studies, the mechanisms of benefit of azithromycin in CF remain unclear. If mechanisms could be elucidated, a designer macrolide, either in nature or synthesised in the laboratory, aimed at the relevant pathway could be a powerful therapeutic tool in CF.

5 Clinical Evidence in CF

5.1 Efficacy

The index case that sparked our interest in the potential benefit of macrolides in CF was a 16yr old male with genotype ΔF508/G551D who had an improvement in forced vital capacity (FVC) from 26% to 65% predicted and forced expiratory volume in one second (FEV_1) from 11% to 26% predicted following empirical treatment with long-term azithromycin. There was also an improvement in baseline oxygen saturations in air from 65% to 93%, resulting in him coming off the heart-lung transplant waiting list for 6 years [195]. This was followed by an open-label study of long-term daily azithromycin; in seven children with CF (median age 12.1

[range 5.8 to 16.8 years]) who were chronically infected with *Pseudomonas aeruginosa* and had end-stage CF lung disease or chronic airflow limitation refractory to conventional therapy, significant improvements in FVC and FEV_1 were demonstrated [195]. Although there was no control group, historical controls and clinical experience suggest that deterioration rather than improvement should have occurred in these patients. The improvements were similar to those seen in patients with DPB [57, 108].

These effects were not replicated in the first single-blind pilot study of ten CF patients (aged 12-26) chronically infected with *Pseudomonas aeruginosa* who were treated with 3 weeks placebo followed by clarithromycin for 6 weeks [196]. No significant change in lung function, sputum neutrophils, CXCL8, free neutrophil elastase, TNF-α or myeloperoxidase were demonstrated, with no correlation between inflammation and lung function. It is likely that clarithromycin was not given for sufficiently long in this study; in DPB clinical benefit is often not seen until at least 6 weeks of treatment. One patient did have an 11% improvement in spirometry, indicating that macrolides might exert their effects in an, as yet undefined, subset of CF patients, something which has been seen in other studies [144, 146, 195, 197].

Since these early studies, there have been several double-blind and placebo-controlled randomised controlled trials (RCTs) of azithromycin with different dosing strategies (daily, thrice weekly, and weekly) undertaken in CF patients. Outcomes are summarised in Table 1. A meta-analysis of some of these studies suggests that azithromycin provides a 4% relative improvement in FEV_1 compared to placebo [194], whilst a recent retrospective cohort study suggests per-year relative FEV_1 decline is reduced by 40% in CF patients with chronic *Pseudomonas aeruginosa* compared to matched controls [198].

As Table 1 demonstrates, the impact of azithromycin therapy on FEV_1 varies across studies. Even in RCTs where the benefit was demonstrated, this was often less than seen in case reports [195], with the caveat that some individuals seemed to respond far better than others. With the advent of newborn screening for CF in many countries [199], there is the opportunity for earlier intervention to try and prevent complications and improve outcomes, particularly in terms of better early weight gain, improved lung function trajectory and delayed onset of chronic *Pseudomonas aeruginosa* infection [200]. This was the premise for undertaking COMBAT-CF; this study showed that, whilst using azithromycin for the first three years of life did not have an impact on structural lung disease on serial CT scans compared to placebo (the primary end point, i.e. this was a negative study), there was a reduction in BAL CXCL8 and neutrophil elastase at 36 months of life [156]. Furthermore, those children who received azithromycin had significantly fewer pulmonary exacerbations with less days in hospital and less exposure to antibiotics. Ongoing follow-up of this cohort of children is planned to see whether this early intervention has had a longer-term effect on structural lung disease and lung function but, given neutrophil elastase has a prominent role in the progression of lung damage in children [201, 202], this could justify starting azithromycin in infants, particularly those who are doing badly or not eligible for CFTR modulators. Reduction in BAL

Table 1 Summary of RCTs of Azithromycin in CF

Design	Intervention	Duration	Age of patients (n)	*PsA* status	Primary outcome	Key results	Ref
RCT Crossover	AZM vs. placebo	6 months for each arm (with a 2-month washout)	8 years – 18 ($n = 41$)	+/-	Change in FEV_1	Median relative improvement FEV_1 5.4% with AZM No change in sputum bacterial density, inflammatory markers, exercise tolerance or subjective well being	[144]
RCT Parallel	AZM vs. placebo	3-months	Adult ($n = 60$)	+/-	Change in FEV_1	Mean difference of 3.6% with AZM Improvement in QoL and fewer courses of IV antibiotics with AZM. Statistically significant but likely clinically insignificant improvement in CRP with AZM	[145]
RCT Parallel	AZM vs. placebo	6 months	6 years – adult ($n = 185$)	+	Change in FEV_1	Mean relative change 6.2% (0.094 litres) with AZM Reduced exacerbations/hospitalisations and mean weight gain of 0.7 kg with AZM. No effect on QoL, microbiology or sputum inflammatory markers	[146]
RCT Parallel	AZM vs. placebo	3 months	6 years – adult ($n = 21$)	+/-	BPI-ANCA levels	No change in BPI-ANCA with AZM compared to controls BPI-ANCA is raised in CF patients compared to healthy controls and higher in patients chronically infected with *PsA*	[147]
RCT Parallel	AZM vs. placebo	12 months	6 years – adult ($n = 82$)	+/-	Change in FEV_1	No benefit in FEV_1 with AZM Reduction in pulmonary exacerbations, time to first exacerbation and additional oral antibiotics (regardless of *PsA* status) with AZM	[148]
RCT Parallel	AZM daily (250mg) vs. AZM weekly (1200mg)	6 months	6 years – adult ($n = 208$)	+/-	Change in FEV_1	Small but similar magnitude of FEV_1 benefit Benefit greater for patients < 14yrs	[149]

(continued)

Table 1 (continued)

Design	Intervention	Duration	Age of patients (*n*)	*PsA* status	Primary outcome	Key results	Ref
RCT Parallel	AZM vs. placebo	2 months	8 years – adult ($n = 38$)	+/-	Change in FEV_1	No benefit in FEV_1 with AZM Reduction in serum IL-8, CRP, LPS binding protein and sputum alginate with AZM. QoL significantly improved with AZM	[150]
RCT Parallel	AZM 5mg vs. 15mg/kg/day	6 months	Children ($n = 47$)	+/-	Change in FEV_1	No improvement in FEV_1 in either dosing group Pulmonary exacerbations increased after discontinuing AZM (both dosing groups, higher in 15mg/kg/day)	[151]
RCT Parallel	AZM vs. placebo	6 months	6–18 years ($n = 260$)	-	Change in FEV_1	No benefit in FEV_1 with AZM 50% reduction in pulmonary exacerbations and increased body weight with AZM. No difference in the use of IV and inhaled antibiotics or hospitalisations with AZM. In a 24-week open-label extension, effect on weight and pulmonary exacerbations was maintained, although use of oral antibiotics increased [152]	[153]
RCT Parallel	AZM vs. placebo	6 months	6–18 years ($n = 260$)	-	Serum inflammatory markers	Reduction in CRP, myeloperoxidase, serum amyloid A calprotectin and neutrophils after 28 days with AZM. Effect was sustained to day 168 for neutrophils, calprotectin and serum amyloid	[154]
RCT Parallel	AZM vs. placebo	18 months	6 months to 18 years ($n = 221$)	+	Time to pulmonary exacerbation	44% reduction in exacerbations with AZM in children with newly acquired *PsA* compared to standard treatment alone Improved weight gain in AZM group. No difference in symptom scores, *Ps*A recurrence or emergence of other pathogens	[155]

RCT Parallel	AZM vs. placebo	Until 3 years of life	3–36 months ($n = 130$)	+/-	Structural lung disease on CT scan	No difference in structural lung disease at 36 months, as assessed by a high-resolution CT scan Fewer days in the hospital for pulmonary exacerbations and fewer courses of inhaled or oral antibiotics with AZM. Reduction in IL-8 and neutrophil elastase in BAL at 36 months (but not at 12 months). No different in parent-reported QoL	[156]

New Abbreviations: *PsA* Pseudomonas aeruginosa; *AZM* Azithromycin, *QoL* Quality of Life; *BPI-ANCA* bactericidal/permeability increasing protein

CXCL8 and neutrophil elastase is particularly relevant as high levels predict future pulmonary exacerbations in children [203], and it is possible that modulation via the mechanisms outlined previously attenuates the inflammatory response to further infective triggers. These findings are mirrored in several RCTs in older people with CF (Table 1) showing azithromycin use led to a reduction in pulmonary exacerbations, which are associated with failure to regain baseline lung function, and long-term respiratory decline [204–207]. However, durability of treatment effect remains unclear [52, 208, 209], and long-term macrolide therapy is currently not universally advised as best practice unlike, for example, recommendations to commence CFTR modulators for patients with specific genotypes or nebulised dornase alfa from 6 years of age [209, 210]. It should also be noted that all therapeutic trials were in patients not on highly effective modulator therapy, and whether macrolides have benefits in those on modulators is currently not known.

The finding that some patients with CF respond better to macrolides than others [144, 146, 195, 197] may be related to the pulmonary microbiome. The lungs,'which were historically considered sterile in the absence of infection, actually harbour diverse microbial communities, even in healthy controls [211], and the microbiome of CF sputum can predict disease course [212]. In a study of the microbiome in CF sputum, 45% of patients had reduced lung function decline (responders) after commencing azithromycin [213]; those who were azithromycin naïve and responded to treatment were found to have relative increased abundance of *Stenotrophomonas* and *Abiotrophia* (but not *Pseudomonas*) in sputum at the end of the study when compared to non-responders. Differences in the baseline microbiome also predict which CF patients respond to inhaled tobramycin [214]. However, unlike in asthma [215] and non-CF bronchiectasis [216], azithromycin does not significantly alter the composition of the CF microbiome [52, 213]; it is possible that the spectrum of treatment benefit observed between individual CF patients treated with macrolides [144, 146, 195, 197] relates to patient-specific characteristics of their unique respiratory microbiome and its interaction with azithromycin, rather than antibacterial properties of the macrolide itself. As recognition and study of the CF microbiome remains an emerging field [217], early clinical trials of azithromycin were not designed to evaluate this possibility and, in an era of personalised therapies, further work is needed to further elucidate these mechanisms.

5.2 *Safety*

Many studies demonstrate that long-term azithromycin is safe and well-tolerated in patients with CF (Table 1). As azithromycin has a long half-life, it continues to accumulate within tissues and does not plateau; the optimum dosing regimen is unclear. RCTs (Table 1) have been conducted using daily, twice weekly or thrice weekly dosing. Studies comparing daily and weekly dosing, and 5mg/kg vs. 15mg/kg, found no difference in change in FEV_1 [149, 151], although gastrointestinal side-effects were more common with 1200mg administered once a week

[149]. Gastrointestinal side-effects are a known side-effect of macrolides, but a metanalysis of RCTs in CF found no difference in abdominal pain, vomiting, diarrhoea or nausea between azithromycin and placebo groups [218]. Increased incidence of wheeze [146] has been described, the mechanism for which is unclear given macrolides reduce expression of ET-1, which is a potent bronchoconstrictor, and other studies describe a reduction in wheeze with azithromycin [219, 220]. It is possible that mobilisation of less viscous mucus into the airways is contributory, but this has not been specifically studied. There is no association between long-term azithromycin use and prolongation of the QT interval in children with CF [221], albeit in a group where very few were on concurrent medications that prolong the QT interval; this needs to be factored in when considering macrolide therapy in adults and children with CF who require polypharmacy.

Macrolide-associated tinnitus and sensorineural hearing loss are reported [222], even at standard oral doses, with the risk of tinnitus thought to be cumulative dose-dependent [223]. Whilst not reported in RCTs (Table 1), the extent of hearing impairment is greater than that which would be expected due to ageing alone in CF patients [224], especially amongst those receiving frequent courses of macrolides or intravenous aminoglycosides [225]. This is a particularly pertinent consideration as the life expectancy of CF patients is improving and should continue to do so with the advent of CFTR modulators [226, 227], so increased lifetime exposure to ototoxic drugs is likely. Macrolides have been associated with hepatic and renal toxicity [226]; whilst not widely reported in CF patients [228], again, this needs to be taken into account in patients receiving polypharmacy.

5.3 Macrolide Use in CF: Concerns

There are concerns about long-term macrolide therapy and emergence of resistant organisms [194]. Prevalence of *Staphylococcus aureus, Haemophilus influenzae* and *Streptococcus pneumoniae* decreases with long-term azithromycin use in CF patients [53], but this also leads to a statistically significant increase in isolation of macrolide-resistant strains of *Staphylococcus aureus* [53, 208]. A significant 3.1% uplift in FEV_1 observed after the first year of azithromycin was reversed after two and three years of therapy, although this was not felt to be related to the emergence of macrolide-resistant *Staphylococcus aureus* [208]. Nevertheless, when considered in relation to the COMBAT-CF trial [156], these findings might discourage early long-term macrolide use, particularly as *Staphylococcus aureus* is the predominant CF pathogen in the early years of life, and increased antibiotic resistance following macrolide treatment can persist even after cessation of treatment [230]. An increase in macrolide-resistant *Haemophilus* species has also been reported in children with CF on long-term azithromycin [231], although other data suggest that this might be offset by a reduced risk of acquiring several CF-related pathogens [51, 53]. In patients with non-CF bronchiectasis without *Pseudomonas aeruginosa* infection, macrolides do not reduce exacerbations and may cause displacement of

Haemophilus influenzae by more troublesome organisms including *Pseudomonas aeruginosa* [216]. This has not been seen in children with CF without *Pseudomonas aeruginosa* [153] but is another factor to bear in mind when considering early intervention with long-term macrolides. A cautionary tale against early use of prophylactic antibiotics is that a trend towards increased *Pseudomonas aeruginosa* isolation has been described in children with CF who receive long-term cephalexin [232] or flucloxacillin [233]; a multicentre trial (CF-START) is currently underway to further delineate the causal nature of the latter relationship.

NTM disease, particularly *Mycobacterium abscessus,* is associated with poor outcomes and can be a relative contraindication to lung transplant in CF [234, 235]. Macrolides are the cornerstone of NTM treatment in CF, and a concern about long-term use prior to isolation of NTM is that they might induce ribosomal methylase resistance proteins encoded by *erm* [41], making NTM more resistant to treatment, even before it has been cultured in sputum [236]. Although no increase in NTM (or MRSA or *Burkholderia cepacia* complex) prevalence has been reported in CF patients on long-term macrolides [51], there are no published data looking at whether patients who isolate NTM have a greater incidence of erm [41] expression if they have previously been on long-term azithromycin. This warrants more investigation.

Intravenous and nebulised tobramycin is widely used to treat *Pseudomonas aeruginosa* and pulmonary exacerbations in CF [237, 238]. It has been shown *in vitro* that azithromycin antagonises the effects of tobramycin [239, 240]. In a cohort study of CF patients, combined use of nebulised tobramycin and azithromycin was associated with a significant decrease in FEV_1, increased need for further antibiotics and a trend towards less reduction in *Pseudomonas aeruginosa* density in sputum when compared with tobramycin monotherapy [240]. In children with CF with chronic *Pseudomonas aeruginosa* infection, the relative improvement in FEV_1 following intravenous tobramycin was lower in patients also receiving azithromycin [207], a finding replicated in a large retrospective registry study that also suggested combined therapy was associated with reduced time to next pulmonary exacerbation [241]. A subsequent RCT demonstrated no difference in clinical outcomes in patients receiving azithromycin or placebo alongside nebulised tobramycin, although there was less reduction in *Pseudomonas aeruginosa* sputum density in the azithromycin group [242], and no inhibitory effect is seen in patients receiving azithromycin along with intravenous colistimethate [243]. Whilst these later studies provide reassurance, the earlier reports highlight a vital point about potential pitfalls of polypharmacy and the importance of tailoring, and rationalising where possible, medication regimens to the individual.

A compelling reason against using macrolides in CF is the advent of CFTR modulators. The first publication in 2011 demonstrated that small molecules are able to potentiate chloride movement across the CFTR channel [244], and subsequent studies showed that correction of other CFTR variants is possible, resulting in the treatment of CF at the cellular level for the first time, with the expectation that this reduces downstream consequences of the disease [227]. CFTR modulators are now able to treat around 90% of known *CFTR* variants, although they are not universally licensed across all age groups or available in all countries due to cost. There is an argument that azithromycin should be used from an early age so that when modulators can be commenced, children start with the best possible lung substrate. However, given long-term azithromycin does not reduce structural lung damage when given in the first three years of life despite reducing inflammation [156] and there are concerns about the durability of benefit [52, 208, 209], we consider it only on a case-by-case basis in patients that are not responding to first-line treatments. A 6- to 12-month trial of therapy to assess response is reasonable; if there is no benefit in terms of FEV_1 (improvement or reduced rate of decline) or fewer exacerbations over this period, discontinuation should be considered as data indicate that not all patients are macrolide responders.

6 Conclusions and Future Directions

Since the last iteration of this chapter, understanding of how macrolides might exert benefits in CF has increased, although it remains unclear why some patients respond better than others, or indeed, what is the mechanism of benefit. This is a key question for future research; in an era of high-cost drugs that are tailored to genotype, we should also be able to identify mechanisms by which patients might achieve benefit from other treatments. Drug-drug interactions are also important; there is little published data on long-term interactions of macrolides with these modulators, some of which are extensively metabolised in the liver, mainly by cytochrome P450 3A (CYP3A), a pathway inhibited by clarithromycin [245]. Longitudinal studies are required to monitor cumulative macrolide and CFTR modulator hepatotoxicity, particularly as patients will likely remain on modulators for life. Long-term follow-up of the infant cohort commenced on azithromycin is planned [156]; it will be fascinating to see if the early attenuation of inflammation seen in the azithromycin group translates into clinical benefits later in life.

There have been monumental advances in CF care since we last wrote this chapter. Aside from CFTR modulation, the rollout of newborn screening in many countries has identified children with CF far earlier, giving an opportunity for earlier intervention which should translate into better outcomes [199] and ever-increased life expectancy [2]. Azithromycin remains an important treatment, though more so now for acute exacerbations than long-term therapy for the majority of patients in our centres. Whilst many novel macrolides with antiviral and anti-inflammatory properties have been identified [246], none are yet commercially available, and further elucidation on the potential benefits of these in CF is urgently needed.

COI Statements AB has no COI.
AJ has no COI.
RP has no COI.

Ethics Compliance Statements Nil relevant.

References

1. Andersen DH. Cystic fibrosis of the pancreas and its relation to celiac disease: a clinical and pathologic study. Am J Dis Child. 1938;56(2):344–99.
2. McBennett KA, Davis PB, Konstan MW. Increasing life expectancy in cystic fibrosis: advances and challenges. Pediatr Pulmonol. 2022;57(Suppl 1):S5–s12.
3. Scotet V, L'Hostis C, Férec C. The changing epidemiology of cystic fibrosis: incidence, survival and impact of the CFTR gene discovery. Genes (Basel). 2020;11(6):589.
4. Wainwright BJ, Scambler PJ, Schmidtke J, Watson EA, Law HY, Farrall M, et al. Localization of cystic fibrosis locus to human chromosome 7cen-q22. Nature. 1985;318(6044):384–5.
5. Riordan JR. Assembly of functional CFTR chloride channels. Annu Rev Physiol. 2005;67: 701–18.
6. Hug MJ, Tamada T, Bridges RJ. CFTR and bicarbonate secretion by [correction of to] epithelial cells. News Physiol Sci. 2003;18:38–42.
7. Tang L, Fatehi M, Linsdell P. Mechanism of direct bicarbonate transport by the CFTR anion channel. J Cyst Fibros. 2009;8(2):115–21.
8. Reddy MM, Light MJ, Quinton PM. Activation of the epithelial Na+ channel (ENaC) requires CFTR Cl- channel function. Nature. 1999;402(6759):301–4.
9. Schwiebert EM, Egan ME, Hwang TH, Fulmer SB, Allen SS, Cutting GR, et al. CFTR regulates outwardly rectifying chloride channels through an autocrine mechanism involving ATP. Cell. 1995;81(7):1063–73.
10. Veit G, Avramescu RG, Chiang AN, Houck SA, Cai Z, Peters KW, et al. From CFTR biology toward combinatorial pharmacotherapy: expanded classification of cystic fibrosis mutations. Mol Biol Cell. 2016;27(3):424–33.
11. Correlation between genotype and phenotype in patients with cystic fibrosis. N Engl J Med. 1993;329(18):1308–13.
12. Tarran R, Button B, Boucher RC. Regulation of normal and cystic fibrosis airway surface liquid volume by phasic shear stress. Annu Rev Physiol. 2006;68:543–61.
13. Regnis JA, Robinson M, Bailey DL, Cook P, Hooper P, Chan HK, et al. Mucociliary clearance in patients with cystic fibrosis and in normal subjects. Am J Respir Crit Care Med. 1994;150 (1):66–71.
14. Robinson M, Bye PT. Mucociliary clearance in cystic fibrosis. Pediatr Pulmonol. 2002;33(4): 293–306.
15. Armstrong D, Grimwood K, Carlin JB, Carzino R, Hull J, Olinsky A, et al. Severe viral respiratory infections in infants with cystic fibrosis. Pediatr Pulmonol. 1998;26(6):371–9.
16. Recchiuti A, Patruno S, Plebani R, Romano M. The resolution approach to cystic fibrosis inflammation. Front Pharmacol. 2020;11:1129.
17. Paemka L, McCullagh BN, Abou Alaiwa MH, Stoltz DA, Dong Q, Randak CO, et al. Monocyte derived macrophages from CF pigs exhibit increased inflammatory responses at birth. J Cyst Fibros. 2017;16(4):471–4.
18. Tarique AA, Sly PD, Holt PG, Bosco A, Ware RS, Logan J, et al. CFTR-dependent defect in alternatively-activated macrophages in cystic fibrosis. J Cyst Fibros. 2017;16(4):475–82.
19. Roesch EA, Nichols DP, Chmiel JF. Inflammation in cystic fibrosis: an update. Pediatr Pulmonol. 2018;53(S3):S30–50.
20. Cohen-Cymberknoh M, Kerem E, Ferkol T, Elizur A. Airway inflammation in cystic fibrosis: molecular mechanisms and clinical implications. Thorax. 2013;68(12):1157.

21. Khan TZ, Wagener JS, Bost T, Martinez J, Accurso FJ, Riches DW. Early pulmonary inflammation in infants with cystic fibrosis. Am J Respir Crit Care Med. 1995;151(4):1075–82.
22. Downey DG, Bell SC, Elborn JS. Neutrophils in cystic fibrosis. Thorax. 2009;64(1):81.
23. Konstan MW, Hilliard KA, Norvell TM, Berger M. Bronchoalveolar lavage findings in cystic fibrosis patients with stable, clinically mild lung disease suggest ongoing infection and inflammation. Am J Respir Crit Care Med. 1994;150(2):448–54.
24. Law SM, Gray RD. Neutrophil extracellular traps and the dysfunctional innate immune response of cystic fibrosis lung disease: a review. J Inflamm (Lond). 2017;14:29.
25. Gray RD, Hardisty G, Regan KH, Smith M, Robb CT, Duffin R, et al. Delayed neutrophil apoptosis enhances NET formation in cystic fibrosis. Thorax. 2018;73(2):134–44.
26. Gramegna A, Amati F, Terranova L, Sotgiu G, Tarsia P, Miglietta D, et al. Neutrophil elastase in bronchiectasis. Respir Res. 2017;18(1):211.
27. Fahy JV, Dickey BF. Airway mucus function and dysfunction. N Engl J Med. 2010;363(23):2233–47.
28. Colom B, Bodkin JV, Beyrau M, Woodfin A, Ody C, Rourke C, et al. Leukotriene B4-neutrophil elastase axis drives neutrophil reverse transendothelial cell migration in vivo. Immunity. 2015;42(6):1075–86.
29. Konstan MW, Döring G, Heltshe SL, Lands LC, Hilliard KA, Koker P, et al. A randomized double blind, placebo controlled phase 2 trial of BIIL 284 BS (an LTB4 receptor antagonist) for the treatment of lung disease in children and adults with cystic fibrosis. J Cyst Fibros. 2014;13(2):148–55.
30. Oglesby IK, Vencken SF, Agrawal R, Gaughan K, Molloy K, Higgins G, et al. miR-17 overexpression in cystic fibrosis airway epithelial cells decreases interleukin-8 production. Eur Respir J. 2015;46(5):1350–60.
31. Linden SK, Sutton P, Karlsson NG, Korolik V, McGuckin MA. Mucins in the mucosal barrier to infection. Mucosal Immunol. 2008;1(3):183–97.
32. Morrison CB, Markovetz MR, Ehre C. Mucus, mucins, and cystic fibrosis. Pediatr Pulmonol. 2019;54(Suppl 3):S84–s96.
33. Niv Y, Ho SB, Rokkas T. Mucin secretion in cystic fibrosis: a systematic review. Dig Dis. 2021;39:375–81.
34. Henke MO, Renner A, Huber RM, Seeds MC, Rubin BK. MUC5AC and MUC5B mucins are decreased in cystic fibrosis airway secretions. Am J Respir Cell Mol Biol. 2004;31(1):86–91.
35. Simonin J, Bille E, Crambert G, Noel S, Dreano E, Edwards A, et al. Airway surface liquid acidification initiates host defense abnormalities in cystic fibrosis. Sci Rep. 2019;9(1):6516.
36. Saiman L, Prince A. Pseudomonas aeruginosa pili bind to asialoGM1 which is increased on the surface of cystic fibrosis epithelial cells. J Clin Invest. 1993;92(4):1875–80.
37. Davies JC, Stern M, Dewar A, Caplen NJ, Munkonge FM, Pitt T, et al. CFTR gene transfer reduces the binding of Pseudomonas aeruginosa to cystic fibrosis respiratory epithelium. Am J Respir Cell Mol Biol. 1997;16(6):657–63.
38. Davies J, Dewar A, Bush A, Pitt T, Gruenert D, Geddes DM, et al. Reduction in the adherence of Pseudomonas aeruginosa to native cystic fibrosis epithelium with anti-asialoGM1 antibody and neuraminidase inhibition. Eur Respir J. 1999;13(3):565–70.
39. Li J, Johnson XD, Iazvovskaia S, Tan A, Lin A, Hershenson MB. Signaling intermediates required for NF-kappa B activation and IL-8 expression in CF bronchial epithelial cells. Am J Physiol Lung Cell Mol Physiol. 2003;284(2):L307–15.
40. Pier GB, Grout M, Zaidi TS, Olsen JC, Johnson LG, Yankaskas JR, et al. Role of mutant CFTR in hypersusceptibility of cystic fibrosis patients to lung infections. Science. 1996;271(5245):64–7.
41. Pier GB, Grout M, Zaidi TS, Goldberg JB. How mutant CFTR may contribute to Pseudomonas aeruginosa infection in cystic fibrosis. Am J Respir Crit Care Med. 1996;154(4 Pt 2):S175–82.

42. Worlitzsch D, Tarran R, Ulrich M, Schwab U, Cekici A, Meyer KC, et al. Effects of reduced mucus oxygen concentration in airway pseudomonas infections of cystic fibrosis patients. J Clin Invest. 2002;109(3):317–25.
43. Moreau-Marquis S, Stanton BA, O'Toole GA. Pseudomonas aeruginosa biofilm formation in the cystic fibrosis airway. Pulm Pharmacol Ther. 2008;21(4):595–9.
44. Høiby N, Ciofu O, Bjarnsholt T. Pseudomonas aeruginosa biofilms in cystic fibrosis. Future Microbiol. 2010;5(11):1663–74.
45. Crull MR, Somayaji R, Ramos KJ, Caldwell E, Mayer-Hamblett N, Aitken ML, et al. Changing rates of chronic Pseudomonas aeruginosa infections in cystic fibrosis: a population-based cohort study. Clin Infect Dis. 2018;67(7):1089–95.
46. Tateda K, Ishii Y, Kimura S, Yamaguchi K, Horikawa M, Miyairi S. Suppression of Pseudomonas aeruginosa quorum-sensing systems by macrolides: a promising strategy or an oriental mystery? J Infect Chemother. 2007;13(6):357–67.
47. Kadota J, Sakito O, Kohno S, Sawa H, Mukae H, Oda H, et al. A mechanism of erythromycin treatment in patients with diffuse panbronchiolitis. Am Rev Respir Dis. 1993;147(1):153–9.
48. Kudoh S, Azuma A, Yamamoto M, Izumi T, Ando M. Improvement of survival in patients with diffuse panbronchiolitis treated with low-dose erythromycin. Am J Respir Crit Care Med. 1998;157(6 Pt 1):1829–32.
49. Akai S, Okayama H, Shimura S, Tanno Y, Sasaki H, Takishima T. Delta F508 mutation of cystic fibrosis gene is not found in chronic bronchitis with severe obstruction in Japan. Am Rev Respir Dis. 1992;146(3):781–3.
50. Wang W, Okayama H, Shirato K. Genotypes of cystic fibrosis (CF) reported in the world and polymorphisms of cystic fibrosis transmembrane conductance regulator (CFTR) gene in Japanese. Nihon Rinsho. 1996;54(2):525–32.
51. Cogen JD, Onchiri F, Emerson J, Gibson RL, Hoffman LR, Nichols DP, et al. Chronic azithromycin use in cystic fibrosis and risk of treatment-emergent respiratory pathogens. Ann Am Thorac Soc. 2018;15(6):702–9.
52. Samson C, Tamalet A, Thien HV, Taytard J, Perisson C, Nathan N, et al. Long-term effects of azithromycin in patients with cystic fibrosis. Respir Med. 2016;117:1–6.
53. Hansen CR, Pressler T, Hoiby N, Johansen HK. Long-term, low-dose azithromycin treatment reduces the incidence but increases macrolide resistance in Staphylococcus aureus in Danish CF patients. J Cyst Fibros. 2009;8(1):58–62.
54. Mikura S, Wada H, Higaki M, Yasutake T, Ishii H, Kamiya S, et al. Erythromycin prevents the pulmonary inflammation induced by exposure to cigarette smoke. Transl Res. 2011;158(1):30–7.
55. Ichikawa Y, Ninomiya H, Koga H, Tanaka M, Kinoshita M, Tokunaga N, et al. Erythromycin reduces neutrophils and neutrophil-derived elastolytic-like activity in the lower respiratory tract of bronchiolitis patients. Am Rev Respir Dis. 1992;146(1):196–203.
56. Ashitani J, Mukae H, Nakazato M, Ihi T, Mashimoto H, Kadota J, et al. Elevated concentrations of defensins in bronchoalveolar lavage fluid in diffuse panbronchiolitis. Eur Respir J. 1998;11(1):104.
57. Sakito O, Kadota J, Kohno S, Abe K, Shirai R, Hara K. Interleukin 1 beta, tumor necrosis factor alpha, and interleukin 8 in bronchoalveolar lavage fluid of patients with diffuse panbronchiolitis: a potential mechanism of macrolide therapy. Respiration. 1996;63(1):42–8.
58. Khair OA, Devalia JL, Abdelaziz MM, Sapsford RJ, Davies RJ. Effect of erythromycin on haemophilus influenzae endotoxin-induced release of IL-6, IL-8 and sICAM-1 by cultured human bronchial epithelial cells. Eur Respir J. 1995;8(9):1451.
59. Kawasaki S, Takizawa H, Ohtoshi T, Takeuchi N, Kohyama T, Nakamura H, et al. Roxithromycin inhibits cytokine production by and neutrophil attachment to human bronchial epithelial cells in vitro. Antimicrob Agents Chemother. 1998;42(6):1499–502.
60. Takizawa H, Desaki M, Ohtoshi T, Kawasaki S, Kohyama T, Sato M, et al. Erythromycin modulates IL-8 expression in normal and inflamed human bronchial epithelial cells. Am J Respir Crit Care Med. 1997;156(1):266–71.

61. Shinkai M, Foster GH, Rubin BK. Macrolide antibiotics modulate ERK phosphorylation and IL-8 and GM-CSF production by human bronchial epithelial cells. Am J Phys Lung Cell Mol Phys. 2006;290(1):L75–85.
62. Pukhalsky AL, Shmarina GV, Kapranov NI, Kokarovtseva SN, Pukhalskaya D, Kashirskaja NJ. Anti-inflammatory and immunomodulating effects of clarithromycin in patients with cystic fibrosis lung disease. Mediat Inflamm. 2004;13(2):111–7.
63. Zimmermann P, Ziesenitz VC, Curtis N, Ritz N. The immunomodulatory effects of macrolides—a systematic review of the underlying mechanisms. Front Immunol. 2018;9:302.
64. Liu T, Zhang L, Joo D, Sun S-C. NF-κB signaling in inflammation. Signal Transduct Target Ther. 2017;2(1):17023.
65. Yu H, Lin L, Zhang Z, Zhang H, Hu H. Targeting NF-κB pathway for the therapy of diseases: mechanism and clinical study. Signal Transduct Target Ther. 2020;5(1):209.
66. Corvol H, Fitting C, Chadelat K, Jacquot J, Tabary O, Boule M, et al. Distinct cytokine production by lung and blood neutrophils from children with cystic fibrosis. Am J Physiol Lung Cell Mol Physiol. 2003;284(6):L997–1003.
67. Everard ML, Sly P, Brenan S, Ryan G. Macrolide antibiotics in diffuse panbronchiolitis and in cystic fibrosis. Eur Respir J. 1997;10(12):2926.
68. Schultz MJ, Speelman P, Zaat S, van Deventer SJ, van der Poll T. Erythromycin inhibits tumor necrosis factor alpha and interleukin 6 production induced by heat-killed Streptococcus pneumoniae in whole blood. Antimicrob Agents Chemother. 1998;42(7):1605–9.
69. Tsai WC, Rodriguez ML, Young KS, Deng JC, Thannickal VJ, Tateda K, et al. Azithromycin blocks neutrophil recruitment in pseudomonas endobronchial infection. Am J Respir Crit Care Med. 2004;170(12):1331–9.
70. Wallwork B, Coman W, Feron F, Mackay-Sim A, Cervin A. Clarithromycin and prednisolone inhibit cytokine production in chronic rhinosinusitis. Laryngoscope. 2002;112(10):1827–30.
71. Abe S, Nakamura H, Inoue S, Takeda H, Saito H, Kato S, et al. Interleukin-8 gene repression by clarithromycin is mediated by the activator protein-1 binding site in human bronchial epithelial cells. Am J Respir Cell Mol Biol. 2000;22(1):51–60.
72. Kikuchi T, Hagiwara K, Honda Y, Gomi K, Kobayashi T, Takahashi H, et al. Clarithromycin suppresses lipopolysaccharide-induced interleukin-8 production by human monocytes through AP-1 and NF-kappa B transcription factors. J Antimicrob Chemother. 2002;49(5):745–55.
73. Desaki M, Takizawa H, Ohtoshi T, Kasama T, Kobayashi K, Sunazuka T, et al. Erythromycin suppresses nuclear factor-kappaB and activator protein-1 activation in human bronchial epithelial cells. Biochem Biophys Res Commun. 2000;267(1):124–8.
74. Joseph T, Look D, Ferkol T. NF-kappaB activation and sustained IL-8 gene expression in primary cultures of cystic fibrosis airway epithelial cells stimulated with Pseudomonas aeruginosa. Am J Physiol Lung Cell Mol Physiol. 2005;288(3):L471–9.
75. Kanoh S, Rubin BK. Mechanisms of action and clinical application of macrolides as immunomodulatory medications. Clin Microbiol Rev. 2010;23(3):590–615.
76. Chalmers JD, Boersma W, Lonergan M, Jayaram L, Crichton ML, Karalus N, et al. Long-term macrolide antibiotics for the treatment of bronchiectasis in adults: an individual participant data meta-analysis. Lancet Respir Med. 2019;7(10):845–54.
77. Tosi MF, Stark JM, Smith CW, Hamedani A, Gruenert DC, Infeld MD. Induction of ICAM-1 expression on human airway epithelial cells by inflammatory cytokines: effects on neutrophil-epithelial cell adhesion. Am J Respir Cell Mol Biol. 1992;7(2):214–21.
78. Aldallal N, McNaughton EE, Manzel LJ, Richards AM, Zabner J, Ferkol TW, et al. Inflammatory response in airway epithelial cells isolated from patients with cystic fibrosis. Am J Respir Crit Care Med. 2002;166(9):1248–56.
79. Hubeau C, Lorenzato M, Couetil JP, Hubert D, Dusser D, Puchelle E, et al. Quantitative analysis of inflammatory cells infiltrating the cystic fibrosis airway mucosa. Clin Exp Immunol. 2001;124(1):69–76.
80. De Rose V, Oliva A, Messore B, Grosso B, Mollar C, Pozzi E. Circulating adhesion molecules in cystic fibrosis. Am J Respir Crit Care Med. 1998;157(4 Pt 1):1234–9.

81. Gorrini M, Lupi A, Viglio S, Pamparana F, Cetta G, Iadarola P, et al. Inhibition of human neutrophil elastase by erythromycin and flurythromycin, two macrolide antibiotics. Am J Respir Cell Mol Biol. 2001;25(4):492–9.
82. Kusano S, Kadota J, Kohno S, Iida K, Kawakami K, Morikawa T, et al. Effect of roxithromycin on peripheral neutrophil adhesion molecules in patients with chronic lower respiratory tract disease. Respiration. 1995;62(4):217–22.
83. Lin HC, Wang CH, Liu CY, Yu CT, Kuo HP. Erythromycin inhibits beta2-integrins (CD11b/CD18) expression, interleukin-8 release and intracellular oxidative metabolism in neutrophils. Respir Med. 2000;94(7):654–60.
84. Okubo Y. Macrolides reduce the expression of surface mac-1 molecule on neutrophil. Kurume Med J. 1997;44(2):115–23.
85. Li Y, Azuma A, Takahashi S, Usuki J, Matsuda K, Aoyama A, et al. Fourteen-membered ring macrolides inhibit vascular cell adhesion molecule 1 messenger RNA induction and leukocyte migration: role in preventing lung injury and fibrosis in bleomycin-challenged mice. Chest. 2002;122(6):2137–45.
86. Dean TP, Dai Y, Shute JK, Church MK, Warner JO. Interleukin-8 concentrations are elevated in bronchoalveolar lavage, sputum, and sera of children with cystic fibrosis. Pediatr Res. 1993;34(2):159–61.
87. Brennan S, Cooper D, Sly PD. Directed neutrophil migration to IL-8 is increased in cystic fibrosis: a study of the effect of erythromycin. Thorax. 2001;56(1):62–4.
88. Torre D, Broggini M, Bottà V, Sampietro C, Busarello R, Garberi C. In vitro and ex vivo effects of recent and new macrolide antibiotics on chemotaxis of human polymorphonuclear leukocytes. J Chemother. 1991;3(4):236–9.
89. Hojo M, Fujita I, Hamasaki Y, Miyazaki M, Miyazaki S. Erythromycin does not directly affect neutrophil functions. Chest. 1994;105(2):520–3.
90. Nguyen GT, Green ER, Mecsas J. Neutrophils to the ROScue: mechanisms of NADPH oxidase activation and bacterial resistance. Front Cell Infect Microbiol. 2017;7:373.
91. Kricker JA, Page CP, Gardarsson FR, Baldursson O, Gudjonsson T, Parnham MJ. Nonantimicrobial actions of macrolides: overview and perspectives for future development. Pharmacol Rev. 2021;73(4):1404.
92. Hull J, Vervaart P, Grimwood K, Phelan P. Pulmonary oxidative stress response in young children with cystic fibrosis. Thorax. 1997;52(6):557–60.
93. Day BJ, van Heeckeren AM, Min E, Velsor LW. Role for cystic fibrosis transmembrane conductance regulator protein in a glutathione response to bronchopulmonary pseudomonas infection. Infect Immun. 2004;72(4):2045–51.
94. Moliteo E, Sciacca M, Palmeri A, Papale M, Manti S, Parisi GF, et al. Cystic fibrosis and oxidative stress: the role of CFTR. Molecules. 2022;27(16):5324.
95. Galli F, Battistoni A, Gambari R, Pompella A, Bragonzi A, Pilolli F, et al. Oxidative stress and antioxidant therapy in cystic fibrosis. Biochim Biophys Acta (BBA) - Mol Basis Dis. 2012;1822(5):690–713.
96. Bernut A, Loynes CA, Floto RA, Renshaw SA. Deletion of cftr leads to an excessive neutrophilic response and defective tissue repair in a zebrafish model of sterile inflammation. Front Immunol. 2020;11:1733.
97. Labro MT, el Benna J, Babin-Chevaye C. Comparison of the in-vitro effect of several macrolides on the oxidative burst of human neutrophils. J Antimicrob Chemother. 1989;24(4):561–72.
98. Anderson R. Erythromycin and roxithromycin potentiate human neutrophil locomotion in vitro by inhibition of leukoattractant-activated superoxide generation and autooxidation. J Infect Dis. 1989;159(5):966–73.
99. Villagrasa V, Berto L, Cortijo J, Perpina M, Sanz C, Morcillo EJ. Effects of erythromycin on chemoattractant-activated human polymorphonuclear leukocytes. Gen Pharmacol. 1997;29(4):605–9.

100. Hand WL, Hand DL, King-Thompson NL. Antibiotic inhibition of the respiratory burst response in human polymorphonuclear leukocytes. Antimicrob Agents Chemother. 1990;34 (5):863–70.
101. Reijnders TDY, Saris A, Schultz MJ, van der Poll T. Immunomodulation by macrolides: therapeutic potential for critical care. Lancet Respir Med. 2020;8(6):619–30.
102. Culić O, Eraković V, Cepelak I, Barisić K, Brajsa K, Ferencić Z, et al. Azithromycin modulates neutrophil function and circulating inflammatory mediators in healthy human subjects. Eur J Pharmacol. 2002;450(3):277–89.
103. Wenisch C, Parschalk B, Zedtwitz-Liebenstein K, Weihs A, el Menyawi I, Graninger W. Effect of single oral dose of azithromycin, clarithromycin, and roxithromycin on polymorphonuclear leukocyte function assessed ex vivo by flow cytometry. Antimicrob Agents Chemother. 1996;40(9):2039–42.
104. Anderson R, Theron AJ, Feldman C. Membrane-stabilizing, anti-inflammatory interactions of macrolides with human neutrophils. Inflammation. 1996;20(6):693–705.
105. Aoshiba K, Nagai A, Konno K. Erythromycin shortens neutrophil survival by accelerating apoptosis. Antimicrob Agents Chemother. 1995;39(4):872–7.
106. Koch CC, Esteban DJ, Chin AC, Olson ME, Read RR, Ceri H, et al. Apoptosis, oxidative metabolism and interleukin-8 production in human neutrophils exposed to azithromycin: effects of Streptococcus pneumoniae. J Antimicrob Chemother. 2000;46(1):19–26.
107. Imperi F, Leoni L, Visca P. Antivirulence activity of azithromycin in Pseudomonas aeruginosa. Front Microbiol. 2014;5:178.
108. Nagai H, Shishido H, Yoneda R, Yamaguchi E, Tamura A, Kurashima A. Long-term low-dose administration of erythromycin to patients with diffuse panbronchiolitis. Respiration. 1991;58 (3–4):145–9.
109. Dupont MJ, Lapointe JR. Effect on Pseudomonas aeruginosa alginate expression of direct plating and culture of fresh cystic fibrosis sputum on to pseudomonas isolation agar containing subinhibitory concentrations of roxithromycin and rifampicin. J Antimicrob Chemother. 1995;36(1):231–6.
110. Baumann U, Fischer JJ, Gudowius P, Lingner M, Herrmann S, Tümmler B, et al. Buccal adherence of Pseudomonas aeruginosa in patients with cystic fibrosis under long-term therapy with azithromycin. Infection. 2001;29(1):7–11.
111. Equi AC, Davies JC, Painter H, Hyde S, Bush A, Geddes DM, et al. Exploring the mechanisms of macrolides in cystic fibrosis. Respir Med. 2006;100(4):687–97.
112. Nakashio S, Susa C, Qiu S, Kijima A, Iwasawa H, Shimomura H, et al. Antimicrobial activity of clarithromycin and its effect on bacterial adherence to medical material. Jpn J Antibiot. 1993;46(6):428–36.
113. Yamasaki T. Adherence of Pseudomonas aeruginosa to mouse tracheal epithelium--the effect of antimicrobial agents. Kansenshogaku Zasshi. 1990;64(5):575–83.
114. Tsang KW, Shum DK, Chan S, Ng P, Mak J, Leung R, et al. Pseudomonas aeruginosa adherence to human basement membrane collagen in vitro. Eur Respir J. 2003;21(6):932–8.
115. Veesenmeyer JL, Hauser AR, Lisboa T, Rello J. Pseudomonas aeruginosa virulence and therapy: evolving translational strategies. Crit Care Med. 2009;37(5):1777–86.
116. Qin S, Xiao W, Zhou C, Pu Q, Deng X, Lan L, et al. Pseudomonas aeruginosa: pathogenesis, virulence factors, antibiotic resistance, interaction with host, technology advances and emerging therapeutics. Signal Transduct Target Ther. 2022;7(1):199.
117. Tanaka E, Kanthakumar K, Cundell DR, Tsang KW, Taylor GW, Kuze F, et al. The effect of erythromycin on Pseudomonas aeruginosa and neutrophil mediated epithelial damage. J Antimicrob Chemother. 1994;33(4):765–75.
118. Govan JR, Deretic V. Microbial pathogenesis in cystic fibrosis: mucoid Pseudomonas aeruginosa and Burkholderia cepacia. Microbiol Rev. 1996;60(3):539–74.
119. Sharma D, Misba L, Khan AU. Antibiotics versus biofilm: an emerging battleground in microbial communities. Antimicrob Resist Infect Control. 2019;8(1):76.

120. Davies D. Understanding biofilm resistance to antibacterial agents. Nat Rev Drug Discov. 2003;2(2):114–22.
121. Kobayashi H. Biofilm disease: its clinical manifestation and therapeutic possibilities of macrolides. Am J Med. 1995;99(6a):26s–30s.
122. Ichimiya T, Yamasaki T, Nasu M. In-vitro effects of antimicrobial agents on Pseudomonas aeruginosa biofilm formation. J Antimicrob Chemother. 1994;34(3):331–41.
123. Ichimiya T, Takeoka K, Hiramatsu K, Hirai K, Yamasaki T, Nasu M. The influence of azithromycin on the biofilm formation of Pseudomonas aeruginosa in vitro. Chemotherapy. 1996;42(3):186–91.
124. Tamaoki J, Nakata J, Takeda Y, Takemura H, Tagaya E, Konno K. Effect of macrolide antibiotics on airway goblet hypersecretion in Guinea pigs. Kansenshogaku Zasshi. 1996;70 (6):591–6.
125. Shimizu T, Shimizu S, Hattori R, Gabazza EC, Majima Y. In vivo and in vitro effects of macrolide antibiotics on mucus secretion in airway epithelial cells. Am J Respir Crit Care Med. 2003;168(5):581–7.
126. Dupont MJ, Lapointe JR. Quantitative effect of roxithromycin and rifampicin on mucoid cultures from directly plated sputum of cystic fibrosis patients chronically colonized with Pseudomonas aeruginosa. Drugs Exp Clin Res. 1990;16(12):597–605.
127. Tai S, Sudo E, Sun F, King M, Sextro W, von der Hardt H, et al. Effect of azithromycin treatment on sputum rheology in cystic fibrosis patients. Pediatr Pulmonol Suppl. 1999;19 (265):2271–5.
128. Kaneko Y, Yanagihara K, Seki M, Kuroki M, Miyazaki Y, Hirakata Y, et al. Clarithromycin inhibits overproduction of muc5ac core protein in murine model of diffuse panbronchiolitis. Am J Physiol Lung Cell Mol Physiol. 2003;285(4):L847–53.
129. Kita E, Sawaki M, Oku D, Hamuro A, Mikasa K, Konishi M, et al. Suppression of virulence factors of Pseudomonas aeruginosa by erythromycin. J Antimicrob Chemother. 1991;27(3): 273–84.
130. Molinari G, Guzmán CA, Pesce A, Schito GC. Inhibition of Pseudomonas aeruginosa virulence factors by subinhibitory concentrations of azithromycin and other macrolide antibiotics. J Antimicrob Chemother. 1993;31(5):681–8.
131. Molinari G, Paglia P, Schito GC. Inhibition of motility of Pseudomonas aeruginosa and Proteus mirabilis by subinhibitory concentrations of azithromycin. Eur J Clin Microbiol Infect Dis. 1992;11(5):469–71.
132. Mizukane R, Hirakata Y, Kaku M, Ishii Y, Furuya N, Ishida K, et al. Comparative in vitro exoenzyme-suppressing activities of azithromycin and other macrolide antibiotics against Pseudomonas aeruginosa. Antimicrob Agents Chemother. 1994;38(3):528–33.
133. Tateda K, Ishii Y, Matsumoto T, Kobayashi T, Miyazaki S, Yamaguchi K. Potential of macrolide antibiotics to inhibit protein synthesis of Pseudomonas aeruginosa: suppression of virulence factors and stress response. J Infect Chemother. 2000;6(1):1–7.
134. Tateda K, Comte R, Pechere JC, Köhler T, Yamaguchi K, Van Delden C. Azithromycin inhibits quorum sensing in Pseudomonas aeruginosa. Antimicrob Agents Chemother. 2001;45 (6):1930–3.
135. Nalca Y, Jänsch L, Bredenbruch F, Geffers R, Buer J, Häussler S. Quorum-sensing antagonistic activities of azithromycin in Pseudomonas aeruginosa PAO1: a global approach. Antimicrob Agents Chemother. 2006;50(5):1680–8.
136. Kawamura-Sato K, Iinuma Y, Hasegawa T, Horii T, Yamashino T, Ohta M. Effect of subinhibitory concentrations of macrolides on expression of flagellin in Pseudomonas aeruginosa and Proteus mirabilis. Antimicrob Agents Chemother. 2000;44(10):2869–72.
137. Wozniak DJ, Keyser R. Effects of subinhibitory concentrations of macrolide antibiotics on Pseudomonas aeruginosa. Chest. 2004;125(2 Suppl):62S–9S. quiz 9S
138. Tateda K, Ishii Y, Matsumoto T, Furuya N, Nagashima M, Matsunaga T, et al. Direct evidence for antipseudomonal activity of macrolides: exposure-dependent bactericidal activity and

inhibition of protein synthesis by erythromycin, clarithromycin, and azithromycin. Antimicrob Agents Chemother. 1996;40(10):2271–5.
139. Schögler A, Kopf BS, Edwards MR, Johnston SL, Casaulta C, Kieninger E, et al. Novel antiviral properties of azithromycin in cystic fibrosis airway epithelial cells. Eur Respir J. 2015;45(2):428 39.
140. Gielen V, Johnston SL, Edwards MR. Azithromycin induces anti-viral responses in bronchial epithelial cells. Eur Respir J. 2010;36(3):646–54.
141. Goffard A, Lambert V, Salleron J, Herwegh S, Engelmann I, Pinel C, et al. Virus and cystic fibrosis: rhinoviruses are associated with exacerbations in adult patients. J Clin Virol. 2014;60 (2):147–53.
142. Vareille M, Kieninger E, Alves MP, Kopf BS, Möller A, Geiser T, et al. Impaired type I and type III interferon induction and rhinovirus control in human cystic fibrosis airway epithelial cells. Thorax. 2012;67(6):517–25.
143. Chattoraj SS, Ganesan S, Faris A, Comstock A, Lee WM, Sajjan US. Pseudomonas aeruginosa suppresses interferon response to rhinovirus infection in cystic fibrosis but not in normal bronchial epithelial cells. Infect Immun. 2011;79(10):4131–45.
144. Equi A, Balfour-Lynn IM, Bush A, Rosenthal M. Long term azithromycin in children with cystic fibrosis: a randomised, placebo-controlled crossover trial. Lancet. 2002;360(9338): 978–84.
145. Wolter J, Seeney S, Bell S, Bowler S, Masel P, McCormack J. Effect of long term treatment with azithromycin on disease parameters in cystic fibrosis: a randomised trial. Thorax. 2002;57 (3):212–6.
146. Saiman L, Marshall BC, Mayer-Hamblett N, Burns JL, Quittner AL, Cibene DA, et al. Azithromycin in patients with cystic fibrosis chronically infected with Pseudomonas aeruginosa: a randomized controlled trial. JAMA. 2003;290(13):1749–56.
147. Rotschild M, Elias N, Berkowitz D, Pollak S, Shinawi M, Beck R, et al. Autoantibodies against bactericidal/permeability-increasing protein (BPI-ANCA) in cystic fibrosis patients treated with azithromycin. Clin Exp Med. 2005;5(2):80–5.
148. Clement A, Tamalet A, Leroux E, Ravilly S, Fauroux B, Jais JP. Long term effects of azithromycin in patients with cystic fibrosis: a double blind, placebo controlled trial. Thorax. 2006;61(10):895.
149. McCormack J, Bell S, Senini S, Walmsley K, Patel K, Wainwright C, et al. Daily versus weekly azithromycin in cystic fibrosis patients. Eur Respir J. 2007;30(3):487–95.
150. Steinkamp G, Schmitt-Grohe S, Döring G, Staab D, Pfründer D, Beck G, et al. Once-weekly azithromycin in cystic fibrosis with chronic Pseudomonas aeruginosa infection. Respir Med. 2008;102(11):1643–53.
151. Kabra SK, Pawaiya R, Lodha R, Kapil A, Kabra M, Vani AS, et al. Long-term daily high and low doses of azithromycin in children with cystic fibrosis: a randomized controlled trial. J Cyst Fibros. 2010;9(1):17–23.
152. Saiman L, Mayer-Hamblett N, Anstead M, Lands LC, Kloster M, Goss CH, et al. Open-label, follow-on study of azithromycin in pediatric patients with CF uninfected with Pseudomonas aeruginosa. Pediatr Pulmonol. 2012;47(7):641–8.
153. Saiman L, Anstead M, Mayer-Hamblett N, Lands LC, Kloster M, Hocevar-Trnka J, et al. Effect of azithromycin on pulmonary function in patients with cystic fibrosis uninfected with Pseudomonas aeruginosa: a randomized controlled trial. JAMA. 2010;303(17):1707–15.
154. Ratjen F, Saiman L, Mayer-Hamblett N, Lands LC, Kloster M, Thompson V, et al. Effect of azithromycin on systemic markers of inflammation in patients with cystic fibrosis uninfected with Pseudomonas aeruginosa. Chest. 2012;142(5):1259–66.
155. Mayer-Hamblett N, Retsch-Bogart G, Kloster M, Accurso F, Rosenfeld M, Albers G, et al. Azithromycin for early pseudomonas infection in cystic fibrosis. The OPTIMIZE Randomized Trial. Am J Respir Crit Care Med. 2018;198(9):1177–87.
156. Stick SM, Foti A, Ware RS, Tiddens H, Clements BS, Armstrong DS, et al. The effect of azithromycin on structural lung disease in infants with cystic fibrosis (COMBAT CF): a phase

3, randomised, double-blind, placebo-controlled clinical trial. Lancet Respir Med. 2022;10(8): 776–84.
157. Lallemand JY, Stoven V, Annereau JP, Boucher J, Blanquet S, Barthe J, et al. Induction by antitumoral drugs of proteins that functionally complement CFTR: a novel therapy for cystic fibrosis? Lancet. 1997;350:711–2.
158. Eisen S, Painter H, Hyde SC, Davies J, Jaffé A. Clinical improvement in cystic fibrosis following anti-tumourous chemotherapy. Arch Dis Child. 2004;89(12):1179.
159. Manavalan P, Smith AE, McPherson JM. Sequence and structural homology among membrane-associated domains of CFTR and certain transporter proteins. J Protein Chem. 1993;12(3):279–90.
160. Gant TW, O'Connor CK, Corbitt R, Thorgeirsson U, Thorgeirsson SS. In vivo induction of liver P-glycoprotein expression by xenobiotics in monkeys. Toxicol Appl Pharmacol. 1995;133(2):269–76.
161. Tamaoki J, Isono K, Sakai N, Kanemura T, Konno K. Erythromycin inhibits Cl secretion across canine tracheal epithelial cells. Eur Respir J. 1992;5(2):234–8.
162. Middleton PG, Geddes DM, Alton EW. Trimethoprim and tetracycline inhibit airway epithelial sodium absorption. Am J Respir Crit Care Med. 1996;154(1):18–23.
163. Davenport AP, Hyndman KA, Dhaun N, Southan C, Kohan DE, Pollock JS, et al. Endothelin. Pharmacol Rev. 2016;68(2):357–418.
164. Takizawa H, Desaki M, Ohtoshi T, Kawasaki S, Kohyama T, Sato M, et al. Erythromycin and clarithromycin attenuate cytokine-induced endothelin-1 expression in human bronchial epithelial cells. Eur Respir J. 1998;12(1):57–63.
165. Blouquit S, Sari A, Lombet A, D'Herbomez M, Naline E, Matran R, et al. Effects of endothelin-1 on epithelial ion transport in human airways. Am J Respir Cell Mol Biol. 2003;29(2):245–51.
166. Pradal U, Delmarco A, Cipolli M, Cazzola G. Chloride transport may be restored by long-term azithromycin treatment in patients with cystic fibrosis. Pediatr Pulmonol. 2000;280
167. Pradal U, Delmarco A, Morganti M, Cipolli M, Mini E, Cazzola G. Long-term azithromycin in cystic fibrosis: another possible mechanism of action? J Chemother. 2005;17(4):393–400.
168. Barker PM, Gillie DJ, Schechter MS, Rubin BK. Effect of macrolides on in vivo ion transport across cystic fibrosis nasal epithelium. Am J Respir Crit Care Med. 2005;171(8):868–71.
169. Oliynyk I, Varelogianni G, Schalling M, Asplund MS, Roomans GM, Johannesson M. Azithromycin increases chloride efflux from cystic fibrosis airway epithelial cells. Exp Lung Res. 2009;35(3):210–21.
170. de Winter-de Groot KM, van der Ent CK. Nitric oxide in cystic fibrosis. J Cyst Fibros. 2005;4 (Suppl 2):25–9.
171. Meng QH, Springall DR, Bishop AE, Morgan K, Evans TJ, Habib S, et al. Lack of inducible nitric oxide synthase in bronchial epithelium: a possible mechanism of susceptibility to infection in cystic fibrosis. J Pathol. 1998;184(3):323–31.
172. Gaston B, Ratjen F, Vaughan JW, Malhotra NR, Canady RG, Snyder AH, et al. Nitrogen redox balance in the cystic fibrosis airway: effects of antipseudomonal therapy. Am J Respir Crit Care Med. 2002;165(3):387–90.
173. Tamaoki J, Kondo M, Kohri K, Aoshiba K, Tagaya E, Nagai A. Macrolide antibiotics protect against immune complex-induced lung injury in rats: role of nitric oxide from alveolar macrophages. J Immunol. 1999;163(5):2909–15.
174. Kohri K, Tamaoki J, Kondo M, Aoshiba K, Tagaya E, Nagai A. Macrolide antibiotics inhibit nitric oxide generation by rat pulmonary alveolar macrophages. Eur Respir J. 2000;15(1): 62–7.
175. Mitsuyama T, Hidaka K, Furuno T, Hara N. Neutrophil-induced endothelial cell damage: inhibition by a 14-membered ring macrolide through the action of nitric oxide. Int Arch Allergy Immunol. 1997;114(2):111–5.
176. Culić O, Eraković V, Parnham MJ. Anti-inflammatory effects of macrolide antibiotics. Eur J Pharmacol. 2001;429(1–3):209–29.

177. Darling KE, Evans TJ. Effects of nitric oxide on Pseudomonas aeruginosa infection of epithelial cells from a human respiratory cell line derived from a patient with cystic fibrosis. Infect Immun. 2003;71(5):2341–9.
178. Zheng S, Xu W, Bose S, Banerjee AK, Haque SJ, Erzurum SC. Impaired nitric oxide synthase-2 signaling pathway in cystic fibrosis airway epithelium. Am J Phys Lung Cell Mol Phys. 2004;287(2):L374–L81.
179. Smith AW, Green J, Eden CE, Watson ML. Nitric oxide-induced potentiation of the killing of Burkholderia cepacia by reactive oxygen species: implications for cystic fibrosis. J Med Microbiol. 1999;48(5):419–23.
180. Bentur L, Gur M, Ashkenazi M, Livnat-Levanon G, Mizrahi M, Tal A, et al. Pilot study to test inhaled nitric oxide in cystic fibrosis patients with refractory mycobacterium abscessus lung infection. J Cyst Fibros. 2020;19(2):225–31.
181. Regamey N, Jeffery PK, Alton EW, Bush A, Davies JC. Airway remodelling and its relationship to inflammation in cystic fibrosis. Thorax. 2011;66(7):624–9.
182. Yatsunami J, Fukuno Y, Nagata M, Tominaga M, Aoki S, Tsuruta N, et al. Antiangiogenic and antitumor effects of 14-membered ring macrolides on mouse B16 melanoma cells. Clin Exp Metastasis. 1999;17(4):361–7.
183. Yatsunami J, Tsuruta N, Fukuno Y, Kawashima M, Taniguchi S, Hayashi S. Inhibitory effects of roxithromycin on tumor angiogenesis, growth and metastasis of mouse B16 melanoma cells. Clin Exp Metastasis. 1999;17(2):119–24.
184. Li A, Dubey S, Varney ML, Dave BJ, Singh RK. IL-8 directly enhanced endothelial cell survival, proliferation, and matrix metalloproteinases production and regulated angiogenesis. J Immunol. 2003;170(6):3369.
185. Fujitani Y, Trifilieff A. In vivo and in vitro effects of SAR 943, a rapamycin analogue, on airway inflammation and remodeling. Am J Respir Crit Care Med. 2003;167(2):193–8.
186. Kramer EL, Hardie WD, Mushaben EM, Acciani TH, Pastura PA, Korfhagen TR, et al. Rapamycin decreases airway remodeling and hyperreactivity in a transgenic model of noninflammatory lung disease. J Appl Physiol (1985). 2011;111(6):1760–7.
187. Hilliard TN, Regamey N, Shute JK, Nicholson AG, Alton EW, Bush A, et al. Airway remodelling in children with cystic fibrosis. Thorax. 2007;62(12):1074–80.
188. Chien KR, Sen A, Reynolds R, Chang A, Kim Y, Gunn MD, et al. Release of arachidonate from membrane phospholipids in cultured neonatal rat myocardial cells during adenosine triphosphate depletion. Correlation with the progression of cell injury. J Clin Invest. 1985;75 (6):1770–80.
189. Travers JB, Rohan JG, Sahu RP. New insights into the pathologic roles of the platelet-activating factor system. Front Endocrinol (Lausanne). 2021;12:624132.
190. Feldman C, Anderson R, Theron AJ, Ramafi G, Cole PJ, Wilson R. Roxithromycin, clarithromycin, and azithromycin attenuate the injurious effects of bioactive phospholipids on human respiratory epithelium in vitro. Inflammation. 1997;21(6):655–65.
191. Tsoupras AB, Chini M, Tsogas N, Lioni A, Tsekes G, Demopoulos CA, et al. In vitro anti-inflammatory and anti-coagulant effects of antibiotics towards platelet activating factor and thrombin. J Inflamm. 2011;8(1):17.
192. Zhanel GG, Walters M, Noreddin A, Vercaigne LM, Wierzbowski A, Embil JM, et al. The ketolides: a critical review. Drugs. 2002;62(12):1771–804.
193. Feldman C, Anderson R, Theron A, Mokgobu I, Cole PJ, Wilson R. The effects of ketolides on bioactive phospholipid-induced injury to human respiratory epithelium in vitro. Eur Respir J. 1999;13(5):1022–8.
194. Southern KW, Barker PM, Solis-Moya A, Patel L. Macrolide antibiotics for cystic fibrosis. Cochrane Database Syst Rev. 2012;11(11):Cd002203.
195. Jaffé A, Francis J, Rosenthal M, Bush A. Long-term azithromycin may improve lung function in children with cystic fibrosis. Lancet. 1998;351(9100):420.

196. Ordoñez CL, Stulbarg M, Grundland H, Liu JT, Boushey HA. Effect of clarithromycin on airway obstruction and inflammatory markers in induced sputum in cystic fibrosis: a pilot study. Pediatr Pulmonol. 2001;32(1):29–37.
197. Saiman L, Mayer-Hamblett N, Campbell P, Marshall BC. Heterogeneity of treatment response to azithromycin in patients with cystic fibrosis. Am J Respir Crit Care Med. 2005;172(8): 1008–12.
198. Nichols DP, Odem-Davis K, Cogen JD, Goss CH, Ren CL, Skalland M, et al. Pulmonary outcomes associated with long-term azithromycin therapy in cystic fibrosis. Am J Respir Crit Care Med. 2020;201(4):430–7.
199. Castellani C, Massie J, Sontag M, Southern KW. Newborn screening for cystic fibrosis. Lancet Respir Med. 2016;4(8):653–61.
200. SchlÃ¼ter DK, Southern KW, Dryden C, Diggle P, Taylor-Robinson D. Impact of newborn screening on outcomes and social inequalities in cystic fibrosis: a UK CF registry-based study. Thorax. 2020;75(2):123–31.
201. Rosenow T, Mok LC, Turkovic L, Berry LJ, Sly PD, Ranganathan S, et al. The cumulative effect of inflammation and infection on structural lung disease in early cystic fibrosis. Eur Respir J. 2019;54(1)
202. Sly PD, Gangell CL, Chen L, Ware RS, Ranganathan S, Mott LS, et al. Risk factors for bronchiectasis in children with cystic fibrosis. N Engl J Med. 2013;368(21):1963–70.
203. Ishak A, Stick SM, Turkovic L, Ranganathan SC, King L, Harrison J, et al. BAL inflammatory markers can predict pulmonary exacerbations in children with cystic fibrosis. Chest. 2020;158 (6):2314–22.
204. Byrnes CA, Vidmar S, Cheney JL, Carlin JB, Armstrong DS, Cooper PJ, et al. Prospective evaluation of respiratory exacerbations in children with cystic fibrosis from newborn screening to 5 years of age. Thorax. 2013;68(7):643–51.
205. Stanford GE, Dave K, Simmonds NJ. Pulmonary exacerbations in adults with cystic fibrosis: a grown-up issue in a changing cystic fibrosis landscape. Chest. 2021;159(1):93–102.
206. Sanders DB, Bittner RC, Rosenfeld M, Hoffman LR, Redding GJ, Goss CH. Failure to recover to baseline pulmonary function after cystic fibrosis pulmonary exacerbation. Am J Respir Crit Care Med. 2010;182(5):627–32.
207. Waters V, Stanojevic S, Atenafu EG, Lu A, Yau Y, Tullis E, et al. Effect of pulmonary exacerbations on long-term lung function decline in cystic fibrosis. Eur Respir J. 2012;40(1): 61–6.
208. Tramper-Stranders GA, Wolfs TF, Fleer A, Kimpen JL, van der Ent CK. Maintenance azithromycin treatment in pediatric patients with cystic fibrosis: long-term outcomes related to macrolide resistance and pulmonary function. Pediatr Infect Dis J. 2007;26(1):8–12.
209. Castellani C, Duff AJA, Bell SC, Heijerman HGM, Munck A, Ratjen F, et al. ECFS best practice guidelines: the 2018 revision. J Cyst Fibros. 2018;17(2):153–78.
210. Mogayzel PJ, Naureckas ET, Robinson KA, Mueller G, Hadjiliadis D, Hoag JB, et al. Cystic fibrosis pulmonary guidelines. Am J Respir Crit Care Med. 2013;187(7):680–9.
211. Morris A, Beck JM, Schloss PD, Campbell TB, Crothers K, Curtis JL, et al. Comparison of the respiratory microbiome in healthy nonsmokers and smokers. Am J Respir Crit Care Med. 2013;187(10):1067–75.
212. Acosta N, Heirali A, Somayaji R, Surette MG, Workentine ML, Sibley CD, et al. Sputum microbiota is predictive of long-term clinical outcomes in young adults with cystic fibrosis. Thorax. 2018;73(11):1016–25.
213. Acosta N, Thornton CS, Surette MG, Somayaji R, Rossi L, Rabin HR, et al. Azithromycin and the microbiota of cystic fibrosis sputum. BMC Microbiol. 2021;21(1):96.
214. Heirali A, Thornton C, Acosta N, Somayaji R, Laforest Lapointe I, Storey D, et al. Sputum microbiota in adults with CF associates with response to inhaled tobramycin. Thorax. 2020;75 (12):1058.
215. Slater M, Rivett DW, Williams L, Martin M, Harrison T, Sayers I, et al. The impact of azithromycin therapy on the airway microbiota in asthma. Thorax. 692014:673–4.

216. Rogers GB, Bruce KD, Martin ML, Burr LD, Serisier DJ. The effect of long-term macrolide treatment on respiratory microbiota composition in non-cystic fibrosis bronchiectasis: an analysis from the randomised, double-blind, placebo-controlled BLESS trial. Lancet Respir Med. 2014;2(12):988–96.
217. Rogers GB, Hart CA, Mason JR, Hughes M, Walshaw MJ, Bruce KD. Bacterial diversity in cases of lung infection in cystic fibrosis patients: 16S ribosomal DNA (rDNA) length heterogeneity PCR and 16S rDNA terminal restriction fragment length polymorphism profiling. J Clin Microbiol. 2003;41(8):3548–58.
218. Cai Y, Chai D, Wang R, Bai N, Liang B-B, Liu Y. Effectiveness and safety of macrolides in cystic fibrosis patients: a meta-analysis and systematic review. J Antimicrob Chemother. 2011;66(5):968–78.
219. Stokholm J, Chawes BL, Vissing NH, Bjarnadóttir E, Pedersen TM, Vinding RK, et al. Azithromycin for episodes with asthma-like symptoms in young children aged 1-3 years: a randomised, double-blind, placebo-controlled trial. Lancet Respir Med. 2016;4(1):19–26.
220. Thorsen J, Stokholm J, Rasmussen MA, Mortensen MS, Brejnrod AD, Hjelmsø M, et al. The airway microbiota modulates effect of azithromycin treatment for episodes of recurrent asthma-like symptoms in preschool children: a randomized clinical trial. Am J Respir Crit Care Med. 2021;204(2):149–58.
221. Magaret AS, Salerno J, Deen JF, Kloster M, Mayer-Hamblett N, Ramsey BW, et al. Long-term azithromycin use is not associated with QT prolongation in children with cystic fibrosis. J Cyst Fibros. 2021;20(2):e16–e8.
222. Ikeda AK, Prince AA, Chen JX, Lieu JEC, Shin JJ. Macrolide-associated sensorineural hearing loss: a systematic review. Laryngoscope. 2018;128(1):228–36.
223. Vanoverschelde A, Oosterloo BC, Ly NF, Ikram MA, Goedegebure A, Stricker BH, et al. Macrolide-associated ototoxicity: a cross-sectional and longitudinal study to assess the association of macrolide use with tinnitus and hearing loss. J Antimicrob Chemother. 2021;76(10): 2708–16.
224. Zettner EM, Gleser MA. Progressive hearing loss among patients with cystic fibrosis and parenteral aminoglycoside treatment. Otolaryngol Head Neck Surg. 2018;159(5):887–94.
225. Cheng AG, Johnston PR, Luz J, Uluer A, Fligor B, Licameli GR, et al. Sensorineural hearing loss in patients with cystic fibrosis. Otolaryngol Head Neck Surg. 2009;141(1):86–90.
226. Balfour-Lynn IM, King JA. CFTR modulator therapies - effect on life expectancy in people with cystic fibrosis. Paediatr Respir Rev. 2022;42:3–8.
227. Lopes-Pacheco M. CFTR modulators: the changing face of cystic fibrosis in the era of precision medicine. Front Pharmacol. 2019;10:1662.
228. Rubinstein E. Comparative safety of the different macrolides. Int J Antimicrob Agents. 2001;18:71–6.
229. Akkerman-Nijland AM, Möhlmann JE, Akkerman OW, Vd Vaart H, Majoor CJ, Rottier BL, et al. The long-term safety of chronic azithromycin use in adult patients with cystic fibrosis, evaluating biomarkers for renal function, hepatic function and electrical properties of the heart. Expert Opin Drug Saf. 2021;20(8):959–63.
230. Abotsi RE, Nicol MP, McHugh G, Simms V, Rehman AM, Barthus C, et al. The impact of long-term azithromycin on antibiotic resistance in HIV-associated chronic lung disease. ERJ Open Res. 2022;8(1)
231. Phaff SJ, Tiddens HA, Verbrugh HA, Ott A. Macrolide resistance of Staphylococcus aureus and Haemophilus species associated with long-term azithromycin use in cystic fibrosis. J Antimicrob Chemother. 2006;57(4):741–6.
232. Stutman HR, Lieberman JM, Nussbaum E, Marks MI. Antibiotic prophylaxis in infants and young children with cystic fibrosis: a randomized controlled trial. J Pediatr. 2002;140(3): 299–305.
233. Smyth AR, Rosenfeld M. Prophylactic anti-staphylococcal antibiotics for cystic fibrosis. Cochrane Database Syst Rev. 2017;4(4):Cd001912.

234. Shaw LP, Doyle RM, Kavaliunaite E, Spencer H, Balloux F, Dixon G, et al. Children with cystic fibrosis are infected with multiple subpopulations of Mycobacterium abscessus with different antimicrobial resistance profiles. Clin Infect Dis. 2019;69(10):1678–86.
235. Degiacomi G, Sammartino JC, Chiarelli LR, Riabova O, Makarov V, Pasca MR. Mycobacterium abscessus, an emerging and worrisome pathogen among cystic fibrosis patients. Int J Mol Sci. 2019;20(23)
236. Richard M, Gutiérrez AV, Kremer L. Dissecting erm(41)-mediated macrolide-inducible resistance in Mycobacterium abscessus. Antimicrob Agents Chemother. 2020;64(2)
237. Ramsey BW, Pepe MS, Quan JM, Otto KL, Montgomery AB, Williams-Warren J, et al. Intermittent administration of inhaled tobramycin in patients with cystic fibrosis. Cystic fibrosis inhaled Tobramycin Study Group. N Engl J Med. 1999;340(1):23–30.
238. Smith S, Rowbotham NJ, Charbek E. Inhaled antibiotics for pulmonary exacerbations in cystic fibrosis. Cochrane Database Syst Rev. 2022;8(8):Cd008319.
239. Nichols DP, Caceres S, Caverly L, Fratelli C, Kim SH, Malcolm K, et al. Effects of azithromycin in Pseudomonas aeruginosa burn wound infection. J Surg Res. 2013;183(2): 767–76.
240. Nick JA, Moskowitz SM, Chmiel JF, Forssén AV, Kim SH, Saavedra MT, et al. Azithromycin may antagonize inhaled tobramycin when targeting Pseudomonas aeruginosa in cystic fibrosis. Ann Am Thorac Soc. 2014;11(3):342–50.
241. Cogen JD, Faino AV, Onchiri F, Gibson RL, Hoffman LR, Kronman MP, et al. Effect of concomitant azithromycin and tobramycin use on cystic fibrosis pulmonary exacerbation treatment. Ann Am Thorac Soc. 2021;18(2):266–72.
242. Nichols DP, Singh PK, Baines A, Caverly LJ, Chmiel JF, Gibson RL, et al. Testing the effects of combining azithromycin with inhaled tobramycin for P. aeruginosa in cystic fibrosis: a randomised, controlled clinical trial. Thorax. 2022;77(6):581–8.
243. Somayaji R, Russell R, Cogen JD, Goss CH, Nick SE, Saavedra MT, et al. Oral azithromycin use and the recovery of lung function from pulmonary exacerbations treated with intravenous tobramycin or Colistimethate in adults with cystic fibrosis. Ann Am Thorac Soc. 2019;16(7): 853–60.
244. Ramsey BW, Davies J, McElvaney NG, Tullis E, Bell SC, Dřevínek P, et al. A CFTR potentiator in patients with cystic fibrosis and the G551D mutation. N Engl J Med. 2011;365(18):1663–72.
245. van der Meer R, Wilms EB, Heijerman HGM. CFTR modulators: does one dose fit all? J Pers Med. [Internet]. 2021;11(6):458.
246. Porter JD, Watson J, Roberts LR, Gill SK, Groves H, Dhariwal J, et al. Identification of novel macrolides with antibacterial, anti-inflammatory and type I and III IFN-augmenting activity in airway epithelium. J Antimicrob Chemother. 2016;71(10):2767–81.

Non-CF Bronchiectasis

Dustin Mills, Anne B. Chang, and Julie M. Marchant

Abstract Bronchiectasis is a disease of recurrent wet cough and acute respiratory exacerbations with objective confirmation by abnormal bronchial dilatation on chest computed tomography scans. There is strong evidence that macrolide maintenance therapy reduces the frequency of respiratory exacerbations in both children and adults. This chapter will focus on the clinical use of macrolides in bronchiectasis in both adults and children, in relation to current guidelines, evidence and key recommendations, as well as exploring risks of long-term therapy and future research priorities.

Keywords Macrolides · Bronchiectasis · Azithromycin · Maintenance antibiotics

D. Mills (✉)
Department of Respiratory and Sleep Medicine, Children's Hospital, Brisbane, QLD, Australia

School of Medicine, The University of Queensland, Brisbane, QLD, Australia
e-mail: Dustin.Mills@health.qld.gov.au

A. B. Chang
Department of Respiratory and Sleep Medicine, Children's Hospital, Brisbane, QLD, Australia

Australian Centre for Health Services Innovation, Queensland University of Technology, Brisbane, QLD, Australia

Child Health Division, Menzies School of Health Research, Darwin City, NT, Australia

J. M. Marchant
Department of Respiratory and Sleep Medicine, Children's Hospital, Brisbane, QLD, Australia

School of Medicine, The University of Queensland, Brisbane, QLD, Australia

Australian Centre for Health Services Innovation, Queensland University of Technology, Brisbane, QLD, Australia

B. K. Rubin, M. Shinkai (eds.), *Macrolides as Immunomodulatory Agents*, Progress in Inflammation Research 92, https://doi.org/10.1007/978-3-031-42859-3_5

1 Introduction

Bronchiectasis, unrelated to cystic fibrosis (hereafter referred to as *bronchiectasis*), is a clinical syndrome of recurrent or persistent wet/productive cough, respiratory exacerbations and abnormal bronchial dilatation on chest computed tomography (CT) scans [1–5]. Bronchiectasis is an increasingly appreciated cause of chronic respiratory–related morbidity worldwide in both adults and children [4, 6–15]. Bronchiectasis is associated with numerous aetiologies that can contribute to the pathophysiologic process [4, 6, 16]. There are various radiological, microbiological, inflammatory and clinical subgroups referred to as phenotypes and endotypes [4, 5, 17]. The pathogenesis of bronchiectasis is complex and is likely to vary depending on the underlying aetiology, patient age and important modifying factors [4, 7, 18–20]. Most evidence supports the "vicious cycle" paradigm, which involves airway infection causing inflammation, impaired mucociliary clearance, obstructive lung disease and lung tissue disruption resulting in a self-perpetuating cycle with a dysregulated immune response [4, 6, 17–20]. (see Fig. 1).

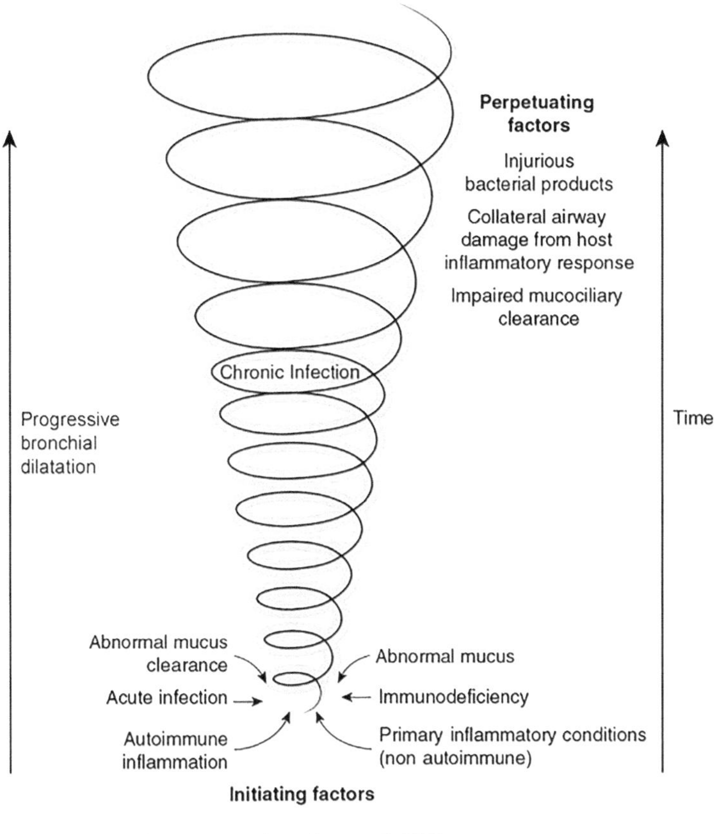

Fig. 1 Vicious vortex of bronchiectasis pathogenesis [19]

Neutrophilic airway infiltration and dysfunction is typically described in bronchiectasis and is observed in stable bronchiectasis in adults with increases during lower airway bacterial infection and exacerbations [21–26]. Less commonly, eosinophilic dominant airway inflammation has also been identified [4, 7]. Neutrophil elastase (NE), a serine protease stored in neutrophil granules and released into neutrophil extracellular traps (NETs) or at times of apoptosis, has been found to increase in quantity during exacerbations of bronchiectasis and decrease after treatment with resolution of symptoms [27–30]. NE impairs ciliary motility and stimulates mucus secretion. Progressive destruction of the elastic, cartilaginous and muscular components of the bronchial wall may be in part related to NE activity [19].

Bacteria, mycobacteria, viruses, and fungi have all been proposed to promote the initiation and perpetuation of bronchiectasis [7]. High bacterial density in the lower airways is associated with more severe and more frequent symptoms, exacerbation frequency, and inflammatory indices [7, 22]. Bronchiectasis patients at greatest risk of acute respiratory exacerbations and lung function decline have reduced lower airway bacterial diversity (i.e., through the loss of important bacterial taxa) or dominance of a single taxon or small group of taxa [31, 32].

Acute respiratory exacerbations in bronchiectasis are characterised by increase in respiratory symptoms, [1, 33] and are particularly important, sustaining the vicious vortex of bronchiectasis and acting as a catalyst for disease progression [34–36]. Bronchiectasis respiratory exacerbations are major determinants of healthcare costs, [37–39] and are associated with worse clinical outcomes; [1–3] impaired quality of life, [40–43] accelerated lung function decline, [44] and in adult studies, increased mortality [2, 35, 45]. In addition, parents of children and patients with bronchiectasis rate exacerbations as one of the most challenging aspects [46]. Thus, impact on acute respiratory exacerbations is a significant outcome measure when assessing efficacy of interventions. Understanding of the pathophysiology of pulmonary exacerbations in bronchiectasis is limited but evolving, with current evidence suggesting respiratory viruses play an initiating role in some but not all exacerbations [47–50].

There is a large variation in prognosis in bronchiectasis, some patients having mild bronchiectasis for many years and others progressing rapidly with frequent exacerbations and accelerated lung function decline [4, 6, 51–53]. An important clinical phenotype of bronchiectasis in adults is the "frequent exacerbator" ($\geq$3 exacerbations/year) as it is the strongest predictor of future exacerbations and is associated with increased 5-year mortality [41]. A paediatric frequent exacerbator phenotype has also been described [54]. Importantly, it has also been shown that bronchiectasis may be reversible, in both children and adults, if treated effectively and early [1, 2, 55–59]. Bronchiectasis management should be focused on interrupting the infection—inflammatory cycle as early as possible to reverse and/or halt disease progression and further lung injury. Clinical outcomes are best optimised through a multi-modality approach involving not only antimicrobial therapies but also airway clearance therapies and anti-inflammatory agents, as well as avoiding lung irritants [1–3, 60, 61].

Antibiotics have a central role in the management of patients with bronchiectasis. Antibiotics aim to reduce airway bacterial loads, [4, 27, 62] thereby interrupting the cycle of infection and inflammation. Antibiotics can be prescribed to prevent and treat acute exacerbations, and to eradicate potentially harmful organisms such as *Pseudomonas aeruginosa* [1–3, 61]. Long-term use of antibiotics (>3 months) is recommended for bronchiectasis patients experiencing frequent exacerbations of more than three per year and could be considered in patients that have infrequent but severe exacerbations, symptoms between exacerbations, radiographic progression of disease or who are at risk of severe exacerbations (e.g. immunocompromised) [1–3, 61]. Three broad approaches are available: macrolides, other oral antibiotics and inhaled antibiotics. Before considering long-term antibiotics it is important to ensure that all other areas of bronchiectasis management have been optimised including addressing underlying conditions and comorbidities that could result in a deterioration of the patients' symptoms [1–3, 61].

2 The History of Macrolide Antibiotic Use in Bronchiectasis

The first published randomised controlled trial (RCT) on using macrolides in bronchiectasis was a double-blind, parallel design study involving 25 children with bronchiectasis and increased airway responsiveness, randomised to 12 weeks of treatment with roxithromycin or placebo [63]. The RCT found a significant reduction in bronchial responsiveness, sputum purulence and leucocyte count as a result of treatment with roxithromycin [63]. While several prior observational studies using macrolides were published in the 1950–60's in adults, the first published adult RCT was the EMBRACE study [64]. Since these first reported RCTs, macrolide antibiotics are now commonly used as long-term treatments to prevent exacerbations in bronchiectasis. Adult data from international bronchiectasis studies and bronchiectasis registries suggests moderate use of long-term azithromycin, generally ranging from 15–30% of patients [65–68]. There is limited data on the prevalence of azithromycin use in paediatric bronchiectasis, with one report on children from the Australian Bronchiectasis Registry in 2021 indicating 47% of patients had 'ever received a macrolide antibiotic' as part of their bronchiectasis management [54].

3 Mechanism of Action of Macrolide Antibiotics in Bronchiectasis

The mechanisms of the action of macrolides are described in Sect. 1 of this book. With respect to its use in people with bronchiectasis, there are numerous possible mechanisms to explain how macrolides may influence bronchiectasis pathophysiology at both the host, and bacterial level. Macrolide antibiotics have well-characterised bacteriostatic activity against a broad range of gram-positive and negative lung pathogens associated with bronchiectasis. Research in the context of inflammatory lung disease has revealed that they also have significant immunomodulatory properties affecting both innate and adaptive immune processes, and both acute and chronic dysregulated airway inflammatory processes, making them an attractive option to interrupt the vicious vortex of bronchiectasis [69–72]. These include mucus-modulating and anti-secretory effects with enhanced mucociliary clearance and lower airway epithelial cell barrier function [69–72]. Azithromycin has also been found to inhibit microbial virulence factors and disrupts microbial quorum sensing and biofilm production [69]. In addition, macrolides have significant anti-viral properties [73].

However, it remains unclear as to which of its properties has the most important effect [74]. The efficacy of azithromycin demonstrated in bronchiectasis patients infected with macrolide-tolerant organisms such as *Pseudomonas aeruginosa* supports the concept that their efficacy is at least partly related to immunomodulatory rather than antibacterial effects [75]. Authors have suggested that the immune modulation provided by macrolides is most accurately viewed as an interplay between improved host response to infection, dampening of dysregulated inflammation and the targeted elimination of several relevant and susceptible airway pathogens and that macrolide-resistant pathogens (e.g. *Pseudomonas aeruginosa*) may be more sensitive in the context of the lung in vivo and associated high tissue drug levels [69, 76].

Further studies of macrolides in patients with bronchiectasis have suggested their mechanism of action includes:

- Low-dose clarithromycin reduces Th17 cell responses [77]
- Long-term roxithromycin reduces airway inflammation, via measuring markers such as Interleukin-8 (IL-8), neutrophil elastase and matrix metalloproteinase-9 [78]
- Erythromycin inhibits of *Pseudomonas aeruginosa* quorum sensing [79]
- Inhibition of the production of the mucus protein MUC5AC in the airway mucosa [80]
- Reduction in sputum neutrophil extracellular traps [81]

4 Recommendations for Long-Term Macrolide Therapy in Bronchiectasis

Several randomised controlled trials have investigated long-term macrolide use in bronchiectasis in both adults [64, 82, 83] and children [84]. These trials were for varying duration (6–24 months), used different types of macrolides (roxithromycin, erythromycin, azithromycin) and different doses and regimes. Yet, all consistently showed a significant reduction in exacerbation frequency when macrolides were used compared to placebo. Whether macrolides are more effective than inhaled long-term therapy for the reduction of exacerbations in bronchiectasis remains unknown in the absence of studies directly comparing oral versus inhaled antibiotics [85].

Eight independently performed systematic reviews and meta-analyses, including these trials, have been completed and confirmed significant reductions in exacerbation frequency with long-term macrolide therapy [86–93].

Hence unsurprisingly, all recent international bronchiectasis guidelines recommend using long-term macrolides for adults and children with three or more respiratory exacerbations in a 12-month period (see Table 1).

Azithromycin is the preferred macrolide in bronchiectasis as most of the supportive data are with this drug. Azithromycin has good oral bioavailability, excellent tissue penetration, prolonged tissue persistence allowing once daily or even one to three times weekly dosing, and favourable side effect profile when administered orally [94–100].

As these systematic reviews and meta-analyses have variably included adult and paediatric data, there is a heterogeneity in analysed studies including in participants' age, aetiology of bronchiectasis as well as macrolide dose and duration of therapy. We will therefore further explore clinical evidence for macrolide use in paediatrics and adults separately below.

4.1 Paediatric Evidence on Long-Term Macrolides in Bronchiectasis Management

While prior guidelines existed, [101] the first global paediatric-specific bronchiectasis management guidelines published by European Respiratory Society in 2021, [1] advises long-term macrolide antibiotics in individuals with recurrent exacerbations (>1 hospitalised or $\geq$ 3 non-hospitalised exacerbations in the previous 12-months). The guidelines recommend a macrolide course for a minimum of 6 months with ongoing evaluation for risk versus benefit, particularly if prescribed for >24-months [1]. Indeed the inflammatory damage may be more important in the developing lung than the matured lung [102].

This guideline recommendation is based on data from three RCTs evaluating long-term macrolide treatment in bronchiectasis specifically in children and adolescents [63, 84, 103]. Two of these RCTs have compared long-term macrolide therapy to placebo with the number of respiratory exacerbations as outcomes. The combined data showed that macrolides reduced the number of individuals experiencing any exacerbations during the trial period (RR 0.86, 95%CI 0.75–0.99) [1].

The largest of these RCTs, described that using long-term azithromycin halves the frequency of exacerbations (incidence rate ratio [IRR] 0.5, 95%CI 0.35–0.70) and also likely reduces hospitalisation (p = 0.06) [84]. This was an international multicentre study which included 89 indigenous children from Australia and New Zealand who were randomised to receive once-weekly azithromycin (30 mg/

Table 1 Recommendations for the use of macrolide therapy in bronchiectasis guidelines

Guideline	Recommendation	Dosage	Duration
European Respiratory Society guidelines for the management of children and adolescents with bronchiectasis, 2021. [1]	Children/adolescents with bronchiectasis and recurrent exacerbations (≥3 non-hospitalised or > 1 hospitalised exacerbations in the previous 12 months)—recommend treatment with long-term macrolide antibiotics to reduce exacerbations (strong recommendation, low-quality of evidence)	Not specified	Course should be for at least 6-months with regular reassessment to determine whether the antibiotic continues to provide a clinical benefit Children/adolescents receiving longer treatment courses (>24-months) should continue to be evaluated for risk versus benefit
European Respiratory Society guidelines for the management of adult bronchiectasis, 2017 [2]	Long-term macrolide (azithromycin, erythromycin) treatment for adults with bronchiectasis who have 3 or more exacerbations per year[a] Not infected with P. aeruginosa (conditional recommendation, moderate quality evidence) Chronic P. aeruginosa infection: Where an inhaled antibiotic is contraindicated, not tolerated, not feasible or high exacerbation frequency despite using an inhaled antibiotic. (conditional recommendation, low-quality evidence)	Not specified Doses used in clinical trials/clinical practice range from 250 mg azithromycin daily, 500 mg or 250 mg three times per week	Not specified Azithromycin duration used in RCT ranged from 6–12 months.
British Thoracic Society guideline for bronchiectasis in adults, 2019 [3]	Long-term macrolide (azithromycin, erythromycin) treatment for adults with bronchiectasis who have 3 or more exacerbations per year[a] Not infected with P. aeruginosa (grade A evidence)	Azithromycin 250 mg three times per week starting dose which can then be increased according to clinical response and adverse events	Not specified Azithromycin duration used in RCT ranged from 6–12 months.

(continued)

Table 1 (continued)

Guideline	Recommendation	Dosage	Duration
	Chronic P. aeruginosa infection: Consider azithromycin or erythromycin as an alternative (e.g., if a patient does not tolerate inhaled antibiotics) (grade B evidence) OR as an additive treatment to an inhaled antibiotic in patients with high exacerbation frequency despite using an inhaled antibiotic. (grade D evidence)		
British Thoracic Society guideline for the use of long-term macrolides in adults with respiratory disease, 2020. [61]	Long-term macrolide treatment could be offered to reduce bronchiectasis exacerbations in those with high exacerbation rate (i.e., 3 or more per year) (strong recommendation)	Dosing regimens with greatest supportive evidence: Azithromycin 500 mg three times per week, azithromycin 250 mg daily and erythromycin 400 mg twice daily starting dose azithromycin 250 mg three times weekly could be considered to minimise adverse effects with subsequent titration according to clinical response.	Therapy should be offered for minimum of 6 months

[a]This threshold may be reduced for adult patients with; a history of severe exacerbation, relevant comorbidities such as immunodeficiency, or those with more severe bronchiectasis

kg) or placebo for up to 24 months. Additional findings included improved mean weight for age z-scores (1.03 vs 0.20; $p = 0.003$) and lower carriage of *H. influenzae* (7 vs 38%, $p = 0.002$) and *M. catarrhalis* (0 vs 24%) at the end of the study. Of note, the azithromycin group developed significantly higher nasal carriage of azithromycin-resistant bacteria (19 of 41, 46%) than those receiving placebo (four of 37, 11%; $p = 0{\cdot}002$), the clinical significance of this being unknown. Adherence was found to be important for efficacy as well as reducing antibiotic resistance. Adherence ≥70% (versus <70%) in the Australian azithromycin group was associated with lower carriage of any pathogen [OR 0.19, 95%CI 0.07–0.53] and fewer macrolide-resistant pathogens (OR 0.34, 95%CI 0.14–0.81). Azithromycin was well tolerated in this study, with no serious adverse events being attributed to the intervention [84].

The ERS guidelines, [1] explained that although the overall quality of evidence was low for long-term macrolide therapy in children, their strong recommendation is from the large effect found on reduction of exacerbations, the panel's clinical experience, consistency of effect with adult based RCTs, well tolerated therapy and preventing exacerbations being key in bronchiectasis management [1].

The most recent paediatric systematic review [93] included 4 RCTs on long-term macrolide treatment for bronchiectasis in children and described a significant decrease in the frequency of exacerbation (OR 0.30; 95%CI 0.10, 0.87), mean number of exacerbations per patient (mean difference, − 1.40; 95%CI − 2.26, − 0.54), and sputum purulence score (mean difference, − 0.78; 95%CI − 1.32, − 0.24). However, long-term macrolide treatment was accompanied by an increased carriage of azithromycin-resistant bacteria (OR 7.13) [93].

4.2 Adult Evidence on Long-Term Macrolides in Bronchiectasis Management

Three RCTs investigating long-term macrolide therapy in adults with bronchiectasis, [64, 82, 83] provided strong evidence on the efficacy of macrolides in reducing respiratory exacerbations frequency, approximately halving the exacerbation rate. In all three studies, a significant increase in macrolide-resistant respiratory pathogens was observed [104].

The EMBRACE study (Effectiveness of Macrolides in patients with Bronchiectasis using Azithromycin to Control Exacerbations) [64] examined 141 patients with at least one exacerbation of bronchiectasis in the prior year who were randomly assigned to take azithromycin 500 mg or placebo, orally three times a week for 6 months. Azithromycin was associated with a decrease in exacerbations compared with placebo (0.59 per patient with azithromycin and 1.57 per patient with placebo, respectively; RR 0.38, 95%CI 0.26–0.54). However, no significant difference was noted in lung function or quality of life [64].

The BAT study (Bronchiectasis and Long-term Azithromycin Treatment), [82] examined 83 patients and included more severely affected patients with at least three pulmonary exacerbations requiring antibiotics and one sputum culture yielding one or more bacterial respiratory pathogens in the year prior to study entry. Azithromycin was given for 12 months at a daily dose of 250 mg significantly reduced the number of exacerbations compared with placebo with a median of 0 versus 2 during treatment. The number of patients with at least one exacerbation during the study was 80% in the placebo group and 46.5% in the azithromycin group, corresponding to an absolute risk reduction of 33.5% (95%CI 14.1–52.9). There was also and longer time to the next exacerbation in the azithromycin group (HR 0.29; 95%CI 0.16, 0.51). Moreover, a significant increase in the forced expiratory volume in 1 second (FEV_1), as well as an improvement in the quality of life, was noted in the treated group [82].

The BLESS study (Bronchiectasis and Low-dose Erythromycin Study), [83] included patients with a history of daily sputum production and two or more infectious exacerbations in the year prior to study entry. There were 117 patients randomly assigned to take erythromycin 400 mg or placebo twice daily for 1 year. The treated group had a modest reduction in exacerbations (mean 1.29 versus 1.97 per patient per year; IRR 0.57, 95%CI 0.42–0.77). The volume of sputum produced and rate of decline in FEV_1 was also decreased, although the clinical importance of these changes appears small [83].

Two of the adult bronchiectasis RCTs later assessed the effects of long-term macrolides on structural lung disease in [105, 106]. They described significant improvement in the structural changes on repeat CT chest scores, mucus plugging and peri bronchial thickening after starting macrolide therapy. However, larger prospective studies are required to confirm the nature, extent and time course of these findings.

A systematic review [107] of the main three RCTs suggested that long-term macrolide therapy is highly effective in reducing the frequency of exacerbations (adjusted IRR 0.49; 95%CI 0.36–0.66). Macrolide treatment improved the time to first exacerbation (adjusted hazard ratio 0·46, 95%CI 0·34 to 0·61; $p < 0{\cdot}0001$). Macrolides were not associated with a significant improvement in FEV_1 (67 mL at 1 year, 95%CI 22 to 112; $p = 0{\cdot}14$). Although the improvement in quality of life measured by the St George respiratory questionnaire (SGRQ) did not exceed the minimum clinically important difference, the proportion of patients who achieved a clinically meaningful improvement in quality of life was increased in the macrolide group compared with the placebo group. Importantly, a reduction in the frequency of exacerbations was evident across all patient subgroups, including a high level of benefit in patients with *P aeruginosa* infection (IRR 0·36, 95%CI 0·18–0·72) and, interestingly, in patients with one to two exacerbations per year (IRR 0·37, 95%CI 0·16–0·88). There was a trend toward decreased quality of life in younger patients (<50 years) and in those with non-frequent exacerbations (one to two per year), which may reflect the increased number of side effects in these particular subgroups [107].

A latter meta-analysis [92] performed a subgroup analysis of the number of patients free from exacerbations and described that azithromycin was superior (RR 2.25, 95%CI 1.67–3.02) compared to erythromycin (RR 1.33, 95%CI 0.92–1.94) and roxithromycin (RR 1.14, 95%CI 0.97–1.35). In the British Thoracic Society guideline [61] their evidence summary was:

- Long-term macrolide treatment reduces exacerbations in bronchiectasis (High).
- There is evidence of an improvement in QoL as measured by SGRQ when azithromycin 250 mg daily is used for 1 year (High).
- The studies with the greatest evidence for reducing exacerbations used therapy for a minimum of 6 months (High).
- Long-term macrolide therapy is not associated with improved exercise capacity.

(High)
- Long-term macrolide therapy may reduce sputum volume and weight (Moderate).
- Long-term macrolide therapy is associated with diarrhoea and abdominal pain (High).
- Long-term macrolide usage can result in increased antimicrobial resistance (High) It is unknown if this has a clinical impact [61].

In addition to the studies targeting all-cause bronchiectasis (other than CF), other disease-specific RCTs have also been published. A European multicentre, double-blind, RCT (BESTCILIA), [108] involving children and adults with primary ciliary dyskinesia (PCD) found that 6 months of azithromycin (versus placebo) significantly reduced exacerbation rates (rate ratio 0.45, 95%CI 0.26–0.78). Limitations of this study was that no definition of exacerbations in PCD was available, and the number of participants with HRCT-defined bronchiectasis was not defined [108].

A double-blind RCT on long-term azithromycin in adults with primary antibody deficiencies and previous respiratory exacerbations (85% had HRCT-confirmed bronchiectasis), [109] found similar results to the aforementioned adult bronchiectasis studies. The number of exacerbations was 3.6 (95%CI 2.5–4.7) per patient-year in the azithromycin arm and 5.2 (95%CI 4.1–6.4) per patient-year in the placebo arm ($p = 0.02$). The rate of additional antibiotic treatment per patient-year was 2.3 (95% CI 2.1–3.4) in the intervention group and 3.6 (95%CI 2.9–4.3) in the placebo group ($p = 0.004$) [109].

5 Recommended Macrolide Dosage and Duration in Bronchiectasis

As most studies in both adults and children have used azithromycin as macrolide of choice, optimal dosage and duration of long-term azithromycin in bronchiectasis will be covered below.

The optimal dosage and duration of long-term azithromycin in bronchiectasis have not been elucidated in adult or paediatric populations [1]. The largest paediatric trial used azithromycin 30 mg/kg once weekly (up to 1500 mg/week), [84] although the typically recommended dosing is 10 mg/kg three times a week [110]. The largest adult trials used azithromycin 250 mg once daily or 500 mg three times weekly [64, 82]. Internationally, the most recommended adult dosing is azithromycin 250 mg or 500 mg three times per week [2, 3, 61].

Based on the available evidence, long-term azithromycin in bronchiectasis, if commenced, should be given for a minimum of 6 months [1–3, 61]. Pragmatically if there is a seasonal approach to the exacerbation frequency, dosing may be limited to the months of the year where exacerbations have been most frequent.

The long half-life of azithromycin allows some flexibility in dosage regimen [4, 74, 99, 100]; hence a dose and regimen within the parameters of the aforementioned clinical trials that is individualised to patient tolerance (particularly gastrointestinal tolerance) and which optimises adherence is preferred. It is particularly important in the knowledge that adherence greater than 70% has been associated with statistically significantly lower carriage of respiratory bacterial pathogens and macrolide-resistant organisms [84].

6 Cost-Effectiveness of Azithromycin in Bronchiectasis

There are currently no cost-effectiveness studies on long-term azithromycin in bronchiectasis [1]. An Australian study, [38] based in a tertiary paediatric hospital, reported that each hospitalised exacerbation cost the health sector in 2016 ~ $AUD31,000 and the patient's parents ~$AUD2,700, indicating large costs associated with hospitalised exacerbations. Therefore, in bronchiectasis patients with recurrent exacerbations, the clear reduction in exacerbations provided by long-term azithromycin therapy (a relatively inexpensive drug) supports the likely cost-effectiveness of long-term azithromycin in bronchiectasis patients with frequent exacerbations. However, with a paucity of studies further research is needed to show cost-effectiveness of maintenance macrolide therapy in bronchiectasis.

7 Safety and Adverse Effects of Long-Term Azithromycin

Long-term azithromycin is generally well tolerated, with discontinuation secondary to adverse effects uncommon in bronchiectasis clinical trials [61, 91]. In a recent meta-analysis, results also showed no higher risk of adverse events (RR 0.98, 95%CI 0.85–1.13), even a lower risk of severe adverse events (RR 0.53, 95%CI 0.33–0.85). However, considerations in prescribing macrolides are that a substantial number of patients will develop gastrointestinal adverse effects, which are likely dose related. Meta-analysis of pooled data shows high-quality evidence for diarrhoea being an adverse event associated with long-term macrolide use. The frequency of patients suffering diarrhoea was 19.3%–20.6% in the treatment groups compared with 4.1%–4.5% in the placebo groups. There was also high-level evidence for abdominal pain/discomfort in meta-analysis data (OR 6.97) [92].

In addition, a higher risk of macrolide resistance respiratory pathogens on oropharyngeal or sputum cultures (RR 3.59, 95%CI 2.6–4.96) was observed [61, 92, 111]. Azithromycin has, compared with other macrolides, significant periods of concentrations below the minimum inhibitory concentration, which likely affects their resistance rates [112]. Currently, there is no evidence that this resistance impacts clinical outcomes, however, this finding does present potential concerns and further studies are needed to evaluate the effect of macrolides on lung microbiome [113].

International guidelines recommend that non-tuberculous mycobacteria (NTM) are excluded from respiratory specimens where possible before commencing long-term azithromycin [1–3, 61]. It is still not clear if chronic macrolide therapy predisposes to NTM infection in individuals with bronchiectasis. There is in vitro evidence that azithromycin can impair autophagic and phagosomal macrophage degradation of NTM [114] and monotherapy with macrolides may increase rates of macrolide-resistant NTM [115].

A further caution is the increased risk of macrolide therapy when prescribed for any indication to cause hepatotoxicity, ototoxicity cardiac arrhythmias (ventricular arrhythmias, torsade des pointes and prolonged QT) and sudden cardiac death [115]. These adverse effects have largely been described in the elderly and those with severe disease, significant other comorbidities and in combination with other QT-prolonging medication [116, 117] and have only rarely been described in adult bronchiectasis studies [118]. However, adult guidelines [61] advise that for safety purposes, an ECG should be performed prior to initiation of macrolide therapy to assess QTc interval and baseline liver function tests. The magnitude of QTc prolongation with azithromycin appears to be less in children [110, 119], and therefore child bronchiectasis management guidelines [1] advise that an ECG is not routinely required before commencing macrolides; however, it should be obtained if there are risk factors (family history of prolonged QT syndrome, arrythmias and acute cardiac events) or indeed other QT-prolonging medications are used.

8 Azithromycin as Acute Management for Acute Respiratory Exacerbations in Bronchiectasis

Antibiotic treatment for acute exacerbations of bronchiectasis is considered standard of care in both adult and child guidelines [1–3, 61] and supported by a high-quality placebo-controlled RCT in children/adolescents [1]. The method of administration (oral, inhaled, or intravenous) depends on the severity of exacerbation. The antibiotic should be selected based on the individual's lower airway microbiology and sensitivities from the most recent sputum or other lower airway specimen culture [1–3, 61].

A recently completed [120] a three-arm, double-dummy, placebo RCT trial of amoxicillin-clavulanate or azithromycin versus placebo in bronchiectasis exacerbations in children found that amoxicillin-clavulanate was superior to placebo at resolving symptoms after 14-days treatment (relative risk for resolution (RR) 1.50, 95%CI 1.08–2.09). Azithromycin was associated with improvement (RR 1.41, 95% CI 1.01–1.97) but did not reach a priori-defined statistical significance of superiority threshold of $p < 0{\cdot}0245$. An earlier RCT, [121] comparing amoxicillin-clavulanate to azithromycin for treating non-severe bronchiectasis exacerbations in children found that by day 21 azithromycin was non-inferior to amoxicillin-clavulanate (within 20% margin). However, symptom resolution in those receiving azithromycin took a median of 4 days longer than those receiving amoxicillin-clavulanate, a statistical and clinically significant result. Therefore, evidence still suggests amoxicillin-clavulanate as the first-line choice for oral antibiotics for an acute respiratory exacerbation, although azithromycin could be considered in particular circumstances of genuine penicillin allergy or the need for directly observed daily therapy [120–122].

No comparable placebo controlled RCTs comparing azithromycin to other oral antibiotics for the management of exacerbations in adults currently exist.

9 Conclusion and Future Perspectives

Bronchiectasis is a heterogenous condition with a wide range of aetiologies and various clinical, microbiological, functional, and radiological features, which presents challenges in providing personalised treatment [6, 74, 123]. The mechanisms of action of macrolides as a maintenance treatment in bronchiectasis, are likely to include immunomodulatory, antiinflammatory and antimicrobial effects. Meta-analyses consistently report a clear beneficial effect of long-term macrolide therapy in bronchiectasis in reducing exacerbations, both in adult and child/adolescent patients. Azithromycin, in particular, has the strongest evidence on effect size, study participants and tolerance. The benefit of maintenance azithromycin on the reduction in number of respiratory exacerbations is significant, given the association of exacerbations with health care costs and clinical outcomes including impaired QoL, parental stress, accelerated lung function decline and in adult studies mortality [1–3, 61].

In each individual patient, the benefit should be balanced with adverse effects and macrolide resistance; for which the impact upon the host microbiome and population health remains uncertain.

Recently, a prospective study [110] indicated that only 31% of respondents (respiratory paediatricians in Australia and New Zealand) would commence azithromycin treatment for three or more pulmonary exacerbations in the preceding 12 months according to international guidelines, indicating the need for ongoing education.

Recognising different phenotypes and endotypes within bronchiectasis could help to decide which individuals would benefit from long-term azithromycin therapy [17, 18, 124]. For example, adults with bronchiectasis and frequent exacerbations ($\geq$3/year) constitute a prognostic group for poor outcomes which is associated with hospitalisation and mortality, and long-term macrolides should be considered for those patients [35, 41]. There is a clear need for large prospective RCTs in bronchiectasis powered for, and with clear exacerbation definitions which assess phenotypes and endotypes that are macrolide responsive.

Other key research priorities include defining the optimum azithromycin dose and duration for bronchiectasis treatment efficacy, continuous vs cyclical regimens, comparison studies of long-term macrolides to other antibiotics and in combination, and establishing the clinical significance of acquiring macrolide-resistant pathogens and effects on the lung microbiome [1, 6, 18, 46, 61, 74, 123–125].

Looking into the future the role of macrolide therapy, with better classification of bronchiectasis using genomics to define those with most benefit, and the development of new macrolides that have separate immunomodulatory actions to minimise the risk of antimicrobial resistance, hold promise [6, 18].

Finally, the timely administration of azithromycin in bronchiectasis, or its precursors of protracted bacterial bronchitis or chronic suppurative lung disease, may halt damage or even reverse existing structural lung damage [126]. Small studies in adult bronchiectasis suggest azithromycin may have a role in improving the structural lung damage associated with bronchiectasis [105, 106]. The role of macrolides in halting the progression of bronchiectasis and its precursors, and aiding in the reversal of structural lung damage warrants further exploration in the future.

Conflict of Interest All authors declare they have no conflict of interest.

Compliance with Ethical Standards This article does not contain any studies with human participants or animals performed by any of the authors.

References

1. Chang AB, Fortescue R, Grimwood K, Alexopoulou E, Bell L, Boyd J, et al. European Respiratory Society guidelines for the management of children and adolescents with bronchiectasis. Eur Respir J. 2021;58(2):2002990.
2. Polverino E, Goeminne PC, McDonnell MJ, Aliberti S, Marshall SE, Loebinger MR, et al. European Respiratory Society guidelines for the management of adult bronchiectasis. Eur Respir J. 2017;50(3):1700629.
3. Hill AT, Welham SA, Sullivan AL, Loebinger MR. Updated BTS adult bronchiectasis guideline 2018: a multidisciplinary approach to comprehensive care. Thorax. 2019;74(1):1–3.
4. Chang AB, Bush A, Grimwood K. Bronchiectasis in children: diagnosis and treatment. Lancet. 2018;392(10150):866–79.
5. Cohen R, Shteinberg M. Diagnosis and evaluation of bronchiectasis. Clin Chest Med. 2022;43 (1):7–22.
6. Chalmers JD, Chotirmall SH. Bronchiectasis: new therapies and new perspectives. Lancet Respir Med. 2018;6(9):715–26.
7. Chalmers JD, Chang AB, Chotirmall SH, Dhar R, McShane PJ. Bronchiectasis. Nat Rev Dis Primers. 2018;4(1):45.
8. Lin JL, Xu JF, Qu JM. Bronchiectasis in China. Ann Am Thorac Soc. 2016;13(5):609–16.
9. Quint JK, Millett ER, Joshi M, Navaratnam V, Thomas SL, Hurst JR, et al. Changes in the incidence, prevalence and mortality of bronchiectasis in the UK from 2004 to 2013: a population-based cohort study. Eur Respir J. 2016;47(1):186–93.
10. Weycker D, Hansen GL, Seifer FD. Prevalence and incidence of noncystic fibrosis bronchiectasis among US adults in 2013. Chron Respir Dis. 2017;14(4):377–84.
11. Aksamit TR, O'Donnell AE, Barker A, Olivier KN, Winthrop KL, Daniels MLA, et al. Bronchiectasis research registry consortium. Adult patients with bronchiectasis: a first look at the US bronchiectasis research registry. Chest. 2017;151(5):982–92.
12. Chandrasekaran R, Mac Aogáin M, Chalmers JD, Elborn SJ, Chotirmall SH. Geographic variation in the aetiology, epidemiology and microbiology of bronchiectasis. BMC Pulm Med. 2018;18(1):83.

13. Henkle E, Chan B, Curtis JR, Aksamit TR, Daley CL, Winthrop KL. Characteristics and health-care utilization history of patients with bronchiectasis in US Medicare enrollees with prescription drug plans, 2006 to 2014. Chest. 2018;154(6):1311–20.
14. Ringshausen FC, Rademacher J, Pink I, de Roux A, Hickstein L, Ploner T, et al. Increasing bronchiectasis prevalence in Germany, 2009-2017: a population-based cohort study. Eur Respir J. 2019;54(6):1900499.
15. Aliberti S, Sotgiu G, Lapi F, Gramegna A, Cricelli C, Blasi F. Prevalence and incidence of bronchiectasis in Italy. BMC Pulm Med. 2020;20(1):15.
16. Araújo D, Shteinberg M, Aliberti S, Goeminne PC, Hill AT, Fardon T, et al. Standardised classification of the aetiology of bronchiectasis using an objective algorithm. Eur Respir J. 2017;50(6):1701289.
17. Boaventura R, Sibila O, Agusti A, Chalmers JD. Treatable traits in bronchiectasis. Eur Respir J. 2018;52(3):1801269.
18. Flume PA, Chalmers JD, Olivier KN. Advances in bronchiectasis: endotyping, genetics, microbiome, and disease heterogeneity. Lancet. 2018;392(10150):880–90.
19. Metersky ML, Barker AF. The pathogenesis of bronchiectasis. Clin Chest Med. 2022;43(1): 35–46.
20. Shteinberg M, Flume PA, Chalmers JD. Is bronchiectasis really a disease? Eur Respir Rev. 2020;29(155):190051.
21. Angrill J, Agustí C, De Celis R, Filella X, Rañó A, Elena M, et al. Bronchial inflammation and colonization in patients with clinically stable bronchiectasis. Am J Respir Crit Care Med. 2001;164(9):1628–32.
22. Chalmers JD, Hill AT. Mechanisms of immune dysfunction and bacterial persistence in non-cystic fibrosis bronchiectasis. Mol Immunol. 2013;55(1):27–34.
23. Osika E, Cavaillon JM, Chadelat K, Boule M, Fitting C, Tournier G, Clement A. Distinct sputum cytokine profiles in cystic fibrosis and other chronic inflammatory airway disease. Eur Respir J. 1999;14(2):339–46.
24. Bedi P, Davidson DJ, McHugh BJ, Rossi AG, Hill AT. Blood neutrophils are reprogrammed in bronchiectasis. Am J Respir Crit Care Med. 2018;198(7):880–90.
25. Tsikrika S, Dimakou K, Papaioannou AI, Hillas G, Thanos L, Kostikas K, et al. The role of non-invasive modalities for assessing inflammation in patients with non-cystic fibrosis bronchiectasis. Cytokine. 2017;99:281–6.
26. Watt AP, Brown V, Courtney J, Kelly M, Garske L, Elborn JS, et al. Neutrophil apoptosis, proinflammatory mediators and cell counts in bronchiectasis. Thorax. 2004;59(3):231–6.
27. Chalmers JD, Smith MP, McHugh BJ, Doherty C, Govan JR, Hill AT. Short- and long-term antibiotic treatment reduces airway and systemic inflammation in non-cystic fibrosis bronchiectasis. Am J Respir Crit Care Med. 2012;186(7):657–65.
28. Chalmers JD, Haworth CS, Metersky ML, Loebinger MR, Blasi F, Sibila O, et al. Phase 2 trial of the DPP-1 inhibitor Brensocatib in bronchiectasis. N Engl J Med. 2020;383(22):2127–37.
29. Keir HR, Shoemark A, Dicker AJ, Perea L, Pollock J, Giam YH, et al. Neutrophil extracellular traps, disease severity, and antibiotic response in bronchiectasis: an international, observational, multicohort study. Lancet Respir Med. 2021;9(8):873–84.
30. Giam YH, Shoemark A, Chalmers JD. Neutrophil dysfunction in bronchiectasis: an emerging role for immunometabolism. Eur Respir J. 2021;58(2):2003157.
31. Mac Aogáin M, Narayana JK, Tiew PY, Ali NABM, Yong VFL, Jaggi TK, et al. Integrative microbiomics in bronchiectasis exacerbations. Nat Med. 2021;27(4):688–99.
32. Mac Aogáin M, Chotirmall SH. Microbiology and the microbiome in bronchiectasis. Clin Chest Med. 2022;43(1):23–34.
33. Hill AT, Haworth CS, Aliberti S, Barker A, Blasi F, Boersma W, et al. EMBARC/BRR definitions working group. Pulmonary exacerbation in adults with bronchiectasis: a consensus definition for clinical research. Eur Respir J. 2017;49(6):1700051.

34. Sheehan RE, Wells AU, Copley SJ, Desai SR, Howling SJ, Cole PJ, Wilson R, et al. A comparison of serial computed tomography and functional change in bronchiectasis. Eur Respir J. 2002;20(3):581–7.
35. Chalmers JD, Goeminne P, Aliberti S, McDonnell MJ, Lonni S, Davidson J, et al. The bronchiectasis severity index. An international derivation and validation study. Am J Respir Crit Care Med. 2014;189(5):576–85.
36. Amati F, Simonetta E, Gramegna A, Tarsia P, Contarini M, Blasi F, et al. The biology of pulmonary exacerbations in bronchiectasis. Eur Respir Rev. 2019;28(154):190055.
37. Lovie-Toon YG, Grimwood K, Byrnes CA, Goyal V, Busch G, Masters IB, et al. Health-resource use and quality of life in children with bronchiectasis: a multi-center pilot cohort study. BMC Health Serv Res. 2019;19(1):561.
38. Goyal V, McPhail SM, Hurley F, Grimwood K, Marchant JM, Masters IB, et al. Cost of hospitalization for bronchiectasis exacerbation in children. Respirology. 2020;25(12):1250–6.
39. de la Rosa D, Martínez-Garcia MA, Olveira C, Girón R, Máiz L, Prados C. Annual direct medical costs of bronchiectasis treatment: impact of severity, exacerbations, chronic bronchial colonization and chronic obstructive pulmonary disease coexistence. Chron Respir Dis. 2016;13(4):361–71.
40. Cox NS, Wilson CJ, Bennett KA, Johnston K, Potter A, Chang AB, et al. Health-related quality of life and psychological wellbeing are poor in children with bronchiectasis and their parents. ERJ Open Res. 2019;5(3):00063–2019.
41. Chalmers JD, Aliberti S, Filonenko A, Shteinberg M, Goeminne PC, Hill AT, et al. Characterization of the "frequent Exacerbator phenotype" in bronchiectasis. Am J Respir Crit Care Med. 2018;197(11):1410–20.
42. Visser SK, Bye PTP, Fox GJ, Burr LD, Chang AB, Holmes-Liew CL, et al. Australian adults with bronchiectasis: the first report from the Australian bronchiectasis registry. Respir Med. 2019;155:97–103.
43. Nathan AM, Muthusamy A, Thavagnanam S, Hashim A, de Bruyne J. Chronic suppurative lung disease in a developing country: impact on child and parent. Pediatr Pulmonol. 2014;49 (5):435–40.
44. Kapur N, Masters IB, Chang AB. Longitudinal growth and lung function in pediatric non-cystic fibrosis bronchiectasis: what influences lung function stability? Chest. 2010;138 (1):158–64.
45. Finch S, McDonnell MJ, Abo-Leyah H, Aliberti S, Chalmers JD. A comprehensive analysis of the impact of Pseudomonas aeruginosa colonization on prognosis in adult bronchiectasis. Ann Am Thorac Soc. 2015;12(11):1602–11.
46. Chang AB, Boyd J, Bell L, Goyal V, Masters IB, Powell Z, et al. Clinical and research priorities for children and young people with bronchiectasis: an international roadmap. ERJ Open Res. 2021;7(3):00122–2021.
47. Gao YH, Guan WJ, Xu G, Lin ZY, Tang Y, Lin ZM, et al. The role of viral infection in pulmonary exacerbations of bronchiectasis in adults: a prospective study. Chest. 2015;147(6): 1635–43.
48. Kapur N, Mackay IM, Sloots TP, Masters IB, Chang AB. Respiratory viruses in exacerbations of non-cystic fibrosis bronchiectasis in children. Arch Dis Child. 2014;99(8):749–53.
49. Crichton ML, Shoemark A, Chalmers JD. The impact of the COVID-19 pandemic on exacerbations and symptoms in bronchiectasis: a prospective study. Am J Respir Crit Care Med. 2021;204(7):857–9.
50. Mallia P, Footitt J, Sotero R, Jepson A, Contoli M, Trujillo-Torralbo MB, et al. Rhinovirus infection induces degradation of antimicrobial peptides and secondary bacterial infection in chronic obstructive pulmonary disease. Am J Respir Crit Care Med. 2012;186(11):1117–24.
51. Loebinger MR, Wells AU, Hansell DM, Chinyanganya N, Devaraj A, Meister M, Wilson R. Mortality in bronchiectasis: a long-term study assessing the factors influencing survival. Eur Respir J. 2009;34(4):843–9.

52. McDonnell MJ, Aliberti S, Goeminne PC, Dimakou K, Zucchetti SC, Davidson J, et al. Multidimensional severity assessment in bronchiectasis: an analysis of seven European cohorts. Thorax. 2016;71(12):1110–8.
53. Goyal V, Chang AB. Bronchiectasis in childhood. Clin Chest Med. 2022;43(1):71–88.
54. Kapur N, Stroil-Salama E, Morgan L, Yerkovich S, Holmes-Liew CL, King P, et al. Factors associated with "frequent Exacerbator" phenotype in children with bronchiectasis: the first report on children from the Australian bronchiectasis registry. Respir Med. 2021;188:106627.
55. Gaillard EA, Carty H, Heaf D, Smyth RL. Reversible bronchial dilatation in children: comparison of serial high-resolution computer tomography scans of the lungs. Eur J Radiol. 2003;47(3):215–20.
56. Eastham KM, Fall AJ, Mitchell L, Spencer DA. The need to redefine non-cystic fibrosis bronchiectasis in childhood. Thorax. 2004;59(4):324–7.
57. Haidopoulou K, Calder A, Jones A, Jaffe A, Sonnappa S. Bronchiectasis secondary to primary immunodeficiency in children: longitudinal changes in structure and function. Pediatr Pulmonol. 2009;44(7):669–75.
58. Foo CT, Karia S, Herre J. Reversible bronchiectasis. Thorax. 2022;77(7):733–4.
59. Zhang J, Wang S, Shao C. Reversible bronchial dilatation in adults. Clin Exp Pharmacol Physiol. 2021;48(7):966–70.
60. Goeminne PC, Cox B, Finch S, Loebinger MR, Bedi P, Hill AT, et al. The impact of acute air pollution fluctuations on bronchiectasis pulmonary exacerbation: a case-crossover analysis. Eur Respir J. 2018;52(1):1702557.
61. Smith D, Du Rand I, Addy CL, Collyns T, Hart SP, Mitchelmore PJ, et al. British Thoracic Society guideline for the use of long-term macrolides in adults with respiratory disease. Thorax. 2020;75(5):370–404.
62. Grimwood K, Bell SC, Chang AB. Antimicrobial treatment of non-cystic fibrosis bronchiectasis. Expert Rev Anti-Infect Ther. 2014;12(10):1277–96.
63. Koh YY, Lee MH, Sun YH, Sung KW, Chae JH. Effect of roxithromycin on airway responsiveness in children with bronchiectasis: a double-blind, placebo-controlled study. Eur Respir J. 1997;10(5):994–9.
64. Wong C, Jayaram L, Karalus N, Eaton T, Tong C, Hockey H, et al. Azithromycin for prevention of exacerbations in non-cystic fibrosis bronchiectasis (EMBRACE): a randomised, double-blind, placebo-controlled trial. Lancet. 2012;380(9842):660–7.
65. Henkle E, Aksamit TR, Barker AF, Curtis JR, Daley CL, Anne Daniels ML, et al. Pharmacotherapy for non-cystic fibrosis bronchiectasis: results from an NTM Info & Research Patient Survey and the bronchiectasis and NTM research registry. Chest. 2017;152(6):1120–7.
66. Haworth CS, Johnson C, Aliberti S, Goeminne PC, Ringhausen F, Boersma W, et al. Management of bronchiectasis in Europe: Data from the European bronchiectasis registry (EMBARC). Eur Respir J. 2016;48(60):OA273.
67. Aliberti S, Lonni S, Dore S, McDonnell MJ, Goeminne PC, Dimakou K, et al. Clinical phenotypes in adult patients with bronchiectasis. Eur Respir J. 2016;47(4):1113–22.
68. Martinez-García MA, Villa C, Dobarganes Y, Girón R, Maíz L, García-Clemente M, Sibila O, et al. RIBRON: the Spanish online bronchiectasis registry. Characterization of the first 1912 patients. Arch Bronconeumol. 2021;57(1):28–35.
69. Pollock J, Chalmers JD. The immunomodulatory effects of macrolide antibiotics in respiratory disease. Pulm Pharmacol Ther. 2021;71:102095.
70. Sun J, Li Y. Long-term, low-dose macrolide antibiotic treatment in pediatric chronic airway diseases. Pediatr Res. 2022;91(5):1036–42.
71. Cramer CL, Patterson A, Alchakaki A, Soubani AO. Immunomodulatory indications of azithromycin in respiratory disease: a concise review for the clinician. Postgrad Med. 2017;129(5):493–9.
72. Parnham MJ, Erakovic Haber V, Giamarellos-Bourboulis EJ, Perletti G, Verleden GM, Vos R. Azithromycin: mechanisms of action and their relevance for clinical applications. Pharmacol Ther. 2014;143(2):225–45.

73. Oliver ME, Hinks TSC. Azithromycin in viral infections. Rev Med Virol. 2021;31(2):e2163.
74. El Boustany P, Gachelin E, Colomban C, Cernoia J, Sudour P, Carsin A, Dubus JC. A review of non-cystic fibrosis bronchiectasis in children with a focus on the role of long-term treatment with macrolides. Pediatr Pulmonol. 2019;54(4):487–96.
75. Steinkamp G, Schmitt-Grohé S, Döring G, Worlitzsch D, Staab D, Schubert R, et al. Clinical and immunomodulatory effects of once weekly azithromycin treatment in Cystic Fibrosis patients chronically infected with Pseudomonas aeruginosa. J Cyst Fibros. 2006;5:S25.
76. Buyck JM, Plésiat P, Traore H, Vanderbist F, Tulkens PM, Van Bambeke F. Increased susceptibility of Pseudomonas aeruginosa to macrolides and ketolides in eukaryotic cell culture media and biological fluids due to decreased expression of oprM and increased outer-membrane permeability. Clin Infect Dis. 2012;55(4):534–42.
77. Fouka E, Lamprianidou E, Arvanitidis K, Filidou E, Kolios G, Miltiades P, et al. Low-dose clarithromycin therapy modulates Th17 response in non-cystic fibrosis bronchiectasis patients. Lung. 2014;192(6):849–55.
78. Liu J, Zhong X, He Z, Wei L, Zheng X, Zhang J, et al. Effect of low-dose, long-term roxithromycin on airway inflammation and remodeling of stable noncystic fibrosis bronchiectasis. Mediat Inflamm. 2014;2014:708608.
79. Burr LD, Rogers GB, Chen AC, Hamilton BR, Pool GF, Taylor SL, et al. Macrolide treatment inhibits Pseudomonas aeruginosa quorum sensing in non-cystic fibrosis bronchiectasis. An analysis from the bronchiectasis and low-dose erythromycin study trial. Ann Am Thorac Soc. 2016;13(10):1697–703.
80. Wang J, Xu L, Lv Y, Sun L. Azithromycin inhibits the production of MUC5AC in the airway mucosa of patients with bronchiectasis induced by Pseudomonas aeruginosa. Pak J Pharm Sci. 2021;34(3 Special):1179–85.
81. Keir H, Shoemark A, Crichton ML, Dicker A, Pollock J, Giam A, et al. T6 Sputum proteomics identifies mechanisms of disease severity and treatment response in bronchiectasis. Thorax. 2021;76(1):A3.
82. Altenburg J, de Graaff CS, Stienstra Y, Sloos JH, van Haren EH, Koppers RJ, et al. Effect of azithromycin maintenance treatment on infectious exacerbations among patients with non-cystic fibrosis bronchiectasis: the BAT randomized controlled trial. JAMA. 2013;309 (12):1251–9.
83. Serisier DJ, Martin ML, McGuckin MA, Lourie R, Chen AC, Brain B, et al. Effect of long-term, low-dose erythromycin on pulmonary exacerbations among patients with non-cystic fibrosis bronchiectasis: the BLESS randomized controlled trial. JAMA. 2013;309(12):1260–7.
84. Valery PC, Morris PS, Byrnes CA, Grimwood K, Torzillo PJ, Bauert PA, et al. Long-term azithromycin for indigenous children with non-cystic-fibrosis bronchiectasis or chronic suppurative lung disease (bronchiectasis intervention study): a multicentre, double-blind, randomised controlled trial. Lancet Respir Med. 2013;1(8):610–20.
85. Spencer S, Felix LM, Milan SJ, Normansell R, Goeminne PC, Chalmers JD, Donovan T. Oral versus inhaled antibiotics for bronchiectasis. Cochrane Database Syst Rev. 2018;3(3): CD012579.
86. Shi ZL, Peng H, Hu XW, Hu JG. Effectiveness and safety of macrolides in bronchiectasis patients: a meta-analysis and systematic review. Pulm Pharmacol Ther. 2014;28(2):171–8.
87. Gao YH, Guan WJ, Xu G, Tang Y, Gao Y, Lin ZY, Lin ZM, Zhong NS, Chen RC. Macrolide therapy in adults and children with non-cystic fibrosis bronchiectasis: a systematic review and meta-analysis. PLoS One. 2014;9(3):e90047.
88. Wu Q, Shen W, Cheng H, Zhou X. Long-term macrolides for non-cystic fibrosis bronchiectasis: a systematic review and meta-analysis. Respirology. 2014;19(3):321–9.
89. Zhuo GY, He Q, Xiang-Lian L, Ya-Nan Y, Si-Te F. Prolonged treatment with macrolides in adult patients with non-cystic fibrosis bronchiectasis: meta-analysis of randomized controlled trials. Pulm Pharmacol Ther. 2014;29(1):80–8.

90. Fan LC, Lu HW, Wei P, Ji XB, Liang S, Xu JF. Effects of long-term use of macrolides in patients with non-cystic fibrosis bronchiectasis: a meta-analysis of randomized controlled trials. BMC Infect Dis. 2015;15:160.
91. Kelly C, Chalmers JD, Crossingham I, Relph N, Felix LM, Evans DJ, et al. Macrolide antibiotics for bronchiectasis. Cochrane Database Syst Rev. 2018;3(3):CD012406.
92. Wang D, Fu W, Dai J. Meta-analysis of macrolide maintenance therapy for prevention of disease exacerbations in patients with noncystic fibrosis bronchiectasis. Medicine (Baltimore). 2019;98(17):e15285.
93. Lee E, Sol IS, Kim JD, Yang HJ, Min TK, Jang GC, et al. Long-term macrolide treatment for non-cystic fibrosis bronchiectasis in children: a meta-analysis. Sci Rep. 2021;11(1):24287.
94. Baldwin DR, Wise R, Andrews JM, Ashby JP, Honeybourne D. Azithromycin concentrations at the sites of pulmonary infection. Eur Respir J. 1990;3(8):886–90.
95. Rodvold KA, George JM, Yoo L. Penetration of anti-infective agents into pulmonary epithelial lining fluid: focus on antibacterial agents. Clin Pharmacokinet. 2011;50(10):637–64.
96. Kryfti M, Bartziokas K, Papaioannou AI, Papadopoulos A, Kostikas K. Clinical effectiveness of macrolides in diseases of the airways: beyond the antimicrobial effects. Pneumonologie. 2013;26(1):33–46.
97. Parnham MJ, Erakovic HV, Giamarellos-Bourboulis EJ, Perletti G, Verleden GM, et al. Azithromycin: mechanisms of action and their relevance for clinical applications. Pharmacol Ther. 2014;143(2):225–45.
98. Lee E, Hong SJ. Pharmacotherapeutic strategies for treating bronchiectasis in pediatric patients. Expert Opin Pharmacother. 2019;20(8):1025–36.
99. Tembo T, Higgins J, Mohammed R, Greenhalgh L, Francis H, Kwong NM. Primary care review of patients on long-term azithromycin for chronic lung conditions. Thorax. 2019;74(2):A232.
100. Kricker JA, Page CP, Gardarsson FR, Baldursson O, Gudjonsson T, Parnham MJ. Nonantimicrobial actions of macrolides: overview and perspectives for future development. Pharmacol Rev. 2021;73(4):233–62.
101. Chang AB, Bell SC, Byrnes CA, Grimwood K, Holmes PW, King PT, et al. Chronic suppurative lung disease and bronchiectasis in children and adults in Australia and New Zealand. Med J Aust. 2010;193(6):356–65.
102. Bush A. Lung development and aging. Ann Am Thorac Soc. 2016;13(5):S438–46.
103. Masekela R, Anderson R, Gongxeka H, Steel HC, Green RJ. Lack of efficacy of erythromycin in children with human immunodeficiency virus-related bronchiectasis–A randomised controlled trial. Paediatr Respir Rev. 2013;14:S82.
104. Barker A, Stoller J, Dieffenbach P. Bronchiectasis in adults: maintaining lung health. In: UpToDate post TW (Ed), UpToDate, Waltham, MA. Accessed May 04, 2022.
105. Goeminne PC, Soens J, Scheers H, De Wever W, Dupont L. Effect of macrolide on lung function and computed tomography (CT) score in non-cystic fibrosis bronchiectasis. Acta clinica belgica. 2012;67(5):338–46.
106. Terpstra LC, Altenburg J, Mohamed Hoesein FA, Bronsveld I, Go S, van Rijin PA, et al. The effect of maintenance azithromycin on radiological features in patients with bronchiectasis–analysis from the BAT randomized controlled trial. Respir Med. 2022;192:106718.
107. Chalmers JD, Boersma W, Lonergan M, Jayaram L, Crichton ML, Karalus N, et al. Long-term macrolide antibiotics for the treatment of bronchiectasis in adults: an individual participant data meta-analysis. Lancet Respir Med. 2019;7(10):845–54.
108. Kobbernagel HE, Buchvald FF, Haarman EG, Casaulta C, Collins SA, Hogg C, et al. Efficacy and safety of azithromycin maintenance therapy in primary ciliary dyskinesia (BESTCILIA): a multicentre, double-blind, randomised, placebo-controlled phase 3 trial. Lancet Respir Med. 2020;8(5):493–505.
109. Milito C, Pulvirenti F, Cinetto F, Lougaris V, Soresina A, Pecoraro A, et al. Double-blind, placebo-controlled, randomized trial on low-dose azithromycin prophylaxis in patients with primary antibody deficiencies. J Allergy Clin Immunol. 2019;144(2):584–593.e7.

110. Chellew N, Chang AB, Grimwood K. Azithromycin prescribing by respiratory pediatricians in Australia and New Zealand for chronic wet cough: a questionnaire-based survey. Front Pediatr. 2020;8:519.
111. Hare KM, Grimwood K, Chang AB, Chatfield MD, Valery PC, Leah AJ, et al. Nasopharyngeal carriage and macrolide resistance in indigenous children with bronchiectasis randomized to long-term azithromycin or placebo. Eur J Clin Microbiol Infect Dis. 2015;34(11):2275–85.
112. Davidson RJ. In vitro activity and pharmacodynamic/pharmacokinetic parameters of clarithromycin and azithromycin: why they matter in the treatment of respiratory tract infections. Infect Drug Resist. 2019;12:585–96.
113. Patel A, Meesters K. Macrolides in children: judicious use, avoiding resistance and reducing adverse effects. Arch Dis Child Educ Pract Ed. 2021;106(4):216–9.
114. Renna M, Schaffner C, Brown K, Shang S, Tamayo MH, Hegyi K, et al. Azithromycin blocks autophagy and may predispose cystic fibrosis patients to mycobacterial infection. J Clin Invest. 2011;121(9):3554–63.
115. Bell SC, Elborn JS, Byrnes CA. Bronchiectasis: treatment decisions for pulmonary exacerbations and their prevention. Respirology. 2018;23(11):1006–22.
116. Ikeda AK, Prince AA, Chen JX, Lieu JEC, Shin JJ. Macrolide-associated sensorineural hearing loss: a systematic review. Laryngoscope. 2018;128(1):228–36.
117. Wong AYS, Chan EW, Anand S, Worsley AJ, Wong ICK. Managing cardiovascular risk of macrolides: systematic review and meta-analysis. Drug Saf. 2017;40(8):663–77.
118. Thomas D, McDonald VM, Simpson JL, Smith A, Gupta S, Majellano E, et al. Patterns of azithromycin use in obstructive airway diseases: a real-world observational study. Intern Med J. 2022;52(6):1016–23.
119. Espadas D, Castillo S, Moreno M, Escribano A. Lack of effect of azithromycin on QT interval in children: a cohort study. Arch Dis Child. 2016;101(11):1079.
120. Goyal V, Grimwood K, Ware RS, Byrnes CA, Morris PS, Masters IB, et al. Efficacy of oral amoxicillin-clavulanate or azithromycin for non-severe respiratory exacerbations in children with bronchiectasis (BEST-1): a multicentre, three-arm, double-blind, randomised placebo-controlled trial. Lancet Respir Med. 2019;7(9):791–801.
121. Goyal V, Grimwood K, Byrnes CA, Morris PS, Masters IB, Ware RW, et al. Amoxicillin-clavulanate versus azithromycin for respiratory exacerbations in children with bronchiectasis (BEST-2): a multicentre, double-blind, non-inferiority, randomised controlled trial. Lancet. 2018;392(10154):1197–206.
122. O'Sullivan B. What's BEST for children with non-cystic fibrosis bronchiectasis? Lancet Respir Med. 2019;7(9):729–30.
123. Sibila O, Laserna E, Shoemark A, et al. Heterogeneity of treatment response in bronchiectasis clinical trials. Eur Respir J. 2022;59(5):2100777.
124. O'Sullivan B. Raising new questions on best care for bronchiectasis. Lancet Respir Med. 2019;7(10):828–9.
125. Wurzel DF, Chang AB. An update on pediatric bronchiectasis. Expert Rev Respir Med. 2017;11(7):517–32.
126. Goyal V, Grimwood K, Marchant JM, Masters IB, Chang AB. Paediatric chronic suppurative lung disease: clinical characteristics and outcomes. Eur J Pediatr. 2016;175(8):1077–84.

Macrolide Use in Chronic Obstructive Pulmonary Disease

Iwein Gyselinck and Wim Janssens

Abstract Chronic obstructive pulmonary disease (COPD) is a progressive inflammatory airway disease characterized by non-reversible airflow limitation and chronic respiratory symptoms. Symptoms may periodically worsen during events called acute exacerbations (AECOPD), which are associated with increased airway inflammation. AECOPD are the main drivers of poor disease outcomes, making their prevention and effective treatment key elements of COPD care. Because a significant proportion of events have an infectious trigger, antibiotics remain a mainstay of exacerbation management. Particularly as prophylaxis, macrolides have been associated with greater benefit compared with other antibiotic classes, possibly due to their additive immunomodulatory actions. However, treatment failures are frequent, the effectivity of long-term administration is unclear, and there is concern for the risk of adverse events and bacterial resistance. Presumably, patients with frequent and bacteria-associated exacerbations benefit most. Yet, a better characterization of the responding disease traits is vital, both for prophylaxis and treatment of exacerbations.

Keywords COPD · Macrolides · Acute COPD exacerbation

1 Introduction and Background

COPD is a clinical syndrome characterized by progressive non-reversible airflow limitation and chronic respiratory symptoms caused by structural pulmonary abnormalities. It is often accompanied by multiple clinically significant comorbid disorders [1]. Over 300 million people worldwide suffer from COPD [2], and it is now the sixth greatest cause of disability-adjusted life years among all causes [3] and the third leading cause of death [4]. It is caused by repetitive inhalational injury, typically

I. Gyselinck (✉) · W. Janssens
Department of Respiratory Diseases, University Hospitals Leuven & BREATHE lab, department CHROMETA, KU, Leuven, Belgium
e-mail: iwein.gyselinck@kuleuven.be

B. K. Rubin, M. Shinkai (eds.), *Macrolides as Immunomodulatory Agents*, Progress in Inflammation Research 92, https://doi.org/10.1007/978-3-031-42859-3_6

from smoking, but also from household air pollution, occupational exposure and ambient air pollution [5]. Pathologically, direct oxidative stress and chronic inflammation result in airway remodelling, narrowing and loss of terminal bronchioles, abnormalities of mucus secretion, loss of alveolar attachments and emphysema. Neutrophilic and eosinophilic inflammation are recognized as major final common inflammatory pathways [6]. Yet, the mechanisms for disease progression are complex and influenced by exposure as well as host factors. This causes considerable individual heterogeneity in the underlying pathology, as well as in the resulting clinical presentation and optimal treatment decisions [1, 7, 8].

The natural disease history of COPD is marked by acute exacerbations (AECOPD). An AECOPD is defined as an acute worsening of symptoms that often requires additional therapy and is usually associated with increased airway inflammation, increased mucus production, and gas trapping [8]. AECOPD are the main driver of poor COPD outcomes. They accelerate disease progression, strongly affect health-related quality of life and carry a high mortality, especially when accompanied by respiratory failure leading to hospitalization. Moreover, patients with frequent AECOPD are at increased risk of cardiovascular events and other acute complications of comorbid diseases, presumably due to concurrent systemic inflammation [9, 10]. Interventions that can prevent exacerbations or improve their outcome are, therefore, of tremendous clinical benefit. In this context, the therapeutic potential of macrolides, with their broad spectrum of antibacterial and immunomodulatory effects, has long been recognized.

About 50% of AECOPD are bacteria-associated, with viral and eosinophilic triggers accounting for most of the remaining events [11]. Evidence supports a causative role for changes in the composition of the microbiome in triggering bacterial exacerbations, like the acquisition of new strains of pathogenic bacteria or antigenic changes in pre-existing strains [12]. Major pathogens involved are nontypeable *Haemophilus influenzae*, *Moraxella catarrhalis*, *Streptococcus pneumoniae* and *Pseudomonas aeruginosa* [13]. Most strains of *H. influenzae*, *M. catarrhalis* and *S. pneumoniae* are susceptible to macrolides. *Pseudomonas* is clinically not susceptible to macrolides, but macrolides have been shown to interfere with many of its major pathogenicity and virulence traits at subinhibitory concentrations. Clinical benefits have been shown in *Pseudomonas*-infected patients with other chronic respiratory diseases, such as non-cystic fibrosis bronchiectasis. The same mechanisms may account for particular responsiveness to macrolides in COPD patients with *Pseudomonas*-dominated airway infections [14, 15].

Besides the potential to treat acute exacerbations, antibiotics may also prevent AECOPD by reducing airway bacterial load or by preventing the acquisition of new strains when they are given prophylactically. Bacterial colonization during a stable state is a risk factor for bacterial exacerbations, and bacterial dysbiosis may also contribute to disease progression during a stable state [11, 16]. This is facilitated by airway damage and altered barrier function, impaired phagocytotic activity of macrophages against *H. influenzae*, muco-obstructive abnormalities and altered immune-responses due to the long-term use of inhaled steroids [17–19]. Bacterial infection is associated with neutrophilic inflammation, attracted through chemokine (C-X-C motif) ligand 8 (CXCL8), previously called interleukin-8. The underlying inflammatory pathways are complex and, in part, determined by the pathogen. Overweight Proteobacteria, *H. influenzae* in particular, has been associated with increased IL-1β and TNFα, while neutrophilic inflammation with a more balanced microbiome has shown a stronger association with T17-regulating cytokines [16]. In response to such pro-inflammatory signals, more inflammatory cells are recruited. There is increased transcription of nuclear factor kappa B (NF-κB), reinforced by cigarette smoke, consequent activation of the NLRP3-inflammasome, and release of IL-1α, IL-33 and IL-18. This leads to a neutrophil influx, with the release of proteases and consequent airway damage [18]. An adaptive T1 immune response may eventually be mounted, with the accumulation of B-cells and organization into tertiary lymphoid follicles in more severe COPD [1, 7].

Macrolides have a long half-life and a large distribution volume. They concentrate intracellularly, and there is a high uptake by leukocytes that ensures effective delivery to sites of infection or inflammation. These favourable pharmacokinetics allow for intermittent dosing and may give them some advantage over other antibiotics for chronic use [20]. Yet, more importantly, macrolides also exert a range of immunomodulatory effects. Macrolides may help restore epithelial barrier function [21]. They curb macrophage signal transducer and activator of transcription 1 (STAT-1) and NF-κB signalling and thereby decrease CXCL8, IL-6 and TNFα release [22–24]. Macrolides promote a switch from M1 to M2 macrophages, thereby restoring their phagocytotic capacities. They are also known to strongly restrain neutrophil recruitment and activation through the down-regulation of chemoattractants and adhesion molecules in activated vascular endothelial cells [20, 25, 26]. Macrolides may also facilitate steroid sensitivity, relevant for both stable and AECOPD treatments [27]. It is noteworthy that trials targeting these inflammatory cascades with stronger and more specific biologic agents like anti-CXCL8-, anti-TNF-, anti-IL17- and anti-IL-1-antibodies, have only yielded marginal successes in COPD [18]. This may in part be explained by the more pleiotropic immunomodulation of macrolides. Yet it may also imply that their antibiotic effect remains indispensable for their clinical benefit.

It is unclear whether macrolides, besides their antibiotic and immunomodulatory actions, exert clinically relevant antiviral effects that would protect against viral AECOPD [11, 28]. The proven in vitro antiviral activity has not translated into clinical benefit during the COVID-19 pandemic, where macrolides have been tested and used on a large scale [29, 30]. Although the setting is different, this questions the relevance of this effect in the prevention and treatment of AECOPD.

Optimal COPD management includes a combination of non-pharmacological (smoking cessation, influenza and pneumococcal vaccination, pulmonary rehabilitation, lung volume reduction) and pharmacological interventions (long-acting beta-agonists, long-acting antimuscarinic agents, inhaled steroids, prophylactic antibiotics), depending on the severity and clinical phenotype [8]. Numerous clinical trials substantiate a place for macrolides as part of a multimodal treatment approach but also raise some safety concerns. These should be weighed against the benefits and warrant careful patient selection. In the following paragraphs, an overview of the existing clinical evidence is given and provides a guide for the rational use of macrolides in routine practice.

2 Macrolides for the Treatment of Acute Exacerbations of COPD

As a significant proportion of AECOPD is caused by bacteria, antibiotics, including macrolides, are expected to improve outcomes during and after such exacerbations. This is supported by clinical trials, but the effect size is often small and inconsistent. A Cochrane metaanalysis [31] showed fewer treatment failures with antibiotic treatment. However, except for ICU patients, there was large heterogeneity in the individual study results. Potential causes for heterogeneity are variable definitions of AECOPD and grading of exacerbation severity, variation in characteristics of inpatient and outpatient treated exacerbations beyond disease severity (regional organization of healthcare, patient's social support). Importantly, several studies did not differentiate exacerbations with bacterial origin from non-bacterial exacerbation phenotypes. Untargeted exposure of patients with non-bacterial exacerbations to the adverse effects of antibiotics will inadvertently affect study outcomes. Also, co-administration of systemic steroids was frequent in the included trials regardless of the exacerbation phenotype and eosinophilia predominance [32]. Moreover, the diagnostic accuracy of clinical signs and routinely available point-of-care tests to identify exacerbations with a bacterial origin is suboptimal. A sputum culture lacks sensitivity and cannot distinguish between colonization and acute infection [33]. CRP and procalcitonin may offer guidance, but cut-offs remain debated [34].

International guidelines support the use of antibiotics in moderate to severe exacerbations, but recommendations remain indistinct as to which patients would benefit [35, 36]. While awaiting more robust predictors of therapeutic responses, the use of antibiotics to treat AECOPD outside of the ICU should only be considered after careful clinical evaluation in patients presenting with: [8, 33, 34, 36, 37].

- moderate to severe acute exacerbations,
- fulfilling at least two out of three clinical Anthonisen criteria (increased dyspnoea, increased sputum volume, increased sputum purulence), and/or
- other biochemical signs that increase the likelihood of bacterial origin (e.g. CRP of >30 mg/l, procalcitonin >0.76 ng/ml) or that decrease the likelihood of an eosinophilic exacerbation (e.g. blood eosinophilia $<2\%$).

When antibiotics are prescribed, adherence to local guidelines based on local sensitivity patterns is advised [35, 36]. For uncomplicated moderate exacerbations, macrolides in monotherapy may be used, yet they are not preferred over other agents [38–40]. Candidates for early and more aggressive antibiotic therapy are older patients (>65 years), patients with more severe airflow limitation or receiving continuous oxygen therapy, patients with a recent history of severe exacerbations, and patients with severe comorbidity. These patients are at increased risk of treatment failure, and second-line agents like amoxicillin/clavulanate or a quinolone may be more appropriate. In patients at risk for *Pseudomonas* or other resistant bacteria, cultures should be obtained before starting treatment, and these bacteria should be covered by the initial antibiotic regimen [8, 35, 36].

The evidence cited above concerns mainly antibiotic monotherapy. Yet, patients with severe AECOPD at high risk for treatment failure might benefit from the broad antibiotic coverage and immunomodulatory effects of adding a macrolide as a combination therapy. This has also been explored for treating community-acquired pneumonia (CAP) [41, 42]. However, in treating COPD, data to support combination regimens is mostly observational. In ICU-admitted patients with AECOPD, macrolide/beta-lactam combination therapy was associated with lower readmission rates compared with quinolone monotherapy [43]. A similar benefit was suggested in COPD patients hospitalized for CAP. Applying a machine learning approach, observational data of 4898 patients hospitalized for CAP were analysed. A survival benefit was suggested for macrolide/beta-lactam combination therapy compared with other regimens in patients with pre-existing chronic respiratory disease, including COPD and with a high leukocyte count in respiratory secretions, regardless of cardiovascular comorbidity [44].

The BACE study is unique in this regard, as it has been the first to examine macrolide add-on in a randomized controlled setting in severe AECOPD [45]. Patients hospitalized for AECOPD and with a history of at least one moderate to severe exacerbation in the previous year were randomized to standard of care—including antibiotics and systemic corticosteroids—or standard of care plus azithromycin. Azithromycin was continued for 3 months after the index exacerbation as post-exacerbation prophylaxis, and patients were followed-up for 6 months after treatment discontinuation. Although the primary composite endpoint, time to treatment failure, was not significantly different (HR: 0.73 (0.53–1.01), $p = 0.052$), a significant reduction in treatment escalation rates (HR: 0.7 (0.51–0.86), $p = 0.02$) and a large reduction in readmission rates was observed (HR: 0.43 (0.25–0.75), $p = 0.003$) at 3 months follow-up. The latter was accompanied by a 24% reduction in hospital days ($p = 0.006$) and 74% reduction in ICU days ($p < 0.0001$). The need for a step-up in hospital care and hospital readmissions within 3 months was significantly reduced in the azithromycin group. A post hoc analysis of the data showed that high CRP (>50 mg/l) and low eosinophil count (<300 cells/µl) were associated with better response to treatment [46]. Once treatment was discontinued, most of the observed effects disappeared over a 6-month follow-up (Fig. 1).

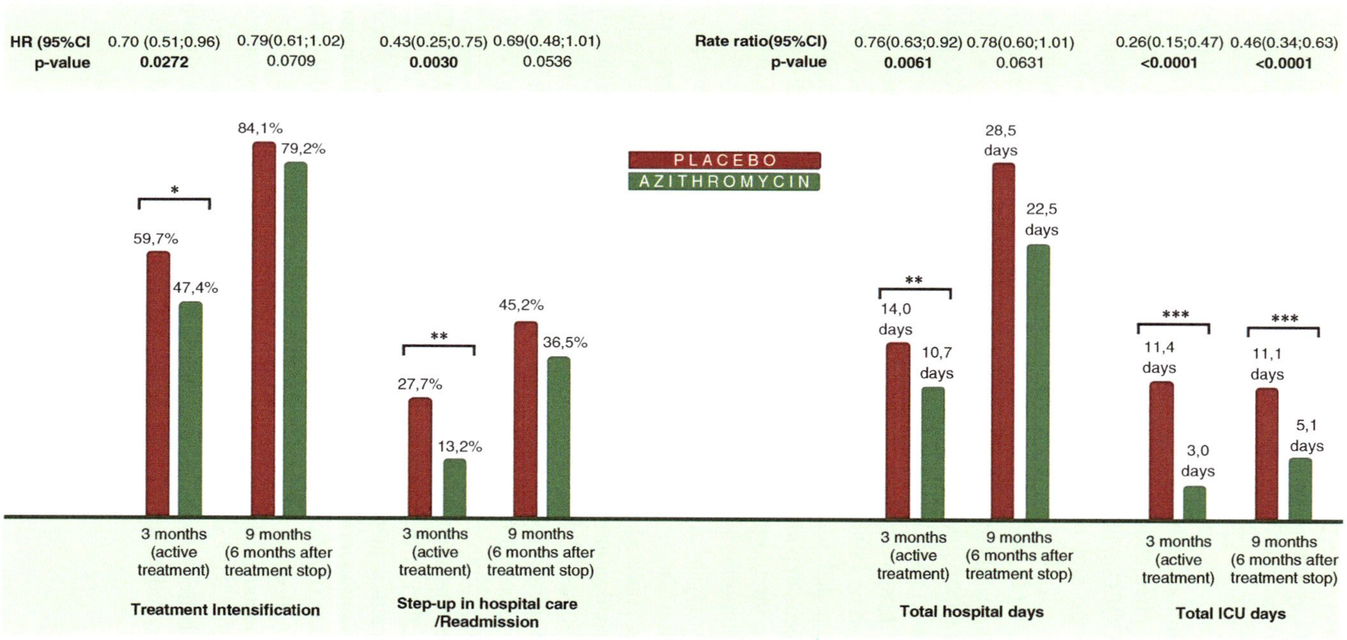

Fig. 1 BACE trial: 3 months of azithromycin treatment after an index hospitalization for an AECOPD was associated with a significant reduction in treatment intensification rate and a step-up in hospital care rate. A total number of hospital and ICU days was reduced. Most of the observed effects waned over a 6-month follow-up period after treatment discontinuation

3 Prophylactic Macrolides for the Prevention of Acute Exacerbations of COPD

There is a long history of testing prophylactic antibiotics, including macrolides, for the prevention of exacerbations of chronic bronchitis. Trials date back to the 1950s, but early studies lack standardization of COPD diagnosis and inclusion criteria [47]. Table 1 [45, 48–64], therefore, provides an overview of randomized controlled trials with macrolides conducted after the year 2000 and four meta-analyses that considered the class effect of macrolides after 2015.

Even when only these more recent trials are considered, there is evident diversity in the study population, intervention and outcome assessments:

- Except for the study of Vermeersch et al. [45] all subjects were randomized during stable disease periods. Most patients presented with at least moderate to severe airflow limitation and a history of exacerbations. Other inclusion criteria, baseline characteristics and clinical phenotypes differed across studies. In the largest trial [53], more than half of the patients received long-term oxygen. In Berkhof et al. [54], Simpson et al. [55] and Brill et al. [57], only patients with chronic cough or neutrophilic airway inflammation were selected. Suzuki et al. [48] excluded patients taking corticosteroids, whereas all patients in Banerjee et al. [49] and most patients in Seemungal et al. [50] received inhaled steroids. All patients in Blasi et al. [51] had a tracheostomy, and all patients in Shafuddin et al. [58] were selected on positive *C. pneumoniae* serology.
- There was variation in treatment regimens in terms of the macrolide (azithromycin, erythromycin, roxithromycin), the total daily doses, the use of intermittent dosing (e.g. azithromycin three times a week) and the duration of treatment. The studies of Suzuki et al. [48] and Blasi et al. [51] were open-label and information regarding blinding was missing in Tan et al. [59].
- Finally, different outcomes were selected. Exacerbation prevention is a key objective of COPD management and, not surprisingly, a main outcome in many of these trials. Still, the assessment of this outcome differed in terms of how exacerbations were defined (only infective exacerbations according to Anthonisen versus all exacerbations, specification of mild versus moderate and severe exacerbations), in terms of outcome estimator (mean or median exacerbation rate versus proportion of patients with one or more exacerbations) and in terms of statistical analysis used (time-to-event analysis, hazard ratios, relative risk and odds ratios). Moreover, while AECOPD are known to be strongly associated with reduced quality of life, mortality and disease progression, it remains unclear if exacerbation prevention effectively impacts on these outcomes. Most studies were grossly underpowered to detect effects on health status, hospitalization rates or mortality and the duration of follow-up would not allow for firm conclusions regarding FEV1-decline.

Despite this diversity, a beneficial effect of macrolides is evident. In the network meta-analysis of Janjua et al., comparing different antibiotic classes for prophylactic

Table 1 Summary of trials assessing azithromycin for the prevention of AECOPD since the year 2000

Study	Design	Intervention	Population and exclusion	PO	Effect on exacerbation (treated versus control)	Effect on hospitalization (treated versus control)	Effect on mortality (treated versus control)	Effect on FEV1 and functional status (treated versus control)	Effect on health-related quality of life (treated versus control)	Effect on bacteriology	Effect on inflammatory markers	Ni 2015	Wedzicha 2017	Cui 2018	Janjua 2021
Suzuki 2001, Japan [48]	RCT, Open label ($n = 109$)	**Antibiotic regimen:** Erythromycin 200 to 400 mg/d,or riboflavin **Treatment duration:** 12 months **Duration of follow-up:** 12 months	– **Diagnosis:** Spirometry confirmed, – **Age (years, mean):** 70.4, – **FEV1 (mean, litres):** 2.64. – **Exacerbation history:** NA, – **Exclusion:** Bronchiectasis, diffuse panbronchiolitis, – **Other:** All study participants were treated with sustained-release theophylline and inhaled anticholinergic agents, but none received corticosteroids.	Number of common colds and exacerbations	**Risk ratio for one or more AECOPD:** 0.20 (0.09; 0.43) **Rate ratio of annualized rate of AECOPD:** 0.21 (0.07; 0.64) **Exacerbation definition:** Acute and sustained Worsening of COPD symptoms requiring changes to regular treatment, including antimicrobial therapy and/or short courses of systemic steroids.	No hospitalized AECOPD in treated group, 11 in control group ($p = 0.0007$) 0 patients hospitalized at least once for severe AECOPD in treated group versus 10 in control group ($p = 0.0004$)	NA	NA	NA	NA	NA				
Banerjee 2005, UK [49]	RCT, Double blind ($n = 67$)	**Antibiotic regimen:** Clarithromycin 500 mg OD, or placebo **Treatment duration:** 3 months **Duration of follow-up:** 3 months	– **Diagnosis:** Spirometry confirmed, – **Age (years, mean):** 66.7, – **FEV1% predicted (mean):** 43.3. – **Exacerbation history:** NA, – **Exclusion:** Reversibility (spirometry), bronchiectasis (clinical),	Health status	**Risk ratio of one or more AECOPD:** 2.90 (0.61; 13.93) **Rate ratio of annualized rate of AECOPD:** 3.27 (0.53; 20.18) **Exacerbation definition:** Infective exacerbation	NA	NA	No significant difference in FEV1 No effect on shuttle walk distance	No difference in total SGRQ[#] or SF-36[$]	No effect on PPM* No multi-resistant gram-negative organisms emerged in treatment clarithromycin group No significant decrease of bacterial load	No effect on CRP				

			uncontrolled ischaemic heart disease, – **Other:** All patients on inhaled steroids,		according to Anthonisen (2 out of 3 present: Increased dyspnoea, increased sputum volume, increased sputum purulence).										
Seemungal 2008, UK [50]	RCT, double blind ($n = 109$)	**Antibiotic regimen:** Erythromycin 250 mg BD, or placebo **Duration of treatment:** 12 months **Follow-up:** 12 months	– **Diagnosis:** Spirometry confirmed, – **Age (years, mean):** 67.2, – **FEV1% predicted (mean):** 49.9. – **Exacerbation history:** 35% of participants had ≥3 exacerbations in the previous 12 months, – **Exclusion:** Reversibility (spirometry), asthma (clinical), bronchiectasis (clinical), unstable cardiac status, prolonged QTc, – **Other:** Most patients on inhaled steroids,	Number of moderate and/or severe exacerbations	**Median time to first AECOPD:** 271 vs 89 days (log rank $p = 0.020$) **Risk ratio of one or more AECOPD:** 0.70 (0.52; 0.95) **Rate ratio of annualized rate of AECOPD:** 0.65 (0.49; 0.86) **Median duration of exacerbation:** 9 vs 13 days ($p = 0.036$) **Exacerbation definition:** Sustained worsening of baseline respiratory symptoms for at least 2 days that required treatment with oral corticosteroids (prednisolone) and/or antibiotics.	Risk ratio for hospitalization 0.66 (no p-value available)	NA	No significant difference in FEV1	NA	No significant differences in sputum flora	No significant differences in serum IL-6, CRP, sputum IL-6, sputum IL-8, sputum myeloperoxidase				

(continued)

Table 1 (continued)

Study	Design	Intervention	Population and exclusion	PO	Effect on exacerbation (treated versus control)	Effect on hospitalization (treated versus control)	Effect on mortality (treated versus control)	Effect on FEV1 and functional status (treated versus control)	Effect on health-related quality of life (treated versus control)	Effect on bacteriology	Effect on inflammatory markers	Ni 2015	Wedzicha 2017	Cui 2018	Janjua 2021
Blasi 2010, Italy [51]	RCT, Open label ($n = 22$)	**Antibiotic regimen:** Azithromycin 500 mg OD, 3 times a weekor SOC **Treatment duration:** 6 months **Duration of follow-up:** 12 months	– **Diagnosis:** Spirometry confirmed severe COPD (severe not otherwise specified), – **Age (years, mean):** 72.5, – **FEV1% predicted (mean):** NA. – **Exacerbation history:** Mean of 3 exacerbations in the previous 12 months, – **Exclusion:** Life expectancy <1 year, – **Other:** All patients were outpatients with a tracheostomy,	Reduction in number of AECOPD and hospitalizations during study duration	**Hazard ratio of having first AECOPD:** 0.18 (0.06; 0.59) **Risk ratio of one or more AECOPD:** NA **Rate ratio of annualized rate of AECOPD:** 0.24 (0.10; 0.59) **NB:** The number of AECOPD in the treated group during the first 6 months of treatment was significantly different from the number of exacerbations experienced in the next 6 months of follow-up **Exacerbation definition:** Worsening of symptoms requiring both a change in regular respiratory medication or medical assistance, or resulting in hospitalization or in an emergency room treatment.	Risk ratio for hospitalization in treated group: 0.38 (0.13–1.08)	Hazard ratio for all-cause mortality 0.49 ($p = 0.33$)	NA	Significant improvement in MRF26[£] score in treated group	Reduction of P. aeruginosa CFU in treated patients compared with baseline Erythromycin-resistant *S. pneumonaie* strain identified in 1 treated patient	A decrease occurred in both TNF-α and IL-6 in the treated but not in the SOC group. Once treatment was discontinued, TNF-α and IL-6 rose back to baseline				

He 2010, China [52]	RCT, Double blind ($n = 36$)	**Antibiotic regimen:** Erythromycin 125 mg TDS, or placebo **Duration of treatment:** 6 months **Follow-up:** 6 months	– **Diagnosis:** Spirometry confirmed, – **Age (years, mean):** 69, – **FEV1% predicted (mean):** 43.2. – **Exacerbation history:** NA, – **Exclusion:** Reversibility (spirometry), exacerbation during last month, history of unstable cardiac disorders, – **Other:** /,	Neutrophil number in sputum and exacerbations	**Median time to first AECOPD:** 155 vs 86 days (log rank $p = 0.032$) **Risk ratio of one or more AECOPD:** 0.64 (0.38; 1.09) **Rate ratio of annualized rate of AECOPD:** 0.5[illegible] (0.31; 0.98) **Exacerbation definition:** Exacerbation was defined as a sustained worsening of baseline respiratory symptoms for at least 2 days that required increased treatment or additional therapy such as oral corticosteroids or antibiotics.	NA	NA	NA	No significant difference in SF-36$^{\$}$ and SGRQ$^{\#}$ scores	No difference in isolated pathogens in sputum	Decrease in sputum neutrophil cell counts at 3 and 6 months compared with baseline and placebo, decrease in neutrophil elastase concentrations, no significant difference in lymphocytes and microphages				
Albert 2011, USA [53]	RCT, Double blind ($n = 1142$)	**Antibiotic regimen:** Azithromycin 250 mg OD, or placebo **Duration of treatment:** 12 months **Follow-up:** 12 months	– **Diagnosis:** Spirometry confirmed, – **Age (years, mean):** 65.5, – **FEV1% predicted (mean):** 39.5. – **Exacerbation history:** 84.5% received systemic glucocorticoids for AECOPD in previous 12 months, 50.2% required	Time to first acute exacerbation	**Median time to first AECOPD:** 266 vs 174 days (log-rank $p < 0.001$) **Hazard ratio for having AECOPD per patient-year:** 0.7[illegible] (0.63; 0.84) **Risk ratio of one or more AECOPD:** 0.84 (0.75; 0.92)	Hazard ratio for hospitalizations per patient year from any cause: 0.94 (0.76–1.15) ($p = 0.52$) (SO) Hazard ratio for hospitalizations per patient year related to COPD: 0.82 (0.64–1.07) ($p = 0.15$) (SO)	All-cause mortality 3% vs 4% ($p = 0.87$)	NA	Significant mean difference in SGRQ$^{\#}$ scores More patients reached MCID$^{¥}$ on SGRQ$^{\#}$: 43% vs. 36% No significant difference in SF-36$^{\$}$	No effect on nasopharyngeal bacterial colonization, assessed through nasopharyngeal swabs Incidence of resistance to macrolides in cultures from nasopharyngeal swabs was 81% treatment and	Post-hoc analysis by O'Reilly et al. [67] showed Proline–glycine–proline (PGP), a neutrophil chemoattractant derived from the enzymatic breakdown of collagen by matrix metalloproteases 8 and 9				

(continued)

Table 1 (continued)

Study	Design	Intervention	Population and exclusion	PO	Effect on exacerbation (treated versus control)	Effect on hospitalization (treated versus control)	Effect on mortality (treated versus control)	Effect on FEV1 and functional status (treated versus control)	Effect on health-related quality of life (treated versus control)	Effect on bacteriology	Effect on inflammatory markers	Ni 2015	Wedzicha 2017	Cui 2018	Janjua 2021
			hospitalization or emergency room visit for AECOPD, – **Excluded:** Exacerbation in last month, asthma (clinical), prolonged QTc and use of QT-prolonging medication, hearing impairment, – **Other:** 60% of patients on long-term oxygen,		**Rate ratio of annualized rate of AECOPD:** 0.83 (0.72; 0.95) **Exacerbation definition:** Complex of respiratory symptoms (increased or new onset) of more than one of the following: Cough, sputum, wheezing, dyspnoea, or chest tightness with a duration of at least 3 days requiring treatment with antibiotics or systemic steroids.					41% in control group ($P < 0.001$)					
Berkhof 2013, The Nether-lands [54]	RCT, Double blind (n = 84)	**Antibiotic regimen:** Azithromycin 250 mg OD three times a week, or placebo **Duration of treatment:** 3 months **Follow-up:** 3 months	– **Diagnosis:** Spirometry confirmed, – **Age (years, mean):** 68, – **FEV1% predicted (mean):** 48.6. – **Exacerbation history:** Median of 1 exacerbation in last year, – **Excluded:**	Cough specific health status (Leicester cough questionnaire)	**Time to first AECOPD** of 20th percentile of most frequent exacerbators: 105 vs 66 days (log-rank $p = 0.13$) **Risk ratio of one or more AECOPD:** 0.59 (0.31; 1.13)	Hospitalization from any cause: 9.5% in treated group vs 11.9% in control group	NA	No significant difference in FEV1	Significant mean difference in SGRQ$^{\#}$ and SF-36$^{\$}$ scores, above MCID$^{¥}$ Improvement of LCQ$^{\Sigma}$	Reduction in sputum PPM	NA				

			Asthma (clinical), exacerbation during last 3 weeks, – **Other:** All patients had chronic cough (cough for at least the last 12 weeks, in two subsequent years),		**Exacerbation definition:** Sustained worsening of the patient's condition, from the stable state and beyond normal day-to-day variations, that necessitates treatment with prednisolone, antibiotics or a combination of both.										
Simpson 2014, Australia [55]	RCT, Double-blind ($n = 30$)	**Antibiotic regimen:** Azithromycin 250 mg OD, or placebo **Duration of treatment:** 3 months **Follow-up:** 6 months	– **Diagnosis:** Spirometry confirmed, – **Age (years, mean):** 70.8, – **FEV1% predicted (mean):** 53.7. – **Exacerbation history:** NA, – **Excluded:** Current smokers, exacerbation during last month, prolonged QTc, – **Other:** All patients had neutrophilic bronchitis (sputum neutrophil proportion > 61% or > 162x104 neutrophils/ml,	Reduction in sputum CXCL8	**Risk ratio of one or more AECOPD:** 0.45 ($p = 0.139$) **Rate ratio of annualized rate of AECOPD:** 0.3[illegible] (0.14–1.05) **Exacerbation definition:** Increase in symptoms requiring unscheduled medical attention and the use of oral corticosteroids and/or antibiotic treatment	NA	NA	No significant difference in FEV1	No significant difference in FEV1	Non-significant reduction in bacterial load on induced sputum	Non-significant reduction in sputum neutrophil count, lymphocyte count, neutrophil elastase levels and CXCL8 levels on induced sputum				
Uzun 2014, The netherlands [56]	RCT, Double-blind ($n = 92$)	**Antibiotic regimen:** Azithromycin 500 mg OD 3x/week, or placebo **Duration of**	– **Diagnosis:** Spirometry confirmed, – **Age (years, mean):** 64.8, – **FEV1% predicted (mean):**	Exacerbation rate	**Median time to first AECOPD:** 130 vs 59 days (log-rank $p = 0.001$) **Risk ratio of one**	No difference in odds for hospitalization or time to first admission	NA	No significant difference in FEV1 and 6MWD	No significant difference in SGRQ[#]	Fewer patients in treated group had positive sputum cultures with new PPM compared with	NA				

(continued)

Table 1 (continued)

Study	Design	Intervention	Population and exclusion	PO	Effect on exacerbation (treated versus control)	Effect on hospitalization (treated versus control)	Effect on mortality (treated versus control)	Effect on FEV1 and functional status (treated versus control)	Effect on health-related quality of life (treated versus control)	Effect on bacteriology	Effect on inflammatory markers	Ni 2015	Wedzicha 2017	Cui 2018	Janjua 2021
		treatment: 12 months **Follow-up:** 12 months	44.6. – **Exacerbation history:** Mean of 4 AECOPD during last 12 months, – **Excluded:** Exacerbation during last month, asthma (clinical), bronchiectasis (on chest CT), heart failure, taking drugs that would interact with azithromycin, – **Other:** NA,		**or more AECOPD:** 0.78 (0.64; 0.94) **Rate ratio of annualized rate of AECOPD:** 0.58 (0.43; 0.78) **Exacerbation definition:** According to Anthonisen criteria (2 out of 3 present: Increased dyspnoea, increased sputum volume, increased sputum purulence), and whether patient needed treatment with steroids or antibiotics					placebo group ($p = 0{\cdot}044$). Acquisition of macrolide-resistant bacteria was 6% treated and 24% in untreated group ($p = 0{\cdot}036$)					
Brill 2015, UK [57]	RCT, placebo-controlled single-blind, ($n = 99$)	**Antibiotic regimen:** Azithromycin 250 mg OD 3 times a week, or moxifloxacin 400 mg OD for 5 days every 4 weeks, or Doxycyclin 100 mg OD, or placebo **Duration of treatment:** 3 months **Follow-up:** 3 months	– **Diagnosis:** Spirometry confirmed, – **Age (years, mean):** 69.4, – **FEV1% predicted (mean):** 50. – Exacerbation history: Mean of 2.22 exacerbations per patient in	Change in sputum bacterial load	**Rate ratio of annualized rate of AECOPD:** – Moxifloxacin: 1.38 (0.62; 3.10). – Doxycyclin: 2.07 (0.99; 4.35). – Azithromycin: 0.72 (0.30; 1.71).	NA	NA	No significant difference in FEV1	No significant differences in SGRQ[#]	Non-significant decrease in sputum bacterial load in all treatment arms (largest decrease with moxifloxacin)	No significant difference in IL-1β, IL-6 or IL-8				

			previous year, – **Excluded:** Prolonged QTc, – **Other:** All patients had chronic productive cough (self-reported sputum expectoration on most days when clinically stable),												
Sha-fuddin 2015, Australia & New Zealand [58]	RCT, Double-blind ($n = 292$)	**Antibiotic regimen:** Roxithromycin 300 mg OD, or Roxithromycin 300 mg + doxycycline 100 mg OD, or placebo **Duration of treatment:** 3 months **Follow-up:** 15 months	– **Diagnosis:** Clinical diagnosis of COPD, – **Age (years, mean):** 67, – **FEV1% predicted (mean):** 34. – **Exacerbation history:** Mean of 5.11 exacerbations per patient in previous 2 years, – **Excluded:** Exacerbation in last month, – **Other:** All patients had positive C. pneumoniae serological status,	Exacerbation rate during post-treatment follow-up	**Time to first AECOPD:** 121 days in roxithromycin/doxycycline group, 140 days in roxithromycin only group and 147 days in placebo group (log-rank $p = 0.254$) **Rate ratio of annualized AECOPD during 3 months of treatment:** 0.73 in the roxithromycin/doxycycline group ($p = 0.1709$), 0.77 in the roxithromycin only group ($p = 0.2545$) **Rate ratio of annualized AECOPD during post-treatment follow-up:** 1.13 in the	NA	NA	No significant difference in FEV1	Significant difference in CRQ, but not reaching MCID[¥], no difference in proportion of patients reaching MCID[¥]	NA	NA				

(continued)

Table 1 (continued)

Study	Design	Intervention	Population and exclusion	PO	Effect on exacerbation (treated versus control)	Effect on hospitalization (treated versus control)	Effect on mortality (treated versus control)	Effect on FEV1 and functional status (treated versus control)	Effect on health-related quality of life (treated versus control)	Effect on bacteriology	Effect on inflammatory markers	Ni 2015	Wedzicha 2017	Cui 2018	Janjua 2021
					roxithromycin/doxycycline group ($p = 0.352$), 1.08 in the roxithromycin only group ($p = 0.5832$) **Exacerbation definition:** Not given										
Tan 2016, China [59]	RCT, Placebo-controlled, no info on blinding ($n = 54$)	**Antibiotic regimen:** Erythromycin 125 mg TDS for 12 months, or erythromycin 125 mg TDS for 6 months, or placebo for 12 months **Duration of treatment:** 6 or 12 months **Follow-up:** 12 months	– **Diagnosis:** Spirometry confirmed, – **Age (years, mean):** 68.4, – **FEV1% predicted (mean):** 44.4. – **Exacerbation history:** NA, – **Excluded:** Asthma, exacerbation during last month, primary diagnosis of bronchiectasis or diffuse panbronchiolitis cardiovascular illness, – **Other:** NA,	Effect on IL17 and IL23 in peripheral blood and induced sputum	NA	NA	NA	No significant difference in FEV1 Significant increase in 6MWD in treated group, effect lost when treatment stopped	NA	NA	Significant decrease in neutrophil cell count on induced sputum and significant decrease in induced sputum and peripheral blood concentrations of IL-17 and IL-23 in both treatment groups after 6 months but not after 3 months compared with placebo. Effect disappeared in erythromycin withdrawal group at months 9 and 12 and fell back to same levels as placebo group				

Wang 2017, China [60]	RCT, Open label ($n = 87$)	**Antibiotic regimen:** Azithromycin 250 mg OD + simvastatin 20 mg OD,or simvastatin monotherapy **Duration of treatment:** 6 months **Follow-up:** 6 months	– **Diagnosis:** Spirometry confirmed, – **Age (years, mean):** 68.4, – **FEV1% predicted (mean):** 44.4. – **Exacerbation history:** NA, – **Excluded:** Asthma, exacerbation during last month, cardiovascular illness, group 1 pulmonary hypertension, – **Other:** All patients had group 3 pulmonary hypertension,	PaO_2, $PaCO_2$ and PH on arterial blood gas	NA	NA	NA	No significant difference in FEV1 Significant increase in 6MWD in combination treatment group Significant improvement in PaO_2 and $PaCO_2$ in combination treatment group	NA	NA	NA				
Ver-meersch 2019, Belgium [45]	RCT, Double blind ($n = 301$)	**Antibiotic regimen:** Azithromycin 500 mg OD for 3 days and then 250 mg every 2 days, or placebo **Duration of treatment:** 3 months **Follow-up:** 9 months	– **Diagnosis:** Spirometry confirmed, – **Age (years, mean):** 66.5, – **FEV1% predicted (mean):** 37.3. – **Exacerbation history:** In previous 12 months 29% had 1, 26% had 2, 17% had 3 and 28% had >3 AECOPD, – **Excluded:** Prolonged QTc, prior use of macrolides, – **Other:** Patients were recruited during hospitalized AECOPD, treated	Treatment failure within 3 months	**Treatment failure rate within 3 months:** 49.5% vs 60.4%, hazard ratio 0.73 (0.53–1.01) **Rate of new exacerbations within 3 months:** 39.6% vs 51.0%, hazard ratio = 0.70 (0.49; 1.00, $p = 0.0497$) **Treatment failure rate within 9 months:** 82.2% vs 84.8%, hazard ratio 0.83 (0.64; 1.08) **Rate of new exacerbations within 9 months:**	Rate ratio of hospital readmissions after hospital discharge of the index AECOPD (post hoc analysis [46]): 0.47 (0.27–0.80)	No significant difference	No significant difference in FEV1	No significant difference in EQ5D[φ]	No significant difference in positive sputum cultures with newly acquired pathogens, nor for the acquisition of macrolide-resistant bacteria	NA				

(continued)

Table 1 (continued)

Study	Design	Intervention	Population and exclusion	PO	Effect on exacerbation (treated versus control)	Effect on hospitalization (treated versus control)	Effect on mortality (treated versus control)	Effect on FEV1 and functional status (treated versus control)	Effect on health-related quality of life (treated versus control)	Effect on bacteriology	Effect on inflammatory markers	Ni 2015	Wedzicha 2017	Cui 2018	Janjua 2021
			with steroids and antibiotics,		75.1% vs 79.5%, hazard ratio = 0.81 (0.62–1.06)										
					Treatment failure definition: Composite of treatment intensification with systemic corticosteroids and/or antibiotics, step-up in hospital care or readmission for respiratory reasons or all-cause mortality **New exacerbation definition:** Composite of a new course of systemic corticosteroids and/or antibiotics, or hospitalization for respiratory reasons, all after the index event										

Ni 2015 [61]					**Risk ratio for one or more exacerbations 0.70 (0.56–0.87)** *Estimated from* [48–50, 52–54, 56] $I^2 > 40\%$ **Risk ratio for one or more exacerbations excluding Suzuki et al 0.80 (0.72–0.88)** *Estimated from* [49, 50, 52–54, 56] $I^2 < 40\%$ **Rate ratio for annualized exacerbation rate per patient 0.58 (0.43–0.78)** *Estimated from* [49–53, 55, 56] $I^2 > 50\%$	Risk ratio of hospitalization 0.89 (0.64–1.24) *Estimated from* [50, 51, 53, 54, 56] $I^2 < 40\%$	Risk ratio 0.66 (0.23–1.85) *Estimated from* [48, 51, 53] $I^2 < 40\%$	NA	Mean difference in SGRQ[#] -2.12 (−3.44; −0.79) *Estimated from* [53, 55, 56] $I^2 < 40\%$	NA	NA				
Wedzicha 2017 [62]					**Time to first exacerbation, mean difference 81.53 days more (53.29–109.77)** *Estimated from* [50, 53, 56] $I^2 < 40\%$ **Rate ratio for exacerbation rate per patient 0.76 (0.68–0.86)** *Estimated from* [50, 53, 56] $I^2 > 50\%$	NA	Risk ratio 0.90 (0.48–1.69) *Estimated from* [48, 53, 56] $I^2 < 40\%$	NA	Mean difference in SGRQ[#] -2.18 (−1.53; 2.82) *Estimated from* [53, 56] $I^2 < 40\%$	NA	NA				

(continued)

Table 1 (continued)

Study	Design	Intervention	Population and exclusion	PO	Effect on exacerbation (treated versus control)	Effect on hospitalization (treated versus control)	Effect on mortality (treated versus control)	Effect on FEV1 and functional status (treated versus control)	Effect on health-related quality of life (treated versus control)	Effect on bacteriology	Effect on inflammatory markers	Ni 2015	Wedzicha 2017	Cui 2018	Janjua 2021
Cui 2018 [63]					**Odds ratio for one or more exacerbations 0.40 (0.24–0.64)** *Estimated from* [48–56, 68] *$I^2 > 50\%$* **Rate ratio for annualized exacerbation rate per patient 0.60 (0.45–0.78)** *Estimated from* [48–53, 55–57] *$I^2 > 50\%$*	Odds ratio for hospitalization 0.60 (0.14–2.65) *Estimated from* [50, 51, 54, 56] *$I^2 < 40\%$*	NA	NA	Mean difference in SGRQ[#] -2.47 (−3.72; −1.22) *Estimated from* [53–57] *$I^2 < 40\%$*	NA	NA				
Janjua 2021 [64]			– .		**Risk ratio for one or more exacerbations 0.85 (0.81–0.90) excluding Suzuki et al** *Estimated from* [50–57] *No significant heterogeneity identified based on unrelated mean effects model* **Hazard ratio for exacerbation (assuming annualized exacerbation rate of**	NA	NA	NA	Mean difference in SGRQ[#] -4.00 (−5.51; −2.68) *Estimated from* [52–57]	NA	NA				

					2 exacerbations per patient per year in placebo) 0.57 (0.60–0.75) *Estimated from* [50–55, 57] *No significant heterogeneity identified based on unrelated mean effects model*										

#SGRQ: St. George's respiratory questionnaire
$SF-36: Short form health survey
£MRF26: Maugeri respiratory failure questionnaire
¥MCID: Minimal clinically important difference
ΣLCQ: Leicester cough questionnaire
φEQ5D: EuroQol-5D questionnaire
*PPM: Potential pathogenic microorganisms (*Haemophilus influenzae*, *Streptococcus pneumoniae*, *Mycobacterium catarrhalis*, *Haemophilus parainfluenzae*, *Staphylococcus aureus*, *Pseudomonas aeruginosa*, *Klebsiella pneumoniae*)

treatment in COPD, continuous treatment with macrolides in intermittent or daily dosing regimens had the largest effect size of all classes assessed. Macrolides were the only class reaching statistical significance on the primary outcome of reduction of exacerbations [64]. This effect of preventing exacerbations is consistent throughout the evidence. The pooled outcome estimates of the meta-analyses generally lay within the confidence intervals of the individual studies. Exceptions are the trials of Suzuki et al. [48] and Blasi et al. [51], which seem to have an overly optimistic estimation of the effect size. Both studies were however open-label and subject to performance bias.

AECOPD reduction remained significant for both azithromycin and erythromycin. Results were more consistent for the studies using azithromycin, but the largest effect size was seen with erythromycin, strongly driven by the open-label study of Suzuki et al. that was not excluded from this analysis. Different treatment regimens were used both for azithromycin and erythromycin. All trials using erythromycin had daily dosing regimens with doses between 200 mg and 500 mg. For azithromycin, trials using higher dosing regimens with intermittent (e.g. 500 mg 3 times a week) or daily (e.g. 250 mg once daily) administration also had longer treatment duration than trials using lower doses and thus more power to detect a significant treatment effect [51, 53, 55, 56]. None of the studies with lower dosing regimens had a treatment duration longer than 3 months [45, 54, 57], and only one was able to show a significant effect on the exacerbation rate [45].

Unadjusted post hoc analyses from the largest trial of Albert et al. [53] suggested differences in treatment effect depending on age, smoking status, concomitant inhaled therapy, oxygen use and GOLD stage. When corrected for potential confounders, only older age, milder GOLD stage and a current non-smoker status remained associated with better treatment response. Notably, no significant treatment interaction effect was observed for a history of chronic bronchitis [65].

While it is clear from the pooled data that macrolides effectively prevent exacerbations, the quality of evidence regarding their effect on the severity of exacerbations is much lower. Effect on the duration of exacerbations was only reported in Seemungal et al., showing a significant reduction from a median of 13 to a median of 9 exacerbation days. Although the setting was slightly different, this is corroborated by the previously mentioned BACE trial, showing a reduction in the total number of days spent in the hospital in the azithromycin-treated group. Most studies that reported the effect on the risk of being admitted to the hospital were underpowered to assess this outcome. Pooled data shows a trend towards lower hospitalization risk, but without reaching significance. However, the BACE trial, with a significant reduction in readmissions in the 3 months following randomization, was not included in the pooled analyses. Equally, a trend towards lower mortality was shown in two of the four meta-analyses, but only based on data from four trials in total [48, 51, 53, 56]. Death-rates were low (e.g. 3% in azithromycin and 4% in the placebo group of Albert et al. [53]), again resulting in a lack of power. Although all of these trials had a relatively long follow-up of 12 months, this may still be too short for an effect of exacerbation reduction on mortality to become manifest.

Exacerbations negatively impact on quality of life [66]. Macrolide treatment may provide a small but statistically significant improvement, as measured by the mean difference in SGRQ-score. However, only in the pooled estimate of Janjua et al. [64] did the point estimate reach the minimal clinically important difference of four points [64], and this was mainly driven by the large effect size reported in Berkhof et al. [54] Yet, one can question if the mean difference in health status and quality of life estimates over the whole study population and study duration are the best estimators for the impact of AECOPD.

A pertinent question is how long prophylactic macrolide treatment should be continued. Except for the BACE trial, [45] all trials with a treatment duration of only 3 months failed to show a statistically significant reduction in exacerbations [49, 54, 57, 58]. Therefore, some authors state that 3 months of treatment is insufficient to gain benefit, and treatment should at least be continued for 6 to 12 months. This may not be the best conclusion. Except for the study with clarithromycin from Banerjee et al. [49], all point estimates for 3-month interventions favoured treatment. More likely, these trials were thus underpowered for the actual treatment effect to show significance over 3 months. What is interesting however, is that all studies with a follow-up longer than the treatment duration suggest a rapid loss of treatment effect when the intervention was stopped [45, 51, 58, 59]. Even in the trial of Blasi et al., where treatment was given for 6 months, the effect was not sustained long after treatment discontinuation [51]. This justifies longer interventions although no published trials have evaluated treatment duration of more than 12 months in a COPD population. No information is thus available on the possible waning of the effect when patients are treated for longer than 1 year. A pragmatic approach may be to continue treatment during periods with the highest risk of infectious exacerbations, for example, during the winter months, and introduce a short 'medication holiday' of 3–4 months during summer. Indirect evidence suggests that even a short therapy break may significantly reduce bacterial resistance (see below).

4 Adverse Effects

Macrolides are generally well tolerated, both for short- and long-term use. The adverse-effect profile of macrolides is well-known and includes mild gastrointestinal side effects, asymptomatic increase of transaminase levels, allergic reactions and drug eruptions and cholestatic jaundice in patients with underlying liver disease. A bitter metallic taste perception has been associated with clarithromycin. Irreversible hearing loss and tinnitus have been associated with erythromycin [69]. Azithromycin has equally been associated with hearing loss that was reversible when treatment was stopped [53]. Drug-drug interactions, mostly due to macrolide induction of hepatic enzymes, are frequent with clarithromycin and erythromycin but less so with azithromycin [69, 70]. The slightly better tolerability and safety profile is probably why most trials with long-term administration of macrolides have used azithromycin. As would be expected, increased odds of adverse events were shown in the pooled data of Ni et al. (odds ratio 1.55, 95% CI 1.00–2.39), [61] but only rarely led to discontinuation of treatment in these COPD-trials [48–52].

One of the most important concerns with long-term macrolide use, from a safety point of view, is probably cardiac toxicity, which is particularly relevant in this vulnerable population with multiple comorbidities and often polypharmacy. However, if macrolides reduce exacerbations, this may be accompanied by a decrease in the incidence of acute cardiovascular events, which are much more common in the peri-exacerbation period [10]. Macrolides affect cardiac delayed rectifier potassium current, which may cause prolongation of repolarization and arrhythmia [71]. Clinical data are conflicting, however, and a large meta-analysis found no increased risk of arrhythmia but rather a small increase in the risk of myocardial infarction, larger with erythromycin and clarithromycin than with azithromycin, for which the mechanism is not clear [71, 72]. In COPD specifically, many of the aforementioned trials reported cardiovascular adverse events but found no significant difference in their incidence in treated patients versus controls [61]. In the pooled analysis of Janjua et al., prophylactic antibiotic use was even associated with decreased odds of serious adverse events (SAE) (odds ratio 0.76, 95% CI 0.62 to 0.93), with the greatest probability of macrolides having the largest risk reduction [64]. Importantly, however, many patients included in these studies had frequent exacerbations. Also, a prolonged QT interval, concomitant use of other QT-prolonging drugs and cardiovascular comorbidity, in general, were very common exclusion criteria. The apparent positive benefit-harm balance may easily shift in populations with other baseline characteristics and with less careful patient selection. Performing an ECG before and during chronic macrolide treatment is advisable, as is a thorough review of medical history and medications for drug-drug interactions.

Increased bacterial resistance is likely with long-term macrolide use and long-term prophylactic antibiotic administration in general but it has been difficult to prove in COPD patients. Trials with both longer duration of therapy (e.g. Albert et al. [53], Seemungal et al. [50]) and shorter duration (e.g. Bril et al. [57]) reported increased resistance of potentially pathogenic microorganisms, while other studies even after 12 months of antibiotic treatment reported a decrease in resistant bacteria. This may be due to low sensitivity and specificity of cultured sputum or nasopharyngeal swabs, and the laboriousness and cost of more accurate techniques. Data about the persistence of resistance after treatment discontinuation in COPD is equally scarce. Indirect data from the AZISAST trial showed increased macrolide resistance of streptococci after 26 weeks of erythromycin treatment in asthma patients but a near halving of the resistant bacteria after a 4 weeks washout period [73]. This may suggest some benefit for a short discontinuation of prophylactic antibiotics, preferably during periods with a lower risk of infectious exacerbations. Despite the conflicting evidence, the concern of increased resistance remains and is clinically relevant both for the individual patient (colonization and overgrowth of resistant pathogens and response to antibiotic therapy during AECOPD) and for the population level. Again, this prompts careful consideration of risks and benefits before treatment is started. The presence of organisms for which macrolides are an essential part of treatment but against which macrolide resistance can emerge, such as atypical mycobacteria, should be tested and adequately treated before therapy is initiated [74].

5 Evidence Summary and Future Directions

Abundant clinical data confirms that macrolides can reduce healthcare utilization in COPD patients. Yet, only some patients are likely to benefit, and concerns about cardiovascular adverse effects and the development of bacterial resistance warrant prudent patient selection. The main body of evidence covers long-term macrolide treatment as antibiotic prophylaxis, with the highest level of evidence for azithromycin in daily or intermittent dosing and a reduced frequency of AECOPD as the key outcome measure. Trials mostly selected patients with a history of frequent exacerbations and excluded patients with important cardiovascular comorbidity, pre-existing QTc abnormalities or concomitant medications that augment the risk of QTc-prolongation. In this particular population, long-term macrolide use is safe and even associated with a reduction of non-respiratory serious adverse events. International guidelines, therefore, support long-term macrolide treatment in patients with moderate to severe airflow limitation, suffering from frequent exacerbations, despite maximal inhalation therapy and optimization of non-pharmacological management [8, 62, 74]. Patients should be screened for cardiovascular comorbidity, hearing impairment and NTM infection before treatment initiation. Follow-up ECG and regular reassessment of sputum cultures are recommended during continued administration. It is uncertain how long the effect from macrolide prophylaxis lasts, but at least it continues during 12 months of treatment, while disappearing quickly after treatment discontinuation. Short therapy holidays during periods with a lower risk of exacerbation may help to maintain a long-term benefit by reducing resistance development. For the treatment of AECOPD, macrolide monotherapy is not preferred over other antibiotic classes. However, severe hospitalized exacerbations with high inflammatory markers and without evidence of eosinophilia may be a good indication to start long-term prophylactic therapy in patients with prior exacerbations. Starting the macrolide as add-on to the standard exacerbation treatment may yield additional benefits in terms of in-hospital morbidity and readmission rates.

Most likely, prophylactic macrolides will only benefit a subset of frequent exacerbators, but identifying patients that are likely to respond is difficult. Guidelines advise assessing treatment effects after 6 to 12 months [74]. Treatable traits that could increase the likelihood of responding to macrolide treatment are co-existent bronchiectasis, *Pseudomonas* infection and repeated non-eosinophilic exacerbations. Greater efficacy is also suggested in older patients and non-smokers [75]. These data are indirect or observational. Another trait that has been considered a classic treatment indication is chronic bronchitis. Chronic bronchitis is a predictor of increased exacerbation frequency and worse outcomes [76]. Yet the point estimates of trials that have specifically targeted patients suffering from chronic cough and sputum production hardly differ, nor has a significant subgroup effect been shown in the largest post hoc analysis. Presumably, this is because chronic bronchitis lacks specificity as a clinical marker and may be related to both eosinophilic and neutrophilic inflammation [6].

Box 1 Practical guidance for macrolide use in COPD

During stable COPD [8, 62, 74]
Consider long-term therapy with azithromycin (or erythromycin) as prophylaxis to reduce the number of AECOPD – In patients with a recent history of frequent exacerbations (2 or more moderate or 1 severe hospitalized AECOPD), – Despite optimal bronchodilator therapy and optimal non-pharmacological management (influenza vaccination, COVID vaccination and pneumococcal-vaccination, rehabilitation), – Especially when evidence of repeated infectious exacerbations, pseudomonas colonization or bronchiectasis.
Prior to initiation of long-term azithromycin (or erythromycin) therapy
• A thorough review of the history of ischaemic vascular disease, heart disease, electrolyte disturbances, known prolonged QT interval should be performed. If present, carefully consider risk–benefit and discuss increased risk of adverse effects with patient.
• A thorough review of drug history to assess risk of drug-drug interactions and agents that may prolong QT interval should be performed and such medication should be stopped. Previous allergy or intolerance to macrolides should be assessed, and treatment should not be started if present.
• An ECG should be performed to assess QT interval, and treatment should not be started in patients with prolonged QTc (> 450 ms for men, >470 ms for women).
• Liver function tests and electrolyte assay should be performed.
• A sputum culture should be performed to test for NTM. When NTM is present, therapy should not be started until patient is successfully treated and NTM is eradicated.
• Hearing problems should be assessed, and audiometry should be considered.
• Potential adverse effects should be discussed with patient (gastrointestinal problems, hearing loss, cardiac adverse effects and bacterial resistance).
Supported treatment regimens (patient preferences should be taken into account) – Azithromycin 500 mg three times week. – Azithromycin 250 mg daily. – Azithromycin 250 mg every 2 days if intolerance for higher doses. – (erythromycin 200–250 mg twice daily)[a].
After treatment intitiation
• A repeat ECG should be considered in high-risk patients within 1 to 4 weeks to reassess the effect of macrolide therapy on QT interval and stop if QTc is prolonged.
• Surveillance cultures should be performed in patients with BRECT or at risk for NTM to assess development of bacterial resistance during long-term macrolide therapy.
• Regular follow-up of liver function tests and electrolyte disturbances is advised.
• Consider treatment holiday during periods with lower exacerbation risk (e.g. 3 month stop during summer months).
During AECOPD [8, 33, 35, 36]

If decided to treat with antibiotics (ICU-admission, moderate to severe exacerbation with suspected infectious origin and/or high risk of treatment failure)
• Adhere to local antibiotic guidelines; macrolides can be used for moderate exacerbations but are not preferred as monotherapy for severe exacerbations.
In patients already on long-term prophylaxis with macrolides
• Another antibiotic class should be chosen if decided to treat AECOPD with antibiotics,
• Macrolides should not be stopped during AECOPD if no other drugs with the potential risk of drug-drug interactions or QT-prolongation are started.
In patients with severe AECOPD not on long-term macrolide therapy and meeting the criteria for prophylaxis
• Starting macrolide therapy during the exacerbation as add-on therapy to standard of care and continue the prophylactic regimen should be considered.

[a]neomacrolides like azithromycin have better absorption, better safety profile, fewer drug-drug interactions compared with erythromycin

Identification of better clinical, radiological and biological markers of response to macrolide treatment remains a major gap in the evidence and an unmet clinical need. Presumably, such markers would be related to bacteria-induced airway damage and consequent neutrophilic inflammation through activation of T1 and T17-related pathways. The available data from randomized trials has been extensively explored, and subgroup and sensitivity analyses have been performed. Little additional inferences can be made with these classic statistical approaches without violating their underlying assumptions. Novel supervised machine learning approaches are able to further mine this existing data, and can identify complex and non-linear relationships [77, 78]. Yet, the depth of data collection is limited with regards to the recent evolution in the understanding of pathobiological processes driving COPD exacerbations and disease progression. Any hope to expand the array of biomarkers requires large prospective studies and extensive biobanking, particularly during exacerbations. Hypotheses generated from such initiatives, should be confirmed in randomized controlled studies with well-defined COPD subgroups [79].

Placebo-controlled trials with follow-up beyond 12 months, or with randomization after 1 year of macrolide treatment are necessary to assess if the effect of long-term treatment on exacerbations remains and how this affects the microbiome. Longer follow-up is also required to evaluate an effect on mortality.

Other future directions include variations on the formulations or on the molecular structure of the macrolide ring, yielding different pharmacokinetic and pharmacodynamic properties. Macrolides have pleiotropic immunomodulatory effects, but it remains unclear how this contributes to the final treatment effect and whether this affects non-infective AECOPD. In vitro and animal data have shown positive effects with macrolides modified to have enhanced immunomodulation but to be devoid of their antibacterial effects (e.g. EM703, EM900), both on viral and bacterial-induced inflammation [80–83]. This would reduce the concern for bacterial resistance. Inhalation of macrolides may be another strategy to optimize the gain while bypassing some of the systemic side effects. Contrary to cystic fibrosis and non-cystic fibrosis bronchiectasis, inhaled antibiotics in general remain largely unexplored in the treatment of COPD. Specifically for macrolides, in vitro and animal studies have demonstrated feasibility of formulating macrolides for inhalation, but no human trials have been performed to date [84–86].

6 Conclusion

Due to their combination of antibiotic and immunomodulatory effects, macrolides can be a valuable addition to the pharmacological management of severe COPD. Solid clinical evidence supports the long-term use of azithromycin and erythromycin in particular, to prevent AECOPD in patients with moderate to severe airflow limitation and a history of frequent exacerbations, despite maximal inhalation therapy and optimization of non-pharmacological management. Presumably, macrolides are the most effective and least expensive drugs to decrease hospital (re)- admission, but larger prospective intervention studies are needed to validate this. In addition, a better characterization of patient subgroups that are most likely to respond is necessary to optimize treatment gain and avoid unnecessary exposure to the adverse effects. Together with the development of novel macrolide derivatives, such as non-antibiotic molecules or inhaled formulations, this may improve the benefit-risk balance and expand future treatment indications.

Authors contributions and acknowledgements Conceptualization of the manuscript was done by WJ and IG. The manuscript was drafted by IG and edited by WJ. We thank Kristina Vermeersch to kindly provide unpublished graphical data from the BACE trial.

Compliance with ethical standards and conflicts of interest IG and WJ declare they have no financial interests that are relevant to the content of this article. IG and WJ are supported by Flemish Research Funds. WJ has received speaker and consultant honoraria from Astra Zeneca, Glaxo-SmithKline, Boerhinger, Chiesi and research funding from Astra Zeneca, Chiesi and PulmonX.

References

1. Agusti A, James CH. Update on the pathogenesis of chronic obstructive pulmonary disease. N Engl J Med. 2019;381(13):1248–56.
2. Quaderi SA, Hurst JR. The unmet global burden of COPD. Glob Heal Epidemiol Genomics. 2018;3:9–11.
3. Abbafati C, Abbas KM, Abbasi-Kangevari M, Abd-Allah F, Abdelalim A, Abdollahi M, et al. Global burden of 369 diseases and injuries in 204 countries and territories, 1990–2019: a systematic analysis for the global burden of disease study 2019. Lancet. 2020;396(10258):1204–22.

4. World Health Organization. Global health estimates: the top 10 causes of death [Internet]. 2019 [cited 2022 Jun 2]. Available from: https://www.who.int/news-room/fact-sheets/detail/the-top-10-causes-of-death
5. Zou J, Sun T, Song X, Liu YM, Lei F, Chen MM, et al. Distributions and trends of the global burden of COPD attributable to risk factors by SDI, age, and sex from 1990 to 2019: a systematic analysis of GBD 2019 data. Respir Res [Internet]. 2022;23(1, 1):–17. Available from: https://respiratory-research.biomedcentral.com/articles/10.1186/s12931-022-02011-y
6. David B, Bafadhel M, Koenderman L, De Soyza A. Eosinophilic inflammation in COPD: from an inflammatory marker to a treatable trait [internet]. Vol. 76, Thorax. BMJ Publishing Group Ltd; 2021 [cited 2022 Sep 9]. p. 188–95. Available from: https://thorax.bmj.com/content/76/2/188.
7. Tanabe N, Vasilescu DM, Kirby M, Coxson HO, Verleden SE, Vanaudenaerde BM, et al. Analysis of airway pathology in COPD using a combination of computed tomography and histology. :1–10. Available from: https://doi.org/10.1183/13993003.01245-2017.
8. Global Initiative for Chronic Obstructive Lung Disease. Global strategy for the diagnosis, management, and prevention of chronic obstructive pulmonary disease: 2022 Report 2022.
9. Rothnie KJ, Müllerová H, Smeeth L, Quint JK. Natural history of chronic obstructive pulmonary disease exacerbations in a general practice-based population with chronic obstructive pulmonary disease. Am J Respir Crit Care Med. 2018;198(4):464–71.
10. Donaldson GC, Hurst JR, Smith CJ, Hubbard RB, Wedzicha JA. Increased risk of myocardial infarction and stroke following exacerbation of COPD. Chest. 2010;137(5):1091–7.
11. Bafadhel M, McKenna S, Terry S, Mistry V, Reid C, Haldar P, et al. Acute exacerbations of chronic obstructive pulmonary disease: identification of biologic clusters and their biomarkers. Am J Respir Crit Care Med [Internet]. 2011 Sep 15 [cited 2021 Feb 4];184(6):662–71. Available from: http://www.atsjournals.org/doi/abs/10.1164/rccm.201104-0597OC
12. Sethi S, Evans N, Grant BJB, Murphy TF. New Strains of bacteria and exacerbations of chronic obstructive pulmonary disease. N Engl J Med [Internet]. 2002 Aug 15 [cited 2022 Aug 29];347(7):465–71. Available from: https://www.nejm.org/doi/10.1056/NEJMoa012561
13. Sethi S, Murphy TF. Infection in the pathogenesis and course of chronic obstructive pulmonary disease. N Engl J Med. 2008;359(22):2355.
14. Burr LD, Rogers GB, Chen ACH, Hamilton BR, Pool GF, Taylor SL, et al. Macrolide treatment inhibits pseudomonas aeruginosa quorum sensing in non-cystic fibrosis bronchiectasis: An analysis from the bronchiectasis and low-dose erythromycin study trial. Ann Am Thorac Soc [Internet]. 2016 Oct 1 [cited 2022 Sep 3];13(10):1697–703. Available from: www.atsjournals.org
15. Polverino E, Dimakou K, Hurst J, Martinez-Garcia MA, Miravitlles M, Paggiaro P, et al. The overlap between bronchiectasis and chronic airway diseases: state of the art and future directions. Eur Respir J [Internet]. 2018 Sep 1 [cited 2022 Sep 9];52(3):1800328. Available from: https://erj.ersjournals.com/content/52/3/1800328
16. Wang Z, Locantore N, Haldar K, Ramsheh MY, Beech AS, Ma W, et al. Inflammatory endotype-associated airway microbiome in chronic obstructive pulmonary disease clinical stability and exacerbations: a multicohort longitudinal analysis [Internet]. Vol. 203, American Journal of Respiratory and Critical Care Medicine. 2021. 1488–1502 p. Available from: https://doi.org/10.1164/rccm.202009-3448OC.
17. Sethi S, Murphy TF. Infection in the pathogenesis and course of chronic obstructive pulmonary disease. N Engl J Med [Internet]. 2008 Nov 27 [cited 2022 Aug 29];359(22):2355–65. Available from: https://www.nejm.org/doi/full/10.1056/nejmra0800353
18. Brightling C, Greening N. Airway inflammation in COPD: progress to precision medicine. Eur Respir J [Internet]. 2019 Aug 1 [cited 2022 Aug 29];54(2). Available from: https://erj.ersjournals.com/content/54/2/1900651
19. Contoli M, Pauletti A, Rossi MR, Spanevello A, Casolari P, Marcellini A, et al. Long-term effects of inhaled corticosteroids on sputum bacterial and viral loads in COPD. Eur Respir J

[Internet]. 2017 Oct 1 [cited 2022 Aug 29];50(4). Available from: https://erj.ersjournals.com/content/50/4/1700451
20. Parnham MJ, Haber VE, Giamarellos-Bourboulis EJ, Perletti G, Verleden GM, Vos R. Azithromycin: mechanisms of action and their relevance for clinical applications. Pharmacol Ther [Internet]. 2014;143(2):225–45. https://doi.org/10.1016/j.pharmthera.2014.03.003.
21. Slater M, Torr E, Harrison T, Forrester D, Knox A, Shaw D, et al. The differential effects of azithromycin on the airway epithelium in vitro and in vivo. Physiol Rep. 2016;4(18):1–15.
22. Stellari FF, Sala A, Donofrio G, Ruscitti F, Caruso P, Topini TM, et al. Azithromycin inhibits nuclear factor-KB activation during lung inflammation : an in vivo imaging study. Pharmacol Res Perspect. 2014;2(5):1–12.
23. Haydar D, Cory TJ, Birket SE, Brian S, Pennypacker KR, Sinai AP, et al. Azithromycin polarizes macrophages to an M2 phenotype via inhibition of the STAT1 and NF- κ B signaling pathways. J Immunol. 2019;203(4):1021–30.
24. Huckle AW, Fairclough LC, Ma IT. Prophylactic antibiotic use in copd and the potential anti-inflammatory activities of antibiotics. Respir Care. 2018;63(5):609–19.
25. Zimmermann P, Ziesenitz VC, Curtis N, Ritz N. The immunomodulatory effects of macrolides-a systematic review of the underlying mechanisms. Front Immunol [Internet]. 2018 Mar 13;9 (302) Available from: https://pubmed.ncbi.nlm.nih.gov/29593707
26. Bystrzycka W, Manda-handzlik A, Sieczkowska S, Moskalik A, Demkow U, Ciepiela O. Azithromycin and chloramphenicol diminish neutrophil extracellular traps (NETs) release. Int J Mol Sci. 2017;18(12):1–9.
27. Barnes PJ. New anti-inflammatory targets for chronic obstructive pulmonary disease. Nat Rev Drug Discov [Internet]. 2013 Jun 14 [cited 2022 Aug 24];12(7):543–59. Available from: https://www.nature.com/articles/nrd4025
28. Gyselinck I, Janssens W, Verhamme P, Vos R. Rationale for azithromycin in COVID-19: an overview of existing evidence. BMJ Open Respir Res. 2021;8(1):1–10.
29. Popp M, Stegemann M, Riemer M, Metzendorf MI, Romero CS, Mikolajewska A, et al. Antibiotics for the treatment of COVID-19. Cochrane Database Syst Rev [Internet] 2021 Oct 22 [cited 2022 Aug 30];2021(10). Available from: https://www.cochranelibrary.com/cdsr/doi/10.1002/14651858.CD015025/full
30. Gyselinck I, Liesenborghs L, Belmans A, Engelen MM, Betrains A, Van Thillo Q, et al. Azithromycin for treatment of hospitalised COVID-19 patients: a randomised, multicentre, open-label clinical trial (DAWn-AZITHRO). ERJ Open Res [Internet] 2022 Jan 1 [cited 2022 Aug 30];8(1). Available from: https://openres.ersjournals.com/content/8/1/00610-2021
31. Vollenweider DJ, Frei A, Steurer-Stey CA, Garcia-Aymerich J, Puhan MA. Antibiotics for exacerbations of chronic obstructive pulmonary disease. Cochrane Database Syst Rev. 2018;2018(10):CD010257.
32. Bafadhel M, McKenna S, Terry S, Mistry V, Pancholi M, Venge P, et al. Blood eosinophils to direct corticosteroid treatment of exacerbations of chronic obstructive pulmonary disease. [Internet]. 2012 Dec 14 [cited 2022 Sep 8];186(1):48–55. Available from: https://doi.org/10.1164/rccm201108-1553OC.; www.controlled-trials.com
33. Jacobs DM, Pandit U, Sethi S. Acute exacerbations in chronic obstructive pulmonary disease: should we use antibiotics and if so, which ones? [Internet]. Vol. 32, Current opinion in infectious diseases. Lippincott Williams and Wilkins; 2019 [cited 2022 Sep 5]. p. 143–151. Available from: https://journals-lww-com.kuleuven.e-bronnen.be/co-infectiousdiseases/Fulltext/2019/04000/Acute_exacerbations_in_chronic_obstructive.10.aspx
34. Hoult G, Gillespie D, Wilkinson TMA, Thomas M, Francis NA. Biomarkers to guide the use of antibiotics for acute exacerbations of COPD (AECOPD): a systematic review and meta-analysis. BMC Pulm Med [Internet] 2022 May 13 [cited 2022 Sep 5];22(1):1–16. Available from: https://bmcpulmmed.biomedcentral.com/articles/10.1186/s12890-022-01958-4
35. National Institute for Health and Clinical Excellence. Chronic obstructive pulmonary disease (acute exacerbation): antimicrobial prescribing. Natl Clin Guidel Cent. 2018;December

36. Wedzicha JA, Miravitlles M, Hurst JR, Calverley PMA, Albert RK, Anzueto A, et al. Management of COPD exacerbations: a European Respiratory Society/American Thoracic Society guideline. Eur Respir J [Internet]. 2017;50(4) https://doi.org/10.1183/13993003.00791-2016.
37. Bafadhel M, McKenna S, Terry S, Mistry V, Pancholi M, Venge P, et al. Blood eosinophils to direct corticosteroid treatment of exacerbations of chronic obstructive pulmonary disease: a randomized placebo-controlled trial. Am J Respir Crit Care Med. 2012;186(1):48–55.
38. Zhang HL, Tan M, Qiu AM, Tao Z, Wang CH. Antibiotics for treatment of acute exacerbation of chronic obstructive pulmonary disease: a network meta-analysis. BMC Pulm Med [Internet]. 2017 Dec 12 [cited 2022 Aug 24];17(1):1–11. Available from: https://bmcpulmmed.biomedcentral.com/articles/10.1186/s12890-017-0541-0
39. Dimopoulos G, Siempos IP, Korbila KG, Manta, Falagas ME. Comparison of first-line with second-line antibiotics for acute exacerbations of chronic bronchitis* A metaanalysis of randomized controlled trials. Chest [Internet]. [cited 2022 Aug 24];132:447–55. Available from: www.chestjournal.org
40. Siempos II, Dimopoulos G, Korbila IP, Manta K, Falagas ME. Macrolides, quinolones and amoxicillin/clavulanate for chronic bronchitis: a meta-analysis. Eur Respir J [Internet] 2007 Jun 1 [cited 2022 Sep 8];29(6):1127–1137. Available from: https://erj.ersjournals.com/content/29/6/1127.
41. Garin N, Genné D, Carballo S, Chuard C, Eich G, Hugli O, et al. β-Lactam monotherapy vs β-lactam–macrolide combination treatment in moderately severe community-acquired pneumonia: a randomized noninferiority trial. JAMA Intern Med [Internet] 2014 Dec 1 [cited 2022 Sep 8];174(12):1894–1901. Available from: https://jamanetwork.com/journals/jamainternalmedicine/fullarticle/1910547
42. Nie W, Li B, Xiu Q. β-Lactam/macrolide dual therapy versus β-lactam monotherapy for the treatment of community-acquired pneumonia in adults: a systematic review and meta-analysis. J Antimicrob Chemother [Internet]. 2014 Jun 1 [cited 2022 Sep 8];69(6):1441–6. Available from: https://academic.oup.com/jac/article/69/6/1441/835189
43. Kiser TH, Reynolds PM, Moss M, Burnham EL, Ho PM, Vandivier RW. Impact of macrolide antibiotics on hospital readmissions and other clinically important outcomes in critically Ill patients with acute exacerbations of chronic obstructive pulmonary disease: a propensity score–matched cohort study. Pharmacotherapy [Internet]. 2019 Mar 1 [cited 2022 Aug 24];39(3):242. Available from: /pmc/articles/PMC6445270/.
44. König R, Cao X, Oswald M, Forstner C, Rohde G, Rupp J, et al. Macrolide combination therapy for patients hospitalised with community-acquired pneumonia? An individualised approach supported by machine learning. Eur Respir J [Internet]. 2019;54(6) Available from::1900824. https://doi.org/10.1183/13993003.00824-2019.
45. Vermeersch K, Gabrivska M, Aumann J, Demedts IK, Corhay JL, Marchand E, et al. Azithromycin during acute chronic obstructive pulmonary disease exacerbations requiring hospitalization (BACE). A multicenter, randomized, double-blind, placebo-controlled trial. Am J Respir Crit Care Med. 2019;200(7):857–68.
46. Vermeersch K, Belmans A, Bogaerts K, Gyselinck I, Cardinaels N, Gabrovska M, et al. Treatment failure and hospital readmissions in severe COPD exacerbations treated with azithromycin versus placebo–a post-hoc analysis of the BACE randomized controlled trial. Respir Res. 2019;20(1):1–12.
47. Murdoch JMC, Leckie WJH, Downie J, Swain RHA. An evaluation of continuous antibiotic therapy in chronic bronchitis. Br Med J. 1959;2(5162):1277–85.
48. Suzuki T, Yanai M, Yamaya M, Satoh-Nakagawa T, Sekizawa K, Ishida S, et al. Erythromycin and common cold in COPD. Chest. 2001;120(3):730–3.
49. Banerjee D, Khair OA, Honeybourne D. The effect of oral clarithromycin on health status and sputum bacteriology in stable COPD. Respir Med. 2005;99(2):208–15.
50. Seemungal TAR, Wilkinson TMA, Hurst JR, Perera WR, Sapsford RJ, Wedzicha JA. Long-term erythromycin therapy is associated with decreased chronic obstructive pulmonary disease

exacerbations. Am J Respir Crit Care Med [Internet]. 2008 Dec 20 [cited 2022 Aug 25];178 (11):1139–47. Available from: www.clinicaltrials.gov
51. Blasi F, Bonardi D, Aliberti S, Tarsia P, Confalonieri M, Amir O, et al. Long-term azithromycin use in patients with chronic obstructive pulmonary disease and tracheostomy. Pulm Pharmacol Ther. 2010;23(3):200–7.
52. He ZY, Ou LM, Zhang JQ, Bai J, Liu GN, Li MH, et al. Effect of 6 months of erythromycin treatment on inflammatory cells in induced sputum and exacerbations in chronic obstructive pulmonary disease. Theatr Res Int 2010 Nov [cited 2022 Aug 25];80(6):445–452. Available from: https://www.karger.com/Article/FullText/321374
53. Albert RK, Connett J, Bailey WC, Casaburi R, Cooper AD, Criner GJ, et al. Azithromycin for prevention of exacerbations of COPD. N Engl J Med. 2011;365(8):689–98.
54. Berkhof FF, Hertog NED, Uil SM, Kerstjens HAM, van den Berg JWK. Azithromycin and cough-specific health status in patients with chronic obstructive pulmonary disease and chronic cough: a randomised controlled trial. Respir Res [Internet]. 2013 Nov 14 [cited 2022 Aug 22];14(1):125. Available from: /pmc/articles/PMC3835397/.
55. Simpson JL, Powell H, Baines KJ, Milne D, Coxson HO, Hansbro PM, et al. The effect of azithromycin in adults with stable neutrophilic COPD: a double blind randomised, placebo controlled trial. PLoS One [Internet] 2014 Aug 22 [cited 2022 Aug 23];9(8). Available from: /pmc/articles/PMC4141795/.
56. Uzun S, Djamin RS, Kluytmans JAJW, Mulder PGH, van't Veer NE, Ermens AAM, et al. Azithromycin maintenance treatment in patients with frequent exacerbations of chronic obstructive pulmonary disease (COLUMBUS): a randomised, double-blind, placebo-controlled trial. Lancet Respir Med [Internet]. 2014;2(5):361–8. Available from:. https://doi.org/10.1016/S2213-2600(14)70019-0.
57. Brill SE, Law M, El-Emir E, Allinson JP, James P, Maddox V, et al. Effects of different antibiotic classes on airway bacteria in stable COPD using culture and molecular techniques: a randomised controlled trial. Thorax [Internet] 2015 Oct 1 [cited 2022 Aug 22];70(10):930–938. Available from: /pmc/articles/PMC4602260/.
58. Shafuddin E, Mills GD, Holmes MD, Poole PJ, Mullins PR, Black PN. A double-blind, randomised, placebo-controlled study of roxithromycin and doxycycline combination, roxithromycin alone, or matching placebo for 12 weeks in adults with frequent exacerbations of chronic obstructive pulmonary disease. J Negat Results Biomed [Internet]. 2015 Sep 7 [cited 2022 Aug 23];14(1). Available from: /pmc/articles/PMC4562194/.
59. Tan C, Huang H, Zhang J, He Z, Zhong X, Bai J. Effects of Low-Dose and Long-Term Treatment with Erythromycin on Interleukin-17 and Interleukin-23 in Peripheral Blood and Induced Sputum in Patients with Stable Chronic Obstructive Pulmonary Disease. Mediators Inflamm [Internet]. 2016 [cited 2022 Aug 23];2016. Available from: /pmc/articles/PMC4834156/.
60. Wang P, Yang J, Yang Y, Ding Z. Effect of azithromycin in combination with simvastatin in the treatment of chronic obstructive pulmonary disease complicated by pulmonary arterial hypertension. Pakistan J Med Sci. 2017;33(2):260–4.
61. Ni W, Shao X, Cai X, Wei C, Cui J, Wang R, et al. Prophylactic use of macrolide antibiotics for the prevention of chronic obstructive pulmonary disease exacerbation: A meta-analysis. PLoS One [Internet]. 2015 Mar 26 [cited 2022 Aug 24];10(3). Available from: https://pubmed.ncbi.nlm.nih.gov/25812085/
62. Wedzicha JA, Calverley PMA, Albert RK, Anzueto A, Criner GJ, Hurst JR, et al. Prevention of COPD exacerbations: a European Respiratory Society/ American Thoracic Society guideline [internet]. Vol. 50, European Respiratory Journal European Respiratory Society; 2017 [cited 2022 Aug 30]. p. 1602265. Available from: https://erj.ersjournals.com/content/50/3/1602265.
63. Cui Y, Luo L, Li C, Chen P, Chen Y. Long-term macrolide treatment for the prevention of acute exacerbations in COPD: a systematic review and meta-analysis. Int J Chron Obstruct Pulmon Dis [Internet]. 2018 Nov 22 [cited 2022 Sep 12];13:3813–29. Available from: https://www.

dovepress.com/long-term-macrolide-treatment-for-the-prevention-of-acute-exacerbation-peer-reviewed-fulltext-article-COPD
64. Janjua S, Ag M, Fortescue R, Rae W, Sharif S, Cjd T, et al. Prophylactic antibiotics for adults with chronic obstructive pulmonary disease: a network meta-analysis (review). Cochrane Database Syst Rev. 2021;1
65. Han MK, Tayob N, Murray S, Dransfield MT, Washko G, Scanlon PD, et al. Predictors of chronic obstructive pulmonary disease exacerbation reduction in response to daily azithromycin therapy. Am J Respir Crit Care Med. 2014;189(12):1503–8.
66. Seemungal TAR, Donaldson GC, Paul EA, Bestall JC, Jeffries DJ, Wedzicha JA. Effect of exacerbation on quality of life in patients with chronic obstructive pulmonary disease. Am J Respir Crit Care Med [Internet]. 1998 [cited 2022 Sep 1];157(5 Pt 1):1418–22. Available from: https://pubmed.ncbi.nlm.nih.gov/9603117/
67. O'Reilly PJ, Jackson PL, Wells JM, Dransfield MT, Scanlon PD, Blalock JE. Sputum PGP is reduced by azithromycin treatment in patients with COPD and correlates with exacerbations. BMJ Open [Internet] 2013 Dec 1 [cited 2022 Aug 25];3(12):e004140. Available from: https://bmjopen.bmj.com/content/3/12/e004140
68. Naderi N, Assayag D, Mostafavi-Pour-Manshadi SMY, Kaddaha Z, Joubert A, Ouellet I, et al. Long-term azithromycin therapy to reduce acute exacerbations in patients with severe chronic obstructive pulmonary disease. Respir Med [Internet]. 2018 May 1 [cited 2022 Sep 14];138: 129–36. Available from: https://pubmed.ncbi.nlm.nih.gov/29724384/
69. Jain R, Danziger L. The macrolide antibiotics: a pharmacokinetic and Pharmacodynamic overview. Curr Pharm Des. 2005;10(25):3045–53.
70. Rubinstein E. Comparative safety of the different macrolides. Int J Antimicrob Agents. 2001;18 (18):71–6.
71. Hansen MP, Scott AM, Mccullough A, Thorning S, Aronson JK, Beller EM, et al. Adverse events in people taking macrolide antibiotics versus placebo for any indication. Cochrane Database Syst Rev [Internet] 2019 Jan 18 [cited 2022 Sep 3];1(1). Available from: https://pubmed.ncbi.nlm.nih.gov/30656650/
72. Gorelik E, Masarwa R, Perlman A, Rotshild V, Muszkat M, Matok I. Systematic review, meta-analysis, and network meta-analysis of the cardiovascular safety of macrolides. Antimicrob Agents Chemother [Internet]. 2018 Jun 1 [cited 2022 Sep 3];62(6). Available from:/pmc/articles/PMC5971614/.
73. Brusselle GG, VanderStichele C, Jordens P, Deman R, Slabbynck H, Ringoet V, et al. Azithromycin for prevention of exacerbations in severe asthma (AZISAST): a multicentre randomised double-blind placebo-controlled trial. Thorax. 2013;68(4):322–9.
74. Smith D, Du Rand I, Addy CL, Collyns T, Hart SP, Mitchelmore PJ, et al. British Thoracic Society guideline for the use of long-term macrolides in adults with respiratory disease. Thorax. 2020;75(5):370–404.
75. Yamaya M, Azuma A, Takizawa H, Kadota JI, Tamaoki J, Kudohe S. Macrolide effects on the prevention of COPD exacerbations. Eur Respir J [Internet]. 2012 Aug 1 [cited 2022 Nov 7];40 (2):485–494. Available from: https://erj.ersjournals.com/content/40/2/485.
76. Kim V, Criner GJ. Chronic bronchitis and chronic obstructive pulmonary disease. Am J Respir Crit Care Med. 2013;187(3):228–37.
77. Castaldi PJ, Boueiz A, Yun J, Estepar RSJ, Ross JC, Washko G, et al. Machine learning characterization of COPD subtypes. Chest. 2019;(February):1–11.
78. Gonem S, Janssens W, Das N, Topalovic M. Applications of artificial intelligence and machine learning in respiratory medicine, vol. 75. Thorax. BMJ Publishing Group; 2020. p. 695–701.
79. Mathioudakis AG, Janssens W, Sivapalan P, Singanayagam A, Dransfield MT, Jensen JUS, et al. Acute exacerbations of chronic obstructive pulmonary disease: in search of diagnostic biomarkers and treatable traits. Thorax. 2020;75(6):520–7.
80. Kalonji NL, Nomura K, Kawase T, Ota C, Kubo H, Sato T, et al. The non-antibiotic macrolide EM900 inhibits rhinovirus infection and cytokine production in human airway epithelial cells.

Physiol Rep [Internet]. 2015 Oct 1 [cited 2022 Sep 12];3(10):e12557. Available from: https://onlinelibrary.wiley.com/doi/full/10.14814/phy2.12557

81. Sugawara A, Sueki A, Hirose T, Nagai K, Gouda H, Hirono S, et al. Novel 12-membered non-antibiotic macrolides from erythromycin A; EM900 series as novel leads for anti-inflammatory and/or immunomodulatory agents. Bioorg Med Chem Lett [Internet]. 2011 Apr 7 [cited 2022 Sep 12];21(11):3373–6. Available from: https://europepmc.org/article/med/21524580
82. Kasetty G, Bhongir RKV, Papareddy P, Herwald H, Egesten A. The nonantibiotic macrolide em703 improves survival in a model of quinolone-treated pseudomonas aeruginosa airway infection. Antimicrob Agents Chemother [Internet]. 2017 Sep 1 [cited 2022 Sep 12];61(9). Available from: https://journals.asm.org/doi/10.1128/AAC.02761-16
83. Gouda H, Sunazuka T, Yoshida K, Sugawara A, Sakoh Y, Omura S, et al. Three-dimensional solution structure of EM703 with potent promoting activity of monocyte-to-macrophage differentiation. Bioorg Med Chem Lett [Internet]. 2006 May 1 [cited 2022 Sep 12];16(9):2496–9. Available from: https://pubmed.ncbi.nlm.nih.gov/16480872/
84. Arauzo B, Lopez-Mendez TB, Lobera MP, Calzada-Funes J, Pedraz JL, Santamaria J. Excipient-free inhalable microparticles of azithromycin produced by electrospray: a novel approach to direct pulmonary delivery of antibiotics. Pharmaceutics [Internet] 2021 Dec 1 [cited 2022 Sep 9];13(12). Available from: https://pubmed.ncbi.nlm.nih.gov/34959270/
85. Manniello MD, Del Gaudio P, Aquino RP, Russo P. Clarithromycin and N-acetylcysteine co-spray-dried powders for pulmonary drug delivery: a focus on drug solubility. Int J Pharm. 2017;533(2):463–9.
86. Siekmeier R, Hofmann T, Scheuch G. Inhalation of Macrolides: A Novel Approach to Treatment of Pulmonary Infections. Adv Exp Med Biol [Internet]. 2015;839:13–24. Available from: https://link.springer.com/chapter/10.1007/5584_2014_50

Macrolides and Asthma Therapy

Krishna Undela, Adil Adatia, Brian H. Rowe, and Giovanni Ferrara

Abstract Asthma is a chronic condition of the airways that is typified by bronchial hyperresponsiveness, variable airflow obstruction, and airway inflammation. Most patients can achieve disease control using inhaled corticosteroids, with some needing adjunct long-acting bronchodilator therapy. However, an important minority of patients have persistent symptoms and exacerbations despite these treatments. The landmark AMAZES study showed that the macrolide azithromycin significantly reduced the exacerbation rate in this population, using a randomized parallel group design. The efficacy of macrolides in chronic asthma was recently confirmed in a Cochrane systematic review, which analyzed 25 randomized controlled trials with a total of 1973 patients. Mechanistic studies have shown that this therapeutic effect is mediated by reduced mucosal inflammation, improved airway mucus clearance, and favorable modulation of host-pathogen interactions.

Keywords Macrolides · Acute asthma · Chronic asthma · Bacterial resistance · Asthma exacerbation

1 Introduction

Asthma is one of the most common respiratory diseases in all age groups, affecting 1–18% of the general population in different countries. The incidence of asthma has been increasing over the past several decades [1]. Asthma is characterized by airway

K. Undela
Department of Pharmacy Practice, National Institute of Pharmaceutical Education and Research (NIPER) Guwahati, Kamrup, Assam, India

A. Adatia · G. Ferrara (✉)
Division of Pulmonary Medicine, Department of Medicine, Faculty of Medicine & Dentistry, College of Health Sciences, University of Alberta, Edmonton, AB, Canada
e-mail: ferrara@ualberta.ca

B. H. Rowe
Department of Emergency Medicine, Faculty of Medicine & Dentistry and School of Public Health, both in the College of Health Sciences, University of Alberta, Edmonton, AB, Canada

B. K. Rubin, M. Shinkai (eds.), *Macrolides as Immunomodulatory Agents*, Progress in Inflammation Research 92, https://doi.org/10.1007/978-3-031-42859-3_7

inflammation, leading to variable symptoms, often in the form of exacerbations, comprising wheezing, shortness of breath, chest tightness, and cough. A hallmark of asthma is variable and reversible expiratory airflow limitation, which is also diagnostic for this condition, although patients with untreated asthma may develop fixed airflow limitation over time [2].

Airway inflammation in asthma can be subclassified based on the presence or absence of type 2 (T2) immune signature. Asthma with elevated T2 immune response (T2-high asthma) is characterized by excessive expression of the cytokines including interleukin (IL)-4, IL-5, and IL-13, and the alarmins thymic stromal lymphopoietin (TSLP), IL-25, and IL-33. Patients with T2-high asthma typically have elevated fractional exhaled nitric oxide measurements, blood and sputum eosinophils, and/or serum immunoglobulin E (IgE). Patients with T2-low asthma are generally identified as those in whom such markers of a T2 immune signature are absent [3].

The main approach to treat asthma and prevent exacerbations is to treat airway inflammation with inhaled corticosteroids (ICS) beginning in the earliest phases of the condition, although the frequency and dosing of this treatment depend on disease severity and symptom burden. Additionally, inhaled short-acting beta 2 agonists (SABA), long-acting beta 2 agonists (LABA) and long-acting muscarinic antagonists (LAMA) can be added to treat persistent or severe airflow limitation and symptoms [1].

The current Global Initiative for Asthma (GINA) guidelines provide guidance on how to diagnose asthma and how to treat patients experiencing different levels of severity by sequentially introducing and increasing the dosage and combination of asthma controller medications [1]. While ICS agents, often combined with LABAs and LAMAs, and novel treatments (e.g., leukotriene receptor antagonists [LTRA], biologic agents) have improved the lives of people living with the disease, symptom control has been elusive for some patients. Despite the progress achieved over the last 30 years, asthma morbidity and mortality remain a problem for national healthcare systems [4, 5]. Moreover, several questions and challenges still exist in the management of patients with asthma, especially in low- and middle-income countries.

First, asthma can present with a variety of clinical phenotypes and variable severity, and, often, inhaled drugs are unavailable or fail to achieve asthma control. In such cases, oral corticosteroids and, in patients with T2-high asthma, biologics targeting T2 inflammation such as IgE, IL-5/5R, IL-4alpha (which inhibits IL-4 and IL-13 signaling), or TSLP may be required [1, 2]. These severe cases account for a significant proportion of asthma-related morbidity and costs [6, 7], and often biologics are unavailable or prohibitively expensive [8]. Second, even inhalers are not always easy to use, especially for children and elderly patients, contributing to the main problem of nonadherence to treatment and suboptimal asthma control [9].

Therefore, there is still a need for new treatment modalities, and macrolide antibiotics have been investigated for several decades, thanks to their interesting properties [10]. Macrolides were initially investigated as potential corticosteroid-sparing agents [11]. Later, the possibility that asthma inflammation and asthma exacerbations could be sustained by intracellular pathogens such as *Chlamydia pneumoniae* triggered interest in testing macrolides in patients with asthma [12, 13]. Finally, a well-designed, well-powered, and well-executed randomized controlled trial (RCT) demonstrated the benefit of treating with azithromycin to reduce asthma exacerbations in patients with moderate-severe asthma [14]. In this chapter, we reviewed the mechanisms behind the effect of macrolides in asthma, and the evidence for their use in acute and chronic forms of asthma.

2 Mechanisms of Action of Macrolides in Asthma

The mechanisms of macrolide therapy in asthma are incompletely understood. Myriad bioactive properties of macrolides have been described and are thought to contribute to their therapeutic effects including the modulation of mucosal inflammation, airway mucus, host-pathogen interactions, and gastrointestinal motility. Please refer to Fig. 1 for summary.

2.1 *Anti-inflammatory and Immunomodulatory Effects*

Macrolides have been shown in multiple small studies to attenuate eosinophilic and neutrophilic airway inflammation in T2-high and T2-low asthma, respectively

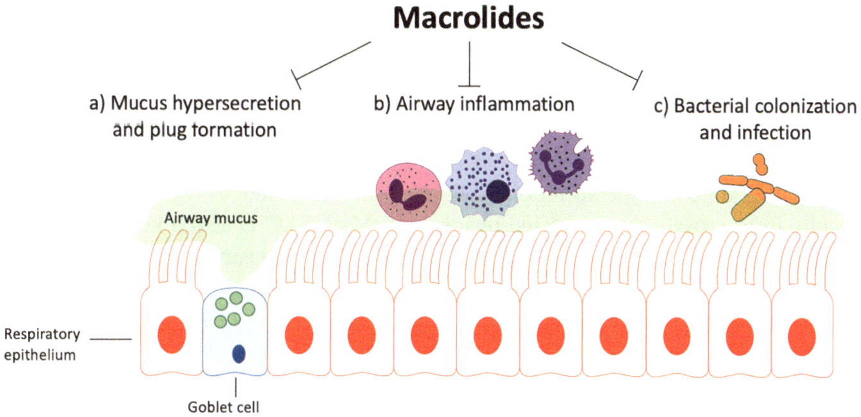

Fig. 1 Mechanisms of macrolides in asthma. Macrolides (**a**) reduce mucus hypersecretion and plug formation by inhibiting IL13-induced goblet cell hyperplasia and mucin glycoprotein MUC5AC production, (**b**) modulate airway inflammation by downregulating inflammatory cytokines (e.g., IL-1β, IL-6) and augmenting neutrophil efferocytosis, (**c**) reduce airway microbial diversity by inhibiting *Haemophilus* spp. and, in colonized patients, blocking biofilm growth of Pseudomonas aeruginosa by interrupting quorum sensing, and (**d**) may reduce asthma symptoms due to gastroesophageal reflux by increasing gastrointestinal motility (not shown). *IL* interleukin

[15]. For example, a small RCT of clarithromycin in T2-low asthma demonstrated a reduction in the neutrophil chemoattractant IL-8 (chemokine (C-X-C motif) ligand 8, CXCL8) and total neutrophils found in sputum. Conversely, in the landmark AMAZES trial [14], a large randomized parallel-group study, azithromycin significantly reduced exacerbation rates with no apparent reduction in sputum eosinophil or neutrophil abundance. Thus, the clinical effects of azithromycin do not appear to be mediated by the amelioration of luminal granulocyte infiltration, although the sputum analysis methods used may not have fully captured the airway inflammatory endotype [16].

Azithromycin has been shown to downregulate inflammatory cytokines in the airway including IL-1β, IL-6, and extracellular DNA [17]. The decrease in sputum extracellular DNA is of particular interest given the emerging role of neutrophil extracellular traps (which are comprised of DNA, histones, and granular proteins) in asthma with sputum neutrophilia [18]. Azithromycin also augments the phagocytic function of alveolar macrophages. It promotes efferocytosis of neutrophils [19] and bronchial epithelial cells [20], and it enhances the phagocytosis of bacteria [21]. Creola bodies, which are clusters of apoptotic epithelial cells, are readily identified in sputa of patients with asthma, and their efficient clearance is important for the control of airway inflammation [22].

2.2 *Effects on Airway Secretions*

Macrolides appear to have significant beneficial effects on airway secretions. Mucus hypersecretion and altered mucus composition are well-established pathologic features of asthma [23], and recent studies have clearly demonstrated that luminal mucus plugging is a major contributor to chronic airflow obstruction in patients with asthma [24, 25]. Macrolides are partial antagonists of neutrophil elastase [26], a neutrophil granule protease that induces mucin glycoprotein MUC5AC production by goblet cells [27], and inhibiting IL13-induced goblet cell hyperplasia [28], thus attenuating mucus hypersecretion [29]. The increased mucus viscoelasticity that results from crosslinking cysteine residues on MUC5AC is also a key mechanism of mucus plug formation in asthma [24], so it is plausible that azithromycin additionally reduces luminal mucus plugging.

2.3 *Antimicrobial Effects*

Macrolides are bacteriostatic antibiotics that block protein synthesis by inhibiting the 50S ribosomal subunit. Azithromycin and clarithromycin are active against gram-positive, gram-negative, and atypical respiratory pathogens including *Streptococcus pneumoniae, Haemophilus* spp., *Mycoplasma pneumoniae, and Chlamydophila pneumoniae* [30]. Chronic azithromycin does not reduce the total bacterial load in patients with asthma, but it does decrease respiratory microbial diversity, particularly by greatly reducing the abundance of *Haemophilus* spp. [31]. This reduction in *Haemophilus* spp. is likely clinically important given that a) the baseline abundance of *Haemophilus influenzae* in sputum appears to predict the efficacy of azithromycin [32] and b) the reduction of *Haemophilus influenzae* is associated with a reduction in pro-inflammatory cytokines, especially in patients with noneosinophilic asthma [17]. Such antimicrobial effects of macrolides are likely to play a larger role in patients predisposed to recurrent infective exacerbations such as those with comorbid primary ciliary dyskinesia and immunodeficiencies [33–35].

Azithromycin also inhibits biofilm growth of *Pseudomonas aeruginosa* by interrupting quorum sensing, the process by which bacteria modulate gene expression in response to population density [36], and by impairing twitching motility, which facilitates the formation of cell aggregates [37]. These mechanisms are thought to partly underlie the benefit of azithromycin in cystic fibrosis and noncystic fibrosis bronchiectasis [38]. Comorbid bronchiectasis and attendant *Pseudomonas* colonization is common in severe asthma [39, 40], and recent studies demonstrated that severe asthma cohorts have a significantly increased pathogenic cystic fibrosis transmembrane conductance regulator (*CFTR*) allele frequency [41, 42], suggesting a possible disease-modifying effect. Hence, the inhibition of biofilm development may be an important mechanism in such patients.

2.4 Effects on Gastrointestinal Motility

Azithromycin and erythromycin ligate the motilin receptor, resulting in increased gastrointestinal motility. Though generally viewed as an adverse off target effect (that causes diarrhea in an important minority of patients), some authors have argued that the increased gastrointestinal motility treats unrecognized gastroesophageal reflux disease (GERD) that triggers asthma symptoms and hence improves asthma control [43]. The role of GERD in triggering asthma symptoms is controversial, and a recent Cochrane review failed to demonstrate that the treatment of GERD significantly improves asthma outcomes [44]. It is plausible, nonetheless, that in a subset of patients, such as those with obesity, this mechanism plays a role.

3 Evidence of Macrolide Treatment Effectiveness

3.1 Acute Asthma

In general, acute asthma exacerbations are the result of exposures to airway irritants (i.e., air pollution, indoor fumes, viruses, environmental allergens, etc.) and/or loss of control due to management nonadherence. Consequently, the focus of treatment in acute asthma is an aggressive approach to reversing the inflammatory cause of the exacerbation. For example, acute severe exacerbations are treated with SABA and short-acting anticholinergic (SAAC) agents, [45] systemic [46] and inhaled corticosteroids [47], and intravenous magnesium sulfate [46]. Since most patients respond to treatment and can avoid admission to hospital, current guidelines recommend the use of systemic [46] and inhaled corticosteroids [47] for all discharged patients and strategies to avoid triggers.

Since bacterial infections are thought to play a negligible role in most acute exacerbations, current guidance recommends against the universal use of antibiotics and restricts their use to cases where there are signs, symptoms, or investigations that confirm a bacterial infection. Despite these recommendations, these therapeutic agents remain prescribed in the management of patients with acute asthma. The anti-inflammatory mechanism of action of macrolides has the potential to contribute to the management of acute asthma and hence the interest in exploring the evidence.

The evidence base for this approach arises from a Cochrane systematic review that was last updated in 2018 involving 6 studies and 681 adults and children with exacerbations of asthma [48]. Importantly, most studies explicitly excluded patients with signs/symptoms of a bacterial infection. Four of the six studies involved macrolides and comparisons were made to standard of care or placebo. Overall, there was significant among-study heterogeneity, poor outcome reporting, and the evidence was imprecise. The authors concluded that there was insufficient evidence to support the use of antibiotics in adults and children with exacerbations of asthma.

An important issue to consider when prescribing antibiotics are the adverse effects such as gastrointestinal side effects, antibiotic-induced diarrhea, rash, and other allergies. The RCTs included in the systematic review reported adverse effects over the short-term and found no difference between those receiving antibiotics and those who did not. These results are imprecise and of low quality.

Given this evidence, in patients experiencing an exacerbation of asthma, we support an approach of seeking confirmation of bacterial infection and treating those patients with antibiotics. In the absence of clear bacterial infection, we recommend maximizing the anti-inflammatory management of all patients experiencing an exacerbation of asthma using systemic [46] and inhaled corticosteroids [47]. Finally, antibiotics might be a reasonable alternative in cases where patients have not fully recovered from their asthma symptoms following aggressive anti-inflammatory treatment.

3.2 Chronic Asthma

The use of macrolides for the management of chronic asthma has been a vigorously debated topic for the past three decades. Preliminary studies on macrolides in people with asthma have suggested a steroid-sparing effect [11, 49], while later reports have demonstrated an anti-inflammatory effect of this class of antibiotics, whereby macrolides also seem to decrease bronchial hyperresponsiveness associated with eosinophilic inflammation [50–53]. Recent studies have identified the effects of macrolides on various clinical outcomes of asthma, such as exacerbations requiring hospitalization, emergency department (ED) visits, use of systemic corticosteroids [54, 55], symptoms, asthma control, quality of life [56, 57], change in rescue medication [58, 59], and/or lung function tests such as forced expiratory volume in 1 second (FEV_1) and peak expiratory flow (PEF) [54, 55, 57, 59].

Most RCTs have evaluated the efficacy of azithromycin [14, 52, 54, 57, 58, 60–63], followed by clarithromycin [50, 51, 53, 59, 62, 64, 65], roxithromycin [66–69], and oleandomycin [11, 49]. A well-designed RCT (AMAZES study) with a large sample size of well-selected participants identified that azithromycin 500 mg three times weekly for 48 weeks reduced asthma exacerbations and improved the quality of life of adults with symptomatic asthma despite the current use of moderate-to-high doses ICS and LABA therapy [14]. In another RCT, children aged 1–3 years with recurrent asthma-like symptoms responded positively to a 3-day course of an azithromycin oral solution (10 mg/kg per day). The mean duration of episodes of asthma-like symptoms after treatment with azithromycin was 3.4 days compared with 7.7 days for children receiving placebo. Evidence suggests that the effect increases with early initiation of therapy [70]. An RCT conducted to evaluate the effect of 16 weeks of clarithromycin in addition to fluticasone in adults with mild-to-moderate persistent asthma suboptimally controlled with low-dose ICS agents alone demonstrated no beneficial effect on asthma control or lung function when clarithromycin was added to fluticasone. A significant reduction in airway hyperresponsiveness, however, was observed with clarithromycin treatment in this study [59].

The most recent Cochrane systematic review on macrolides for chronic asthma included 25 RCTs and involved 1973 patients. The primary findings were that macrolides likely reduce exacerbations requiring hospitalizations, ED visits, and/or treatment with systemic corticosteroids compared with placebo, and may reduce asthma symptoms, resulting in slightly improved asthma control [10]. Another systematic review of three RCTs identified that children treated with macrolides had a significantly lower time to symptom resolution and a decrease in the severity of symptoms than controls. No difference was detected, however, in hospitalization and time to the next exacerbation between groups [71].

Overall, the current evidence suggests that macrolides provide a potential benefit to patients with moderate-severe asthma. International guidelines and consensus statements suggest adding azithromycin if a patient has persistent, uncontrolled asthma despite high-dose ICS and LABA therapy, as an alternative to biologics [1, 72, 73]. Hence, macrolide therapy may be especially useful in resource limited settings where biologics are not widely available. Macrolide therapy is also one of the only evidence-based treatments available for patients with T2-low asthma who do not adequately respond to high-dose ICS, LABA, and LAMA treatment and is thus widely used in this patient population [74].

4 Conclusions

Macrolides have been investigated in different asthma populations and in different clinical settings. There is no convincing evidence for the use of macrolides to treat acute asthma exacerbations in the absence of concurrent bacterial infection. Conversely, a large, well-designed RCT in chronic asthma clearly demonstrated that azithromycin reduces asthma exacerbation rates in patients who are inadequately controlled despite ICS and LABA therapy [14]. This finding was confirmed by a Cochrane systematic review [10] and a meta-analysis of individual patient data [75].

International guidelines and position statements recommend considering chronic azithromycin therapy in uncontrolled patients already treated with high-dose ICS and LABA therapies as an alternative to biologics [1, 72, 73]. Hence, it may be particularly useful in resource-constrained healthcare settings where the cost of biologics is prohibitive. Macrolides are generally considered to be safe, although this aspect has not been widely studied in resource-limited settings where older classes of drugs (e.g., digoxin) are still widely used.

Chronic use of antibiotics may increase the development of antibiotic-resistant bacterial strains that cause respiratory and systemic infections. Whether the use of macrolides for the treatment of asthma aggravate this problem, particularly in areas where antibiotic resistance is already a serious issue, is a question that needs to be addressed with properly designed studies and surveillance strategies. A clear risk/benefit assessment and strict patient selection criteria for the use of macrolides in chronic asthma are paramount to secure individual benefit and to avoid potential detrimental consequences for the patient and the community.

Ethical Approval This article does not contain any studies with human participants or animals performed by any of the authors.

Conflict of Interest All authors declare they have no conflict of interest.

References

1. Global Initiative for Asthma. Global Strategy for Asthma Management and Prevention (Updated 2022). Available at ginasthma.org
2. Papi A, Brightling C, Pedersen SE, Reddel HK. Asthma. Lancet (London, England). 2018;391 (10122):783–800.
3. Adatia A, Vliagoftis H. Challenges in severe asthma: do we need new drugs or new biomarkers? Front Med. 2022;9:921967.
4. Engelkes M, de Ridder MA, Svensson E, Berencsi K, Prieto-Alhambra D, Lapi F, et al. Multinational cohort study of mortality in patients with asthma and severe asthma. Respir Med. 2020;165:105919.
5. Shaw DE, Gaynor CM, Fogarty AW. Changes in asthma mortality in England and Wales since 2001. Thorax. 2019;74(12):1174–5.

6. Jansson SA, Backman H, Andersson M, Telg G, Lindberg A, Stridsman C, et al. Severe asthma is related to high societal costs and decreased health related quality of life. Respir Med. 2020;162:105860.
7. Janson C, Lisspers K, Ställberg B, Johansson G, Telg G, Thuresson M, et al. Health care resource utilization and cost for asthma patients regularly treated with oral corticosteroids–a Swedish observational cohort study (PACEHR). Respir Res. 2018;19(1):168.
8. Caminati M, Morais-Almeida M, Bleecker E, Ansotegui I, Canonica GW, Bovo C, et al. Biologics and global burden of asthma: a worldwide portrait and a call for action. World Allergy Org J. 2021;14(2):100502.
9. Usmani OS, Lavorini F, Marshall J, Dunlop WCN, Heron L, Farrington E, et al. Critical inhaler errors in asthma and COPD: a systematic review of impact on health outcomes. Respir Res. 2018;19(1):10.
10. Undela K, Goldsmith L, Kew KM, Ferrara G. Macrolides versus placebo for chronic asthma. Cochrane Database Syst Rev. 2021;11(11):Cd002997.
11. Nelson HS, Hamilos DL, Corsello PR, Levesque NV, Buchmeier AD, Bucher BL. A double-blind study of troleandomycin and methylprednisolone in asthmatic subjects who require daily corticosteroids. Am Rev Respir Dis. 1993;147(2):398–404.
12. Kraft M, Cassell GH, Henson JE, Watson H, Williamson J, Marmion BP, et al. Detection of mycoplasma pneumoniae in the airways of adults with chronic asthma. Am J Respir Crit Care Med. 1998;158(3):998–1001.
13. Gencay M, Rüdiger JJ, Tamm M, Solér M, Perruchoud AP, Roth M. Increased frequency of chlamydia pneumoniae antibodies in patients with asthma. Am J Respir Crit Care Med. 2001;163(5):1097–100.
14. Gibson PG, Yang IA, Upham JW, Reynolds PN, Hodge S, James AL, et al. Effect of azithromycin on asthma exacerbations and quality of life in adults with persistent uncontrolled asthma (AMAZES): a randomised, double-blind, placebo-controlled trial. Lancet. 2017;390(10095):659–68.
15. Zimmermann P, Ziesenitz VC, Curtis N, Ritz N. The immunomodulatory effects of macrolides-a systematic review of the underlying mechanisms. Front Immunol. 2018;9:302.
16. Kjarsgaard M, Adatia A, Bhalla A, LaVigne N, Radford K, Huang C, et al. Underestimation of airway luminal eosinophilia by quantitative sputum cytometry. Allergy Asthma Clin Immunol. 2021;17(1):63.
17. Shukla SD, Taylor SL, Gibson PG, Barker D, Upham JW, Yang IA, et al. Add-on azithromycin reduces sputum cytokines in non-eosinophilic asthma: an AMAZES substudy. Thorax. 2021;76(7):733–6.
18. Twaddell SH, Baines KJ, Grainge C, Gibson PG. The emerging role of neutrophil extracellular traps in respiratory disease. Chest. 2019;156(4):774–82.
19. Yamaryo T, Oishi K, Yoshimine H, Tsuchihashi Y, Matsushima K, Nagatake T. Fourteen-member macrolides promote the phosphatidylserine receptor-dependent phagocytosis of apoptotic neutrophils by alveolar macrophages. Antimicrob Agents Chemother. 2003;47(1):48–53.
20. Hodge S, Hodge G, Brozyna S, Jersmann H, Holmes M, Reynolds PN. Azithromycin increases phagocytosis of apoptotic bronchial epithelial cells by alveolar macrophages. Eur Respir J. 2006;28(3):486–95.
21. Hodge S, Reynolds PN. Low-dose azithromycin improves phagocytosis of bacteria by both alveolar and monocyte-derived macrophages in chronic obstructive pulmonary disease subjects. Respirology (Carlton, Vic). 2012;17(5):802–7.
22. Penberthy KK, Juncadella IJ, Ravichandran KS. Apoptosis and engulfment by bronchial epithelial cells. Implications for allergic airway inflammation. Ann Am Thorac Soc. 2014;11(Suppl 5):S259–62.
23. Fahy JV, Dickey BF. Airway mucus function and dysfunction. N Engl J Med. 2010;363(23):2233–47.

24. Dunican EM, Elicker BM, Gierada DS, Nagle SK, Schiebler ML, Newell JD, et al. Mucus plugs in patients with asthma linked to eosinophilia and airflow obstruction. J Clin Invest. 2018;128 (3):997–1009.
25. Tang M, Elicker BM, Henry T, Gierada DS, Schiebler ML, Huang BK, et al. Mucus plugs persist in asthma, and changes in mucus plugs associate with changes in airflow over time. Am J Respir Crit Care Med. 2022;205(9):1036–45.
26. Gorrini M, Lupi A, Viglio S, Pamparana F, Cetta G, Iadarola P, et al. Inhibition of human neutrophil elastase by erythromycin and flurythromycin, two macrolide antibiotics. Am J Respir Cell Mol Biol. 2001;25(4):492–9.
27. Shao MX, Nadel JA. Neutrophil elastase induces MUC5AC mucin production in human airway epithelial cells via a cascade involving protein kinase C, reactive oxygen species, and TNF-alpha-converting enzyme. J Immunol. 2005;175(6):4009–16.
28. Nagashima A, Shinkai M, Shinoda M, Shimokawaji T, Kimura Y, Mishina K, et al. Clarithromycin suppresses Chloride Channel accessory 1 and inhibits Interleukin-13-induced goblet cell hyperplasia in human bronchial epithelial cells. Antimicrob Agents Chemother. 2016;60(11):6585–90.
29. Shimizu T, Shimizu S. Azithromycin inhibits mucus hypersecretion from airway epithelial cells. Mediat Inflamm. 2012;2012:265714.
30. Davidson RJ. In vitro activity and pharmacodynamic/pharmacokinetic parameters of clarithromycin and azithromycin: why they matter in the treatment of respiratory tract infections. Infect Drug Resist. 2019;12:585–96.
31. Taylor SL, Leong LEX, Mobegi FM, Choo JM, Wesselingh S, Yang IA, et al. Long-term azithromycin reduces Haemophilus influenzae and increases antibiotic resistance in severe asthma. Am J Respir Crit Care Med. 2019;200(3):309–17.
32. Taylor SL, Ivey KL, Gibson PG, Simpson JL, Rogers GB. Airway abundance of Haemophilus influenzae predicts response to azithromycin in adults with persistent uncontrolled asthma. Eur Respir J. 2020;56(4):2000194.
33. Gibson PG, McDonald VM, Granchelli A, Olin JT. Asthma and comorbid conditions-pulmonary comorbidity. J Allergy Clin Immunol Pract. 2021;9(11):3868–75.
34. Petrov AA, Adatia A, Jolles S, Nair P, Azar A, Walter JE. Antibody deficiency, chronic lung disease, and comorbid conditions: a case-based approach. J Allergy Clin Immunol Pract. 2021;9 (11):3899–908.
35. Adatia A, Allen CJ, Wald J, Richards CD, Waserman S, Nair P. Benralizumab for prednisone-dependent eosinophilic asthma associated with novel STAT3 loss of function mutation. Chest. 2021;159(4):e181–e4.
36. Hoffmann N, Lee B, Hentzer M, Rasmussen TB, Song Z, Johansen HK, et al. Azithromycin blocks quorum sensing and alginate polymer formation and increases the sensitivity to serum and stationary-growth-phase killing of Pseudomonas aeruginosa and attenuates chronic P. aeruginosa lung infection in Cftr(−/−) mice. Antimicrob Agents Chemother. 2007;51(10): 3677–87.
37. Nalca Y, Jansch L, Bredenbruch F, Geffers R, Buer J, Haussler S. Quorum-sensing antagonistic activities of azithromycin in Pseudomonas aeruginosa PAO1: a global approach. Antimicrob Agents Chemother. 2006;50(5):1680–8.
38. Spagnolo P, Fabbri LM, Bush A. Long-term macrolide treatment for chronic respiratory disease. Eur Respir J. 2013;42(1):239–51.
39. Gupta S, Siddiqui S, Haldar P, Raj JV, Entwisle JJ, Wardlaw AJ, et al. Qualitative analysis of high-resolution CT scans in severe asthma. Chest. 2009;136(6):1521–8.
40. Mao B, Yang JW, Lu HW, Xu JF. Asthma and bronchiectasis exacerbation. Eur Respir J. 2016;47(6):1680–6.
41. Izquierdo ME, Marion CR, Moore WC, Raraigh KS, Taylor-Cousar JL, Cutting GR, et al. DNA sequencing analysis of cystic fibrosis transmembrane conductance regulator gene identifies cystic fibrosis-associated variants in the severe asthma Research program. Pediatr Pulmonol. 2022;57(7):1782–8.

42. Priel E, Adatia A, Kjarsgaard M, Nair P. CFTR heterozygosity in severe asthma with recurrent airway infections: a retrospective review. Allergy Asthma Clin Immunol. 2022;18(1):46.
43. Crooks MG, Faruqi S, Morice AH. How does azithromycin improve asthma exacerbations? Lancet. 2018;391(10115):28.
44. Kopsaftis Z, Yap HS, Tin KS, Hnin K, Carson-Chahhoud KV. Pharmacological and surgical interventions for the treatment of gastro-oesophageal reflux in adults and children with asthma. Cochrane Database Syst Rev. 2021;5(5):Cd001496.
45. Kirkland SW, Vandenberghe C, Voaklander B, Nikel T, Campbell S, Rowe BH. Combined inhaled beta-agonist and anticholinergic agents for emergency management in adults with asthma. Cochrane Database Syst Rev. 2017;1(1):Cd001284.
46. Cates CJ, Welsh EJ, Rowe BH. Holding chambers (spacers) versus nebulisers for beta-agonist treatment of acute asthma. Cochrane Database Syst Rev. 2013;2013(9):Cd000052.
47. Edmonds ML, Camargo CA, Pollack CV, Rowe BH. Early use of inhaled corticosteroids in the emergency department treatment of acute asthma. Cochrane Database Syst Rev. 2000;3: Cd002308.
48. Normansell R, Sayer B, Waterson S, Dennett EJ, Del Forno M, Dunleavy A. Antibiotics for exacerbations of asthma. Cochrane Database Syst Rev. 2018;6(6):Cd002741.
49. Kamada AK, Hill MR, Iklé DN, Brenner AM, Szefler SJ. Efficacy and safety of low-dose troleandomycin therapy in children with severe, steroid-requiring asthma. J Allergy Clin Immunol. 1993;91(4):873–82.
50. Amayasu H, Yoshida S, Ebana S, Yamamoto Y, Nishikawa T, Shoji T, et al. Clarithromycin suppresses bronchial hyperresponsiveness associated with eosinophilic inflammation in patients with asthma. Ann Allergy Asthma Immunol. 2000;84(6):594–8.
51. Kostadima E, Tsiodras S, Alexopoulos EI, Kaditis AG, Mavrou I, Georgatou N, et al. Clarithromycin reduces the severity of bronchial hyperresponsiveness in patients with asthma. Eur Respir J. 2004;23(5):714–7.
52. Piacentini GL, Peroni DG, Bodini A, Pigozzi R, Costella S, Loiacono A, et al. Azithromycin reduces bronchial hyperresponsiveness and neutrophilic airway inflammation in asthmatic children: a preliminary report. Allergy Asthma Proc. 2007;28(2):194–8.
53. Simpson J, Powell H, Boyle M, Scott R, Gibson PJR. Anti-inflammatory effects of clarithromycin in refractory non-eosinophilic asthma. Am J Respir Crit Care Med. 2007;12: A11.
54. Brusselle GG, Vanderstichele C, Jordens P, Deman R, Slabbynck H, Ringoet V, et al. Azithromycin for prevention of exacerbations in severe asthma (AZISAST): a multicentre randomised double-blind placebo-controlled trial. Thorax. 2013;68(4):322–9
55. Gibson PG, Upham J, Reynolds P, James A, McElduff P, Tyler G, et al. The amazes study: asthma and macrolides: the azithromycin efficacy and safety study research protocol.
56. Hahn D, Grasmick M, Hetzel S. Pragmatic controlled trial of azithromycin for asthma in adults. Eur Respiratory Soc. 2011;
57. Cameron EJ, Chaudhuri R, Mair F, McSharry C, Greenlaw N, Weir CJ, et al. Randomised controlled trial of azithromycin in smokers with asthma. Eur Respir J. 2013;42(5):1412–5.
58. Hahn DL, Plane MB, Mahdi OS, Byrne GI. Secondary outcomes of a pilot randomized trial of azithromycin treatment for asthma. PLoS Clinical Trials. 2006;1(2):e11.
59. Sutherland ER, King TS, Icitovic N, Ameredes BT, Bleecker E, Boushey HA, et al. A trial of clarithromycin for the treatment of suboptimally controlled asthma. J Allergy Clin Immunol. 2010;126(4):747–53.
60. He J, Zhu N, Chen X. Clinical impacts of azithromycin on lung function and cytokines for athmatic patients. 2009:719–722.
61. Strunk RC, Bacharier LB, Phillips BR, Szefler SJ, Zeiger RS, Chinchilli VM, et al. Azithromycin or montelukast as inhaled corticosteroid–sparing agents in moderate-to-severe childhood asthma study. J Allergy Clin Immunol. 2008;122(6):1138–44. e4.
62. Wang Y, Zhang S, Qu Y. Effect of clarithromycin on non-eosinophilic refractory asthma 2012;17(11):1948–1951.

63. Zhang L, Qian Q. Clinical effect of azithromycin combined with Seretide for asthma 2013;25: 159–160.
64. Kraft M, Cassell GH, Pak J, Martin RJ. Mycoplasma pneumoniae and chlamydia pneumoniae in asthma: effect of clarithromycin. Chest. 2002;121(6):1782–8.
65. Wan K-S, Liu Y-C, Huang C-S, Su Y-M. Effects of low-dose clarithromycin added to fluticasone on inflammatory markers and pulmonary function among children with asthma: a randomized clinical trial. Allergy Rhinol. 2016;7(3):131.
66. Black PN, Blasi F, Jenkins CR, Scicchitano R, Mills GD, Rubinfeld AR, et al. Trial of roxithromycin in subjects with asthma and serological evidence of infection with chlamydia pneumoniae. Am J Respir Crit Care Med. 2001;164(4):536–41.
67. Shoji T, Yoshida S, Sakamoto H, Hasegawa H, Nakagawa H, Amayasu HJC, et al. Anti-inflammatory effect of roxithromycin in patients with aspirin-intolerant asthma 1999;29(7): 950–956.
68. Xiao KA. The study on effect of roxithromycin combined with budesonide in therapy in patients with asthma 2013;11:119–120.
69. YAN X-q, WU L-q, Lin J, Xia X-D, Dai Y-R. Clinical study on efficacy of roxithromycin combined with inhaled budesonide dry powder inhalation on asthma 2008;13(2):184.
70. Stokholm J, Chawes BL, Vissing NH, Bjarnadóttir E, Pedersen TM, Vinding RK, et al. Azithromycin for episodes with asthma-like symptoms in young children aged 1-3 years: a randomised, double-blind, placebo-controlled trial. Lancet Respir Med. 2016;4(1):19–26.
71. Pincheira MA, Bacharier LB, Castro-Rodriguez JA. Efficacy of macrolides on acute asthma or wheezing exacerbations in children with recurrent wheezing: a systematic review and meta-analysis. Paediatr Drugs. 2020;22(2):217–28.
72. Smith D, Du Rand IA, Addy C, Collyns T, Hart S, Mitchelmore P, et al. British Thoracic Society guideline for the use of long-term macrolides in adults with respiratory disease 2020;7 (1):e000489.
73. FitzGerald JM, Lemiere C, Lougheed MD, Ducharme FM, Dell SD, Ramsey C, et al. Recognition and management of severe asthma: a Canadian thoracic society position statement. Can J Respir Crit Care Sleep Med. 2017;1(4):199–221.
74. Hinks TSC, Levine SJ, Brusselle GG. Treatment options in type-2 low asthma. Eur Respir J. 2021;57(1):2000528.
75. Hiles SA, McDonald VM, Guilhermino M, Brusselle GG, Gibson PG. Does maintenance azithromycin reduce asthma exacerbations? An individual participant data meta-analysis. Eur Respir J. 2019;54(5):1901381.

Macrolides and Interstitial Lung Diseases

Yu Hara and Takeshi Kaneko

Abstract Macrolide antibiotics are well known for their antibacterial properties, but extensive research in inflammatory lung diseases such as diffuse panbronchiolitis, cystic fibrosis, bronchiectasis, and chronic obstructive pulmonary disease has revealed that they also have powerful immunomodulatory properties. Interstitial lung diseases (ILD) are a group of diffuse parenchymal lung disorders associated with substantial morbidity and mortality. There is accumulating evidence of the clinical usefulness of macrolides for various ILDs, including idiopathic pulmonary fibrosis and cryptogenic and secondary organizing pneumonias, although antifibrotic agents or immunosuppressants are currently the most widely accepted treatment strategies for these diseases.

Keywords Autophagy capacity · Interstitial lung disease · Macrophage polarization · Microbiota · Surfactant homeostasis

Abbreviations

AE	acute exacerbation
BAL	bronchoalveolar lavage
BALF	bronchoalveolar lavage fluid
CHP	chronic hypersensitivity pneumonitis
COP	cryptogenic organizing pneumonia
ER	endoplasmic reticulum
HO-1	heme oxygenase-1
IL	interleukin
ILD	interstitial lung disease
IPF	idiopathic pulmonary fibrosis

Y. Hara (✉) · T. Kaneko
Department of Pulmonology, Yokohama City University Graduate School of Medicine, Yokohama, Japan
e-mail: yhara723@yokohama-cu.ac.jp; takeshi@yokohama-cu.ac.jp

B. K. Rubin, M. Shinkai (eds.), *Macrolides as Immunomodulatory Agents*, Progress in Inflammation Research 92, https://doi.org/10.1007/978-3-031-42859-3_8

LPS	lipopolysaccharide
MCC	mucociliary clearance
NSIP	nonspecific interstitial pneumonia
OP	organizing pneumonia
SASP	senescence-associated secretory phenotype
TGF	Transforming growth factor
sTNFR	soluble TNF receptor
TNF	tumor necrosis factor

1 Introduction

Macrolide antibiotics contain a macrocyclic lactone ring and are classified as 14-, 15-, or 16-membered based on the number of carbon atoms within this structure. Macrolide antibiotics have powerful immunomodulatory properties. The discovery of the immunoregulatory effects of macrolides is based on the findings by Kudo et al. that administration of low-dose erythromycin to patients with diffuse panbronchiolitis dramatically improved their prognosis [1].

Interstitial lung disease (ILD) is a group of diffuse parenchymal lung disorders associated with substantial morbidity and mortality. Among these, idiopathic pulmonary fibrosis (IPF) has the worst prognosis in adults, and is characterized as having a chronic and progressive course characterized by aberrant accumulation of fibrotic tissue in the lung parenchyma. Antifibrotic drugs including nintedanib and pirfenidone have been associated with a significant slowing of respiratory deterioration in IPF and perhaps prolonged survival [2, 3]. Non-IPF ILD patients with progressive fibrosing ILD (PF-ILD) have generally been treated with a combination of antifibrotic agents and immunosuppressants [4].

Macrolides may be a therapeutic option in ILDs due to their immunomodulatory effects; however, there is currently no established evidence of their efficacy. In this section, the possible mechanism of macrolide therapy in ILD is introduced, and recent reports of macrolide efficacy are discussed for each ILD subtype.

2 Possible Mechanisms for Macrolide Action in ILD

2.1 *Promotion of Autophagy Capacity and Regulation of Surfactant Homeostasis*

Epithelial proteins are susceptible to misfolding, which can occur with disease. The endoplasmic reticulum (ER) has control mechanisms that recognize misfolded proteins. Tissue homeostasis is then restored via activation of the unfolded protein response, which facilitates the processing, export, and degradation of these proteins.

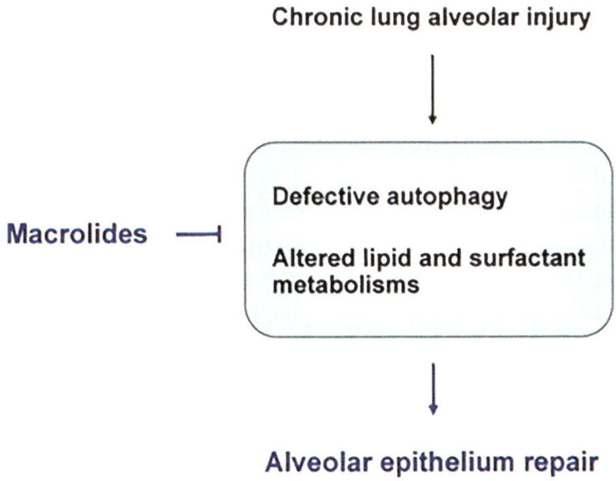

Fig. 1 Therapeutic potential of macrolides in the context of chronic lung alveolar injury. Reproduced from Guillot et al [11]. Emerging potential therapeutic targets of macrolides for restoring the proper repair of alveolar structure include the autophagic pathway and lipid and surfactant metabolisms

If the client protein load is excessive compared with the reserve of ER chaperones, the cell is said to be experiencing ER stress [5]. Ineffective reconstitution of the epithelium is a key factor in the inappropriate tissue regeneration observed in pulmonary fibrosis. The underlying pathologic mechanisms involve ER stress and its participation in cell death through both apoptosis and autophagic pathways [6]. Defects in the autophagocytotic mechanism have been found in many pathological conditions associated with tissue damage and inflammation [7]. Rapamycin, a type of macrolide that is not used for antibiotic purposes, induces autophagy by inactivating mTOR (mammalian target of rapamycin), a protein kinase that has been shown to have an inhibitory effect on autophagy [8]. Macrolide antibiotics such as azithromycin have also shown this effect, supporting the hypothesis that they protect against the toxic effect of excessive amounts of intracellular protein aggregates [9]. Macrolides may also act on lipid metabolism and surfactant homeostasis by interacting with the regulating molecules of lipid homeostasis [10, 11]. This role is of particular importance when considering that lipids account for almost 90% of surfactant mass. Chronic injury of the alveolar epithelium is associated with the accumulation of damaged cellular components including proteins and lipids that could progressively overwhelm the autophagic capacity of the cells and alter lipid and surfactant homeostasis. Emerging potential therapeutic targets of macrolides for proper restoration and repair of the alveolar structure include the autophagic pathway and the lipid and surfactant metabolisms (Fig. 1).

2.2 *Eliminating Senescent Alveolar Epithelial Cells*

Cellular senescence is a state of irreversible cell cycle arrest occurring naturally or in response to exogenous stressors [12]. Senescent cells remain metabolically active, secreting inflammatory cytokines, growth factors, chemokines, and extracellular matrix proteins, collectively known as senescence-associated secretory phenotype (SASP) [13]. Studies have shown that increased senescence markers are detected in IPF-derived cells and IPF tissues harvested from humans or animal models [14]. SASP such as matrix metalloproteinases MMP2 and MMP9 and collagen type I alpha 1, are more highly expressed in IPF lungs [14]. Increased expression of p16, along with increased pro-fibrotic SASP, has been reported in bleomycin-induced pulmonary fibrosis mouse models [14]. Because of this, efforts to develop drugs that eliminate senescent alveolar epithelial cells (senolytic) without affecting normal cells have become a focus [15]. The ability of roxithromycin to selectively kill senescent cells by inducing apoptosis and inhibiting the expression of senescence-associated secretory phenotype factors suggests the potential role of a “senolytic” drug. As well, transforming growth factor (TGF)-β- and senescent cell-induced lung fibroblast activation was inhibited by roxithromycin treatment [16], suggesting that roxithromycin may have clinical benefits in treating IPF.

2.3 Modulation of Microbiota

The microbiome refers to the community of microbes that share a particular environment. Based on the results of classical, culture-based studies, the lungs of healthy humans were previously believed to be sterile; however, using techniques such as 16S rRNA sequencing, it is now known that the lungs of healthy never-smokers are inhabited by communities of bacteria that are few in number but composed of diverse types of bacteria [17]. Recent evidence suggests that the lung microbiome might influence the progression of ILDs. In patients with IPF, in particular, alterations in lung microbiome composition have been reported to play key roles in disease progression. The composition of the lung microbiome has been reported to depend on the balance of several factors, including instillation of microbiota originating from the mouth, gastric contents, and inhaled air; the ability of the lung to clear micro-organisms through mucocilliary clearance and cough; and local environmental conditions such as oxygen partial pressure and fluctuations in temperature and pH. A shift in the balance of these factors, as occurs in lung diseases, can alter the microbiome (Fig. 2) [18]. In the Correlating Outcomes with Biochemical Markers to Estimate Time-progression in Idiopathic Pulmonary Fibrosis (COMET-IPF) study, the most commonly identified bacteria from 55 samples of bronchoalveolar lavage (BAL) were *Prevotella*, *Veillonella*, and *Escherichia spp*, and there was a strong association between the presence of specific species of *Streptococcus* and *Staphylococcus* and disease progression [19]. In a prospective study that included 65 patients with IPF, Molyneaux et al. reported that subjects with IPF had twice the number of bacteria in BAL fluid compared with 44 control subjects, and the baseline bacterial burden predicted the rate of decline in lung volume and risk of death [20]. They also demonstrated that *Haemophilus*, *Streptococcus*, *Neisseria*, and *Veillonella* spp. were more abundant in subjects with IPF than in control subjects. In an investigation of the composition of microbial communities

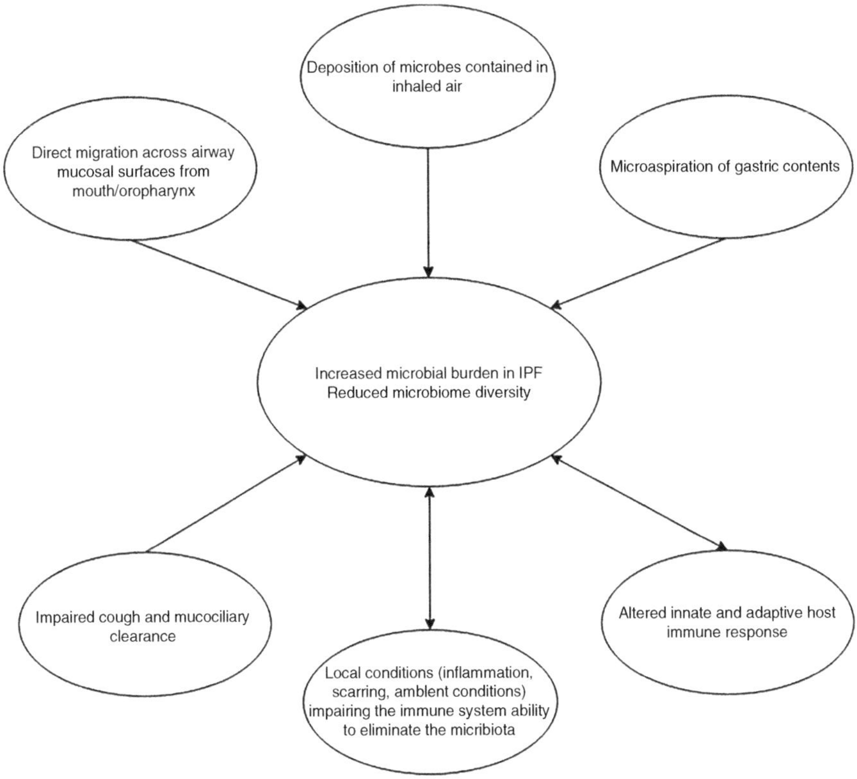

Fig. 2 Mechanisms that lead to increased microbial burden and reduced diversity of microbiota in lungs with idiopathic pulmonary fibrosis (IPF). Reproduced from Ntolios P et al [13]. Composition of the lung microbiome has been reported to depend on the balance of several factors, including instillation of microbiota originating from the mouth, gastric contents, and inhaled air; the ability of the lung to clear micro-organisms through mucociliary clearance and coughing; and local environmental conditions such as oxygen partial pressure, temperature, and pH fluctuations. A shift in the balance of these factors, as occurs in lung diseases, can alter the microbiome

in the lower airways between chronic hypersensitivity pneumonitis (CHP) and IPF, Invernizzi R et al. demonstrated that at the genus level, the *Staphylococcus* burden was increased in both CHP and IPF and that *Actinomyces* and *Veillonella* burdens were increased in IPF. However, in contrast to IPF, there was no association between bacterial burden and survival in CHP [21]. In a single-center retrospective study conducted by Takahashi et al. that included 34 patients with IPF, it was shown that an abundance of *Streptococcaceae*, *Veillonellaceae*, and *Prevotellaceae* families and a decrease in the phylum Proteobacteria in the lower airways of IPF patients led to reduced microbiota diversity and was associated with disease progression [22]. These results suggest that bacterial burden may be an important treatable trait in IPF and may be an important therapeutic target for macrolides. However, the serial changes in microbiota due to the use of macrolides and the prognosis of IPF treated with macrolides are unknown.

2.4 Macrophage Polarization

Oxidative/nitrosative stress results from an imbalance between cellular production of reactive oxygen species/reactive nitrogen species and endogenous antioxidants such as stress response protein (heme oxygenase-1 (HO-1)) and classic antioxidant enzymes (superoxide dismutase, catalase, glutathione peroxidase) [23]. Several clinical studies have suggested that increased oxidative/nitrosative stress might play a role in the progression of IPF [24–26]. Macrophages play key roles in each of the inflammation, proliferation, and remodeling phases of adult wound healing. Human peripheral monocytes are differentiated uncommitted macrophages (M0) that can be broadly divided into pro-inflammatory M1 macrophages and anti-inflammatory M2 macrophages [27]. M2 macrophages, hemorrhage-specialist macrophages, and macrophages generated with oxidized phospholipids (as novel macrophage subsets) highly express HO-1 [28, 29]. The interaction between M1 and M2 macrophages is reported to be closely correlated with disease progression in patients with idiopathic interstitial pneumonia, including IPF [30, 31]. Early in vitro evidence has suggested that macrolides might impair the oxidative burst and they are consistently reported to direct macrophage precursors and existing M1 cells toward an M2 phenotype in vitro, and subsequently alter macrophage cytokine production [32–35].

2.5 Reducing MUC5B in the Distal Airway

MUC5B is a major gel-forming mucin in the lung that plays a key role in mucociliary clearance (MCC) and host defense [36]. A MUC5B promoter polymorphism is reported to be the strongest and the most replicated genetic risk factor for IPF. This polymorphism appears to be protective and predictive in this disease and is likely involved in disease pathogenesis through an increase in MUC5B expression in terminal bronchi and honeycombed cysts [37]. Hancock LA et al. demonstrated that *MUC5B*, a mucin thought to be restricted to conducting airways, is co-expressed with surfactant protein C in type 2 alveolar epithelia and in epithelial cells lining honeycomb cysts, indicating that cell types involved in lung fibrosis in distal airspace express *MUC5B* [38]. Also, MUC5B concentration in bronchoalveolar epithelia proved to be related to impaired MCC and to the extent and persistence of bleomycin-induced lung fibrosis [38]. In IPF distal airways, the proportion of MUC5B positive cells is more than twofold greater compared with control, idiopathic nonspecific interstitial pneumonia (NSIP), and systemic sclerosis-associated NSIP distal airways and the distal airways, rather than honeycomb cysts, appear to be the primary site of MUC5B overexpression in IPF lungs [39]. In a murine asthma model, treatment with azithromycin significantly decreased IL-13, mucus secretion, and gene expression of IL-33, MUC5AC, and MUC5B; compared to the nontreated asthma group [40]. Other research showed that azithromycin inhibited ATP-induced mucin secretion and airway inflammation in house dust mite-exposed mice [41]. From these observations, mucociliary dysfunction might play a role in pulmonary fibrosis in mice overexpressing MUC5B, and MUC5B in distal airspaces is a potential therapeutic target in humans with IPF.

3 Clinical Evidence of Macrolide Efficacy in Patients with ILD (Table 1)

3.1 *IPF*

3.1.1 Inhibition of IPF Progression

IPF is a form of chronic fibrosing ILD of unknown etiology that occurs predominantly in older adults [42, 43]. Radiologic and/or histopathologic patterns are consistent with usual interstitial pneumonia. The clinical course and rate of progression of IPF is extremely variable among patients. With therapy, the median survival of patients with IPF is generally in the range of 2.5–3.5 years from the time of diagnosis. Some patients have acute exacerbation (AE) of IPF that causes a more rapid progression of disease, potentially resulting in respiratory failure and death [44]. In October 2014, the antifibrotic medications pirfenidone and nintedanib were concurrently approved by the Food and Drug Administration (FDA) following the results of two phase III, multicenter, placebo-randomized controlled trials (Assessment of Pirfenidone to Confirm Efficacy and Safety in Idiopathic Pulmonary Fibrosis [ASCEND] and INPULSIS 1 and 2) that demonstrated that these medications slowed the decline in lung function in patients with IPF [45, 46]. Since the "conditional recommendation" of these antifibrotic agents for IPF treatment in the 2015 American Thoracic Society IPF clinical practice guideline statement, there has been increasing real-world evidence of their efficacy [47, 48]. The treatment strategy in IPF patients is to introduce antifibrotic agents as early as possible [49].

Although recent evidence suggests that macrolide antibiotics may improve survival in AE of IPF, to date, few studies have examined the potential role of prophylactic macrolides in reducing these emergency admissions or disease progression [50]. In a retrospective study that included 108 IPF subjects who received prophylactic azithromycin 250 mg three times a week, a total of 31 hospital admissions (0.29 ± 0.62 per patient-year) were recorded in the pretreatment 12-month period, but only seven hospital admissions in the same cohort at 1 year after starting azithromycin (0.08 ± 0.3 per patient-year). Treatment conferred a relative risk reduction in all-cause nonelective hospitalization rates of 0.72 (0.67–0.88, $P < 0.001$); this was the first study to report the possible benefits of prophylactic

Table 1 Summary of clinical evidence of macrolide efficacy in patients with ILD

Diagnosis	Study design	Patient number	Types of macrolide	Description of outcomes	Ref.
IPF					
Stable condition	Retrospective	108	AZM	**Reduction of hospital admission and therapeutic antibiotic courses** without significant impact on rate of decline in lung function	[51]
	Retrospective (two arms)	29 with MAC vs. 23 without MAC	Not defined	**Reduction of AE** (4 of 29 cases (13.8%) treated with MAC and 8 of 23 cases (34.8%) treated without MAC, respectively, for 36 months)	[52]
	Double-blind randomized controlled crossover trial	25 were randomized	AZM	No significant change in the Leicester Cough Questionnaire score or the visual analog scale score with AZM or with placebo.	[53]
AE	A prospective, open-label study with historical controls	20 with AZM vs. 56 with fluoroquinolone	AZM	**Reduction of mortality at 60 days** (20 vs. 69.6%) ($p < 0.001$)	[63]
	Retrospective	97	Not defined	**The MAC use (+) group displayed a better 6-month survival rate than the MAC use (−) group**.	[64]
	Retrospective from a nationwide inpatient database	209	Not defined	**Survivors received co-trimoxazole ($p \leq 0.001$) and MAC ($p = 0.02$) more frequently than nonsurvivors.**	[65]
Non-IPF					
OP	Case reports	3: Cryptogenic 3: Radiation induced	CAM	**Improvement of clinical symptoms and pulmonary involvements.**	[77]
RP	Retrospective (two arms)	445 with CAM era vs. 136 with non-CAM era	CAM	**The rates of RP ≥ grade 2 and ≥ grade 3 were significantly lower in CAM group**	[78]

(continued)

Table 1 (continued)

Diagnosis	Study design	Patient number	Types of macrolide	Description of outcomes	Ref.
				(grade ≥ 2, 16% vs. 9.6%, $P = 0.047$; grade ≥ 3, 3.8% vs. 0.73%, $P = 0.037$).	
COP	Retrospective (two arms)	40 with CAM vs. 22 with PRE	CAM	Although s complete response was achieved in 35(88%) patients treated with CAM and in all treated with PRE, **patients treated with PRE relapsed more frequently than those treated with CAM (54.5% vs. 10%; $p \leq 0.0001$).**	[79]

Footnotes:
Abbreviations: *AE* acute exacerbation; *AZM* azithromycin; *CAM* clarithromycin; *COP* cryptogenic organizing pneumonia; *ILD* interstitial lung disease; *IPF* idiopathic pulmonary fibrosis; *MAC* macrolide; *OP* organizing pneumonia; *RP* radiation pneumonitis; *PRE* prednisolone

macrolides for reducing the burden of unplanned hospitalizations in patients with IPF [51]. Kuse et al. retrospectively reviewed data on 52 IPF patients who were treated with a combination of conventional agents with or without macrolides. There were AE in 4 of 29 (13.8%) treated with macrolides and in 8 of 23 (34.8%) treated without macrolides over 36 months. The AE-free survival rate was significantly higher in the macrolide group than in the nonmacrolide group (log-rank test $P = 0.027$) [52]. However, these preliminary data need to be considered with caution, not only because of their retrospective nature but also because they were collected over a period of time (2003–2008) during which "conventional therapy" for IPF has changed profoundly. In a double-blind, randomized controlled crossover trial, 20 patients with IPF underwent two 12-week intervention periods (azithromycin 500 mg three times per week or placebo three times per week) to determine the safety and efficacy of azithromycin for the treatment of chronic cough. There was no significant change in the Leicester Cough Questionnaire score or the cough visual analog scale score with azithromycin or with placebo (NCT02173145) [53]. The trial did not support the use of low-dose azithromycin for chronic cough in patients with IPF, although the number of cases was extremely small and the duration of therapy was short. Therefore, the clinical efficacy of macrolides in IPF is unclear, and prospective randomized placebo-controlled studies are needed to confirm these observations.

3.1.2 Treatment of AE (Including Other ILDs)

Prognosis is poor in patients who have AE of ILD because the histological pattern typically involves diffuse alveolar damage superimposed upon lung fibrosis without obvious clinical causes such as fluid overload, left heart failure, or pulmonary embolism [43, 54]. The subtypes of underlying ILD comprise idiopathic interstitial pneumonias (IIPs), including IPF and nonspecific interstitial pneumonia; and ILDs of known etiology such as collagen vascular disease and CHP [55, 56]. The in-hospital mortality rate in patients with AE of IPF is reported to be in excess of 50% [57]. A retrospective cohort study that included IPF and non-IPF patients showed overall survival rates for AE of 67% at 30 days, 43% at 60 days, and 40% at 90 days after admission [58]. Other reports have shown mortality rates for AE of collagen vascular disease-associated IP (CVD-IP) ranging from 34% to 83% [59].

Corticosteroid pulse therapy is the current mainstay of treatment for AE of ILD. Potential therapies for AE of IPF specified by the International Working Group Report include nintedanib, pirfenidone, and anti-acid drugs as preventative therapy; and corticosteroid monotherapy, cyclophosphamide, cyclosporine, polymyxin-B immobilized fiber column hemoperfusion, rituximab, plasma exchange, and intravenous immunoglobulin, tacrolimus, and thrombomodulin as additional treatment options [60]. However, evidence is lacking regarding the efficacy of these treatments and of macrolides in patients with AE of ILD, though administration of macrolide antibiotics has been reported to be associated with improved outcomes in patients with acute lung injury [61].

Despite the scant evidence, macrolides tend to be used frequently in the treatment of AE-IPF patients in the clinical setting [62]. Kawamura et al. conducted a prospective, open-label study (Clinical trial JMA-IIA00095) in patients with AE of chronic fibrosing interstitial pneumonia, including 20 in an azithromycin group and 56 in a fluoroquinolone group (historical controls), and reported that mortality was significantly lower in patients treated with azithromycin than in those treated with fluoroquinolone (mortality rate at 60 days: 20 vs. 69.6%, $P < 0.001$; median survival time: not reached vs. 29.5 days, $P < 0.001$) [63]. Kawamura et al. also conducted another single-center retrospective study that included 85 consecutive patients hospitalized in our department for idiopathic AE of IPF. They reported that mortality was significantly lower in patients treated with azithromycin than in those treated with fluoroquinolone (azithromycin, 26% vs. control, 70%; $P < 0.001$)0.40 Nagasawa et al. reviewed 97 patients with acute exacerbation of ILD that required corticosteroid pulse therapy and found significantly worse 6-month mortality among patients without macrolide use (22 of 97, 23%: azithromycin, $n = 14$; clarithromycin, $n = 6$; and erythromycin, $n = 2$) than among those with macrolide use ($P = 0.020$) [64]. In a retrospective epidemiologic and prognostic analysis that included IPF patients who received mechanical ventilation and high-dose corticosteroids, the administration of co-trimoxazole (OR = 0.28, 95%Cl 0.132–0.607; $P = 0.001$) and macrolides (OR = 0.37, 95%Cl 0.155–0.867; $P = 0.033$) was associated with better survival [65]. Papiris et al. measured blood levels of interleukin (IL)-4, IL-6, CXCL8, IL-10, and IL-13, as well as active TGF-β of both stable and exacerbated patients with IPF and found that high levels of IL-6 and CXCL8 characterized early-onset AE of IPF. In addition, an increase in the levels of IL-6 and CXCL8 was associated with worse outcomes in all patients [66]. The use of macrolides in addition to conventional treatment for patients with AE of ILD has been reported to improve prognosis, perhaps by suppressing local pulmonary IL-6 and CXCL8 production [67–69].

3.2 *Cryptogenic Organizing Pneumonia*

Organizing pneumonia (OP) is characterized pathologically by the presence of buds of granulation tissue that consist of fibroblasts and myofibroblasts intermixed with loose connective matrix within the lumen of distal pulmonary airspaces [70]. OP is associated with connective tissue disorders, infections, drug and radiation reactions, hypersensitivity pneumonitis, and aspiration. OP that cannot be linked to an associated condition and appears to be idiopathic is termed cryptogenic organizing pneumonia (COP) [71]. Corticosteroid treatment in COP results in rapid clinical improvement and clearing of opacities on chest imaging without significant sequelae. However, relapses are common upon stopping or decreasing corticosteroids, thus often leading to prolonged treatment. Lazor et al. reported one or more relapses in 58% of a 48-patient cohort with biopsy-proven COP and found that 68% of relapsing patients were still receiving treatment for their initial episode of COP when their first relapse occurred (length of follow-up, 35 ± 31 months; time to relapse, 8 ± 9 months) [72].

Hyperactivation of proinflammatory mediators from alveolar macrophages in both COP and OP appears to be a main reason for using anti-inflammatory therapies [73–76]. Because the clinical characteristics of OP correlate with an increase in the risk of steroid-related side effects, it is common to use steroid-sparing agents such as macrolides. In a 1996 study of biopsy-proven COP patients who showed neutrophilia on BAL, Hotta observed a reduction in CXCL8 and neutrophilic chemotactic activity in BAL after 600 mg/day erythromycin for 2–3 months, which is consistent with a beneficial effect of low-dose macrolides on neutrophil-mediated inflammation [74]. In COP patients, response to clarithromycin treatment was associated with decreases in serum concentrations of IL-6, CXCL8, and TGF-β and the BAL concentration of IL-6 [75]. Analysis of alveolar macrophages of OP patients revealed that clarithromycin and azithromycin significantly attenuated the lipopolysaccharide (LPS)-stimulated production of soluble TNF receptor (sTNFR)1, sTNFR2, CXCL8, and CCL18 in a dose-dependent manner. Clarithromycin also inhibited LPS-stimulated production of TNF-α, IL-1β, IL-6, and IL-10 [76]. Related to these cytokines and chemokines in OP, studies have reported the usefulness of macrolide treatment as a first-line alternative to steroids. Stover and Mangino reported six patients (three with COP and three with OP secondary to radiation therapy) who responded to clarithromycin [77], suggesting that long-term macrolide therapy can be considered as adjuvant therapy in patients receiving steroids or those who cannot tolerate steroids, even those with minimal symptoms or minimal physiological impairment. In a retrospective cohort study, clarithromycin mitigated radiation pneumonitis including organizing pneumonia and acute lung injury following stereotactic body radiotherapy for lung cancer [78]. In an observational study of COP patients, of whom 40 were treated with clarithromycin (500 mg twice daily orally for 3 months) and 22 were treated with prednisone (mean initial dose of 0.67 ± 0.24 mg/kg/d for a mean of 8.59 ± 3.05 months), complete response was reported in 35 (88%) of the patients treated with clarithromycin and in all of those treated with prednisone. Unexpectedly, patients treated with prednisone relapsed more frequently than those treated with clarithromycin (54.5% vs. 10%; $P < 0.0001$) [79]. However, it is unknown which patients are likely to respond to macrolide therapy, as well as appropriate dose and treatment duration.

4 Conclusion

In general, antifibrotic drugs are the principal treatment for IPF, and anti-inflammatory drugs such as steroids are used for AE-ILDs and COP. Although macrolides are not the first choice in these ILDs, they can be effective as supportive treatment options. From an ethical point of view, however, it is difficult to plan a clinical trial of macrolides alone, and validation is therefore based mainly on accumulated evidence from retrospective studies.

5 Ethical Approval

All procedures performed in studies involving human participants were in accordance with the ethical standards of the institutional and/or national research committee and with the 1964 Helsinki declaration and its later amendments or comparable ethical standards.

Conflict of Interest There is no conflict of interest about this manuscript.

References

1. Kudoh S, Azuma A, Yamamoto M, Izumi T, Ando M. Improvement of survival in patients with diffuse panbronchiolitis treated with low-dose erythromycin. Am J Respir Crit Care Med. 1998;157(6 Pt 1):1829–32.
2. Richeldi L, Varone F, Bergna M, de Andrade J, Falk J, Hallowell R, et al. Pharmacological management of progressive-fibrosing interstitial lung diseases: a review of the current evidence. Eur Respir Rev. 2018;27:180074.

3. Kolb M, Bonella F, Wollin L. Therapeutic targets in idiopathic pulmonary fibrosis. Respir Med. 2017;131:49–57.
4. Flaherty KR, Wells AU, Cottin V, Devaraj A, Walsh SLF, Inoue Y, et al. Nintedanib in progressive fibrosing interstitial lung diseases. N Engl J Med. 2019;381:1718–27.
5. Yoshida H. ER stress and diseases. FEBS J. 2007;274:630–58.
6. Korfei M, Ruppert C, Mahavadi P, Henneke I, Markart P, Koch M, et al. Epithelial endoplasmic reticulum stress and apoptosis in sporadic idiopathic pulmonary fibrosis. Am J Respir Crit Care Med. 2008;178:838–46.
7. Monick MM, Powers LS, Walters K, Lovan N, Zhang M, Gerke A, et al. Identification of an autophagy defect in smokers' alveolar macrophages. J Immunol. 2010;185:5425–35.
8. Thomson AW, Turnquist HR, Raimondi G. Immunoregulatory functions of mTOR inhibition. Nat Rev Immunol. 2009;9:324–37.
9. Stamatiou R, Paraskeva E, Boukas K, Gourgoulianis KI, Molyvdas PA, Hatziefthimiou AA. Azithromycin has an antiproliferative and autophagic effect on airway smooth muscle cells. Eur Respir J. 2009;34:721–30.
10. Zhong Q, Zhou B, Ann DK, Minoo P, Liu Y, Banfalvi A, et al. Role of ER stress in EMT of alveolar epithelial cells: effects of misfolded surfactant protein. Am J Respir Cell Mol Biol. 2011;45:498–509.
11. Guillot L, Tabary O, Nathan N, Corvol H, Clement A. Macrolides: new therapeutic perspectives in lung diseases. Int J Biochem Cell Biol. 2011;43:1241–6.
12. Aghali A, Koloko Ngassie ML, Pabelick CM, Prakash YS. Cellular senescence in aging lungs and diseases. Cell. 2022;11:1781.
13. Coppé JP, Desprez PY, Krtolica A, Campisi J. The senescence-associated secretory phenotype: the dark side of tumor suppression. Annu Rev Pathol. 2010;5:99–118.
14. Schafer MJ, White TA, Iijima K, Haak AJ, Ligresti G, Atkinson EJ, et al. Cellular senescence mediates fibrotic pulmonary disease. Nat Commun. 2017;8:14532.
15. Kirkland JL, Tchkonia T. Senolytic drugs: from discovery to translation. J Intern Med. 2020;288:518–36.
16. Zhang X, Dong Y, Li WC, Tang BX, Li J, Zang Y. Roxithromycin attenuates bleomycin-induced pulmonary fibrosis by targeting senescent cells. Acta Pharmacol Sin. 2021;42:2058–68.
17. Erb-Downward JR, Thompson DL, Han MK, Freeman CM, McCloskey L, Schmidt LA, et al. Analysis of the lung microbiome in the "healthy" smoker and in COPD. PLoS One. 2011;6:e16384.
18. Ntolios P, Tzilas V, Bouros E, Avdoula E, Karakasiliotis I, Bouros D, et al. The role of microbiome and virome in idiopathic pulmonary fibrosis. Biomedicine. 2021;9:442.
19. Han MK, Zhou Y, Murray S, Tayob N, Noth I, Lama VN, et al. Lung microbiome and disease progression in idiopathic pulmonary fibrosis: an analysis of the COMET study. Lancet Respir Med. 2014;2:548–56.
20. Molyneaux PL, Cox MJ, Willis-Owen SA, Mallia P, Russell KE, Russell AM, et al. The role of bacteria in the pathogenesis and progression of idiopathic pulmonary fibrosis. Am J Respir Crit Care Med. 2014;190:906–13.
21. Invernizzi R, Wu BG, Barnett J, Ghai P, Kingston S, Hewitt RJ, et al. The respiratory microbiome in chronic hypersensitivity pneumonitis is distinct from that of idiopathic pulmonary fibrosis. Am J Respir Crit Care Med. 2021;203:339–47.
22. Takahashi Y, Saito A, Chiba H, Kuronuma K, Ikeda K, Kobayashi T, et al. Impaired diversity of the lung microbiome predicts progression of idiopathic pulmonary fibrosis. Respir Res. 2018;19:34.
23. Hosseinzadeh A, Javad-Moosavi SA, Reiter RJ, Yarahmadi R, Ghaznavi H, Mehrzadi S. Oxidative/nitrosative stress, autophagy and apoptosis as therapeutic targets of melatonin in idiopathic pulmonary fibrosis. Expert Opin Ther Targets. 2018;22:1049–61.
24. Cameli P, Carleo A, Bergantini L, Landi C, Prasse A, Bargagli E. Oxidant/antioxidant disequilibrium in idiopathic pulmonary fibrosis pathogenesis. Inflammation. 2020;43:1–7.

25. Cameli P, Bergantini L, Salvini M, Refini RM, Pieroni M, Bargagli E, et al. Alveolar concentration of nitric oxide as a prognostic biomarker in idiopathic pulmonary fibrosis. Nitric Oxide. 2019;89:41–5.
26. Walters DM, Cho H, Kleeberger SR. Oxidative stress and antioxidants in the pathogenesis of pulmonary fibrosis: a potential role of Nrf2. Antiox Redox Signal. 2008;10:321–31.
27. Gordon S. Alternative activation of macrophages. Nat Rev Immunol. 2003;3:23–35.
28. Boyle JJ, Harrington HA, Piper E, Elderfield K, Stark J, Landis RC, et al. Coronary intraplaque hemorrhage evokes a novel atheroprotective macrophage phenotype. Am J Pathol. 2009;174: 1097–108.
29. Kadl A, Meher AK, Sharma PR, Lee MY, Doran AC, Johnstone SR, et al. Identification of a novel macrophage phenotype that develops in response to atherogenic phospholipids via Nrf2. Circ Res. 2010;107:737–46.
30. Nouno T, Okamoto M, Ohnishi K, Kaieda S, Tominaga M, Zaizen Y, Ichiki M, et al. Elevation of pulmonary CD163+ and CD204+ macrophages is associated with the clinical course of idiopathic pulmonary fibrosis patients. J Thorac Dis. 2019;11:4005–17.
31. Yamashita M, Saito R, Yasuhira S, Fukuda Y, Sasamo H, Sugai T, et al. Distinct profiles of CD163-positive macrophages in idiopathic interstitial pneumonias. J Immunol Res. 2018;1436236:1.
32. Labro MT, el Benna J, Babin-Chevaye C. Comparison of the in-vitro effect of several macrolides on the oxidative burst of human neutrophils. J Antimicrob Chemother. 1989;24: 561–72.
33. Murphy BS, Sundareshan V, Cory TJ, Hayes D Jr, Anstead MI, Feola DJ. Azithromycin alters macrophage phenotype. J Antimicrob Chemother. 2008;61:554–60.
34. Wang J, Xie L, Wang S, Lin J, Liang J, Xu J. Azithromycin promotes alternatively activated macrophage phenotype in systematic lupus erythematosus via PI3K/Akt signaling pathway. Cell Death Dis. 2018;9:1080.
35. Zhang B, Kopper TJ, Liu X, Cui Z, Van Lanen SG, Gensel JC. Macrolide derivatives reduce proinflammatory macrophage activation and macrophage-mediated neurotoxicity. CNS Neurosci Ther. 2019;25:591–600.
36. Evans CM, Fingerlin TE, Schwarz MI, Lynch D, Kurche J, Warg L, et al. Idiopathic pulmonary fibrosis: a genetic disease that involves mucociliary dysfunction of the peripheral airways. Physiol Rev. 2016;96:1567–91.
37. Yang IV, Fingerlin TE, Evans CM, Schwarz MI, Schwartz DA. MUC5B and idiopathic pulmonary fibrosis. Ann Am Thorac Soc. 2015;12(Suppl 2):S193–9.
38. Hancock LA, Hennessy CE, Solomon GM, Dobrinskikh E, Estrella A, Hara N, et al. Muc5b overexpression causes mucociliary dysfunction and enhances lung fibrosis in mice. Nat Commun. 2018;9:5363.
39. Conti C, Montero-Fernandez A, Borg E, Osadolor T, Viola P, De Lauretis A, et al. Mucins MUC5B and MUC5AC in distal airways and honeycomb spaces: comparison among idiopathic pulmonary fibrosis/usual interstitial pneumonia, fibrotic nonspecific interstitial pneumonitis, and control lungs. Am J Respir Crit Care Med. 2016;193:462–4.
40. Wang Z, Xin L, Zhang W. Study effect of azithromycin and doxycycline in mucus producing and inflammatory signaling pathways of allergic asthma. Iran J Allergy Asthma Immunol. 2022;21:119–27.
41. Mann TS, Larcombe AN, Wang KCW, Shamsuddin D, Landwehr KR, Noble PB, et al. Azithromycin inhibits mucin secretion, mucous metaplasia, airway inflammation, and airways hyperresponsiveness in mice exposed to house dust mite extract. Am J Physiol Lung Cell Mol Physiol. 2022;322:L683–98.
42. Raghu G, Collard HR, Egan JJ, Martinez FJ, Behr J, Brown KK, et al. ATS/ERS/JRS/ALAT committee on idiopathic pulmonary fibrosis. An official ATS/ERS/JRS/ALAT statement: idiopathic pulmonary fibrosis: evidence-based guidelines for diagnosis and management. Am J Respir Crit Care Med. 2011;183:788–824.

43. Ryu JH, Moua T, Daniels CE, Hartman TE, Yi ES, Utz JP, et al. Idiopathic pulmonary fibrosis: evolving concepts. Mayo Clin Proc. 2014;89:1130–42.
44. Hyzy R, Huang S, Myers J, Flaherty K, Martinez F. Acute exacerbation of idiopathic pulmonary fibrosis. Chest. 2007;132:1652–8.
45. King TE Jr, Bradford WZ, Castro-Bernardini S, Fagan EA, Glaspole I, Glassberg MK, et al. A phase 3 trial of pirfenidone in patients with idiopathic pulmonary fibrosis. N Engl J Med. 2014;370:2083–92.
46. Richeldi L, du Bois RM, Raghu G, Azuma A, Brown KK, Costabel U, et al. Efficacy and safety of nintedanib in idiopathic pulmonary fibrosis. N Engl J Med. 2014;370:2071–82.
47. Raghu G, Rochwerg B, Zhang Y, Garcia CA, Azuma A, Behr J, et al. An official ATS/ERS/JRS/ALAT clinical practice guideline: treatment of idiopathic pulmonary fibrosis. An update of the 2011 clinical practice guideline. Am J Respir Crit Care Med. 2015;192:e3–19.
48. Dempsey TM, Sangaralingham LR, Yao X, Sanghavi D, Shah ND, Limper AH. Clinical effectiveness of antifibrotic medications for idiopathic pulmonary fibrosis. Am J Respir Crit Care Med. 2019;200:168–74.
49. Wijsenbeek M, Cottin V. Spectrum of fibrotic lung diseases. N Engl J Med. 2020;383:958–68.
50. Kawamura K, Ichikado K, Yasuda Y, Anan K, Suga M. Azithromycin for idiopathic acute exacerbation of idiopathic pulmonary fibrosis: a retrospective single-center study. BMC Pulm Med. 2017;17:94.
51. Macaluso C, Maritano Furcada J, Alzaher O, Chaube R, Chua F, Wells AU, et al. The potential impact of azithromycin in idiopathic pulmonary fibrosis. Eur Respir J. 2019;53:1800628.
52. Kuse N, Abe S, Hayashi H, Kamio K, Saito Y, Usuki J, et al. Long-term efficacy of macrolide treatment in idiopathic pulmonary fibrosis: a retrospective analysis. Sarcoidosis Vasc Diffuse Lung Dis. 2016;33:242–6.
53. Guler SA, Clarenbach C, Brutsche M, Hostettler K, Brill AK, Schertel A, et al. Azithromycin for the treatment of chronic cough in idiopathic pulmonary fibrosis: a randomized controlled crossover trial. Ann Am Thorac Soc. 2021;18:2018–26.
54. Collard HR, Moore BB, Flaherty KR, Brown KK, Kaner RJ, King TE Jr, et al. Acute exacerbations of idiopathic pulmonary fibrosis. Am J Respir Crit Care Med. 2007;176:636–43.
55. Park IN, Kim DS, Shim TS, Lim CM, Lee SD, Koh Y, et al. Acute exacerbation of interstitial pneumonia other than idiopathic pulmonary fibrosis. Chest. 2007;132:214–20.
56. Suda T, Kaida Y, Nakamura Y, Enomoto N, Fujisawa T, Imokawa S, et al. Acute exacerbation of interstitial pneumonia associated with collagen vascular diseases. Respir Med. 2009;103:846–53.
57. Kim DS, Park JH, Park BK, Lee JS, Nicholson AG, Colby T. Acute exacerbation of idiopathic pulmonary fibrosis: frequency and clinical features. Eur Respir J. 2006;27:143–50.
58. Usui Y, Kaga A, Sakai F, Shiono A, Komiyama K, Hagiwara K, et al. A cohort study of mortality predictors in patients with acute exacerbation of chronic fibrosing interstitial pneumonia. BMJ Open. 2013;3:e002971.
59. Tachikawa R, Tomii K, Ueda H, Nagata K, Nanjo S, Sakurai A, et al. Clinical features and outcome of acute exacerbation of interstitial pneumonia: collagen vascular diseases-related versus idiopathic. Respiration. 2012;83:20–7.
60. Collard HR, Ryerson CJ, Corte TJ, Jenkins G, Kondoh Y, Lederer DJ, et al. Acute exacerbation of idiopathic pulmonary fibrosis. An international working group report. Am J Respir Crit Care Med. 2016;194:265–75.
61. Walkey AJ, Wiener RS. Macrolide antibiotics and survival in patients with acute lung injury. Chest. 2012;141:1153–9.
62. Polke M, Kondoh Y, Wijsenbeek M, Cottin V, Walsh SLF, Collard HR, et al. Management of acute exacerbation of idiopathic pulmonary fibrosis in specialised and non-specialised ILD centres around the world. Front Med (Lausanne). 2021;8:699644.
63. Kawamura K, Ichikado K, Suga M, Yoshioka M. Efficacy of azithromycin for treatment of acute exacerbation of chronic fibrosing interstitial pneumonia: a prospective, open-label study with historical controls. Respiration. 2014;87:478–84.

64. Nagasawa R, Hara Y, Murohashi K, Saigusa Y, Nishikawa Y, Tanaka M, et al. Additional efficacy of macrolide for patients with acute deterioration of interstitial lung disease requiring corticosteroid pulse therapy. Am J Ther. 2021;30(Jan 7):170. https://doi.org/10.1097/MJT.0000000000001321.
65. Oda K, Yatera K, Fujino Y, Ishimoto H, Nakao H, Hanaka T, et al. Efficacy of concurrent treatments in idiopathic pulmonary fibrosis patients with a rapid progression of respiratory failure: an analysis of a national administrative database in Japan. BMC Pulm Med. 2016;16:91.
66. Papiris SA, Tomos IP, Karakatsani A, Spathis A, Korbila I, Analitis A, et al. High levels of IL-6 and IL-8 characterize early-on idiopathic pulmonary fibrosis acute exacerbations. Cytokine. 2018;102:168–72.
67. Shinkai M, Henke MO, Rubin BK. Macrolide antibiotics as immunomodulatory medications: proposed mechanisms of action. Pharmacol Ther. 2008;117:393–405.
68. Oishi K, Sonoda F, Kobayashi S, Iwagaki A, Nagatake T, Matsushima K, et al. Role of interleukin-8 (IL-8) and an inhibitory effect of erythromycin on IL-8 release in the airways of patients with chronic airway diseases. Infect Immun. 1994;62:4145–52.
69. Takizawa H, Desaki M, Ohtoshi T, Kawasaki S, Kohyama T, Sato M, et al. Erythromycin modulates IL-8 expression in normal and inflamed human bronchial epithelial cells. Am J Respir Crit Care Med. 1997;156:266–71.
70. Cordier JF. Cryptogenic organising pneumonia. Eur Respir J. 2006;28:422–46.
71. Raghu G, Meyer KC. Cryptogenic organising pneumonia: current understanding of an enigmatic lung disease. Eur Respir Rev. 2021;30:210094.
72. Lazor R, Vandevenne A, Pelletier A, Leclerc P, Court-Fortune I, Cordier JF. Cryptogenic organizing pneumonia. Characteristics of relapses in a series of 48 patients. The Groupe d'Etudes et de Recherche sur les Maladles “Orphelines” Pulmonaires (GERM"O"P). Am J Respir Crit Care Med. 2000;162:571–7.
73. Carré PC, King TE Jr, Mortensen R, Riches DW. Cryptogenic organizing pneumonia: increased expression of interleukin-8 and fibronectin genes by alveolar macrophages. Am J Respir Cell Mol Biol. 1994;10:100–5.
74. Hotta M. Neutrophil chemotactic activity in cryptogenic organizing pneumonia and the response to erythromycin. Kurume Med J. 1996;43:207–17.
75. Radzikowska E, Roży A, Jagus P, Polubiec-Kownacka M, Wiatr E, Chorostowska-Wynimko J, et al. Clarithromycin decreases IL-6 concentration in serum and BAL fluid in patients with cryptogenic organizing pneumonia. Adv Clin Exp Med. 2016;25:871–8.
76. Cai M, Bonella F, Dai H, Sarria R, Guzman J, Costabel U. Macrolides inhibit cytokine production by alveolar macrophages in bronchiolitis obliterans organizing pneumonia. Immunobiology. 2013;218:930–7.
77. Stover DE, Mangino D. Macrolides: a treatment alternative for bronchiolitis obliterans organizing pneumonia? Chest. 2005;128:3611–7.
78. Takeda A, Tsurugai Y, Sanuki N, Enomoto T, Shinkai M, Mizuno T, et al. Clarithromycin mitigates radiation pneumonitis in patients with lung cancer treated with stereotactic body radiotherapy. J Thorac Dis. 2018;10:247–61.
79. Radzikowska E, Wiatr E, Langfort R, Bestry I, Skoczylas A, Szczepulska-Wójcik E, et al. Cryptogenic organizing pneumonia-results of treatment with clarithromycin versus corticosteroids-observational study. PLoS One. 2017;12:e0184739.

Macrolides in Acute Respiratory Distress Syndrome and Acute Lung Injury

Kodai Kawamura

Abstract Acute respiratory distress syndrome (ARDS) is a life-threatening condition caused by injury to the lungs. Despite increased knowledge of the immunopathogenesis and advances and improvements in supportive care in clinical management (e.g., lung protection strategies), the mortality remains high at approximately 40%. Despite over 55 years of preclinical and clinical trials, there are no effective pharmacotherapies to improve the outcomes in patients with ARDS, thus necessitating novel therapeutic agents. Macrolides are antibiotics with potent immunomodulatory properties and may be beneficial in ARDS by reversing the dysregulated immune response in ARDS.

Keywords Acute lung injury · Acute respiratory distress syndrome · Azithromycin · Acute exacerbation of pulmonary fibrosis

1 Introduction

Acute respiratory distress syndrome (ARDS) is a life-threatening form of respiratory failure driven by an uncontrolled inflammatory host response induced by direct (pulmonary inflammation) or indirect (systemic inflammation) insults [1]. It presents as acute hypoxemia with pulmonary infiltrates on chest imaging, which is not fully explained by cardiac failure or fluid overload [2]. A previous international study demonstrated a 46% mortality in patients with severe ARDS [3]. Treating the underlying cause and providing supportive care is the mainstay of therapy [4]. Since its first description in 1967, and despite over 50 years of research, there are no clearly effective pharmacological therapies for ARDS. Supportive care remains the primary treatment, and this includes lung-protective ventilation and conservative fluid management [5].

K. Kawamura (✉)
Division of Respiratory Medicine, Social Welfare Organization Saiseikai Imperial Gift Foundation, Inc., Saiseikai Kumamoto Hospital, Kumamoto, Japan

B. K. Rubin, M. Shinkai (eds.), *Macrolides as Immunomodulatory Agents*, Progress in Inflammation Research 92, https://doi.org/10.1007/978-3-031-42859-3_9

Macrolides exert pleiotropic immunomodulatory effects that may reverse the uncontrolled immune response in critically ill patients. Their beneficial effects have been reported for chronic pulmonary diseases, such as asthma [6], chronic obstructive pulmonary disease (COPD) [7, 8], and diffuse pan-bronchiolitis [9]. Evidence suggests that macrolides could be potentially beneficial in ARDS [10–13].

This chapter provides an overview of current studies on the immunomodulatory effects of macrolides in ARDS and acute lung injury (ALI) and we discuss potential mechanisms underlying the immunomodulatory properties of macrolides in ARDS, ALI, and ARDS-related conditions.

2 ARDS

2.1 Overview of ARDS

ARDS is a common cause of respiratory failure in critically ill patients. It is defined by the acute onset of noncardiogenic pulmonary edema, hypoxemia, and the need for respiratory support [4, 14]. Risk factors for ARDS may include pneumonia, aspiration, smoke inhalation, drowning, sepsis, and systemic inflammatory reactions (e.g., pancreatitis, trauma, surgery, blood transfusion, and toxic drugs). ARDS predominantly occurs in the setting of pneumonia, sepsis, the aspiration of gastric contents, or severe trauma [15]. Its prevalence was confirmed in 10% and 23% of the patients in intensive care and on mechanical ventilation, respectively, in a cross-sectional analysis of 29,144 patients from 50 countries conducted in the winter of 2014 [3]. Since it was first described by Ashbaugh et al. 56 years ago [16], the mortality has decreased in clinical trials, but remains high at approximately 40% in observational studies. Pathological specimens from patients with ARDS frequently reveal diffuse alveolar damage. Laboratory studies have demonstrated alveolar epithelial and lung endothelial injury, resulting in the accumulation of protein-rich inflammatory edematous fluid in the alveolar space. The diagnosis is usually based on the Berlin definition (Table 1) [2]. The management of ARDS focuses on the diagnosis

Table 1 Berlin definition

Timing	Within 1 week of a known clinical insult or new or worsening respiratory symptoms
Chest imaging	Bilateral opacities—Not fully explained by effusions, lobar/lung collapse, or nodules
Origin of edema	Respiratory failure not fully explained by cardiac dysfunction or fluid overload
Oxygenation	
Mild	200 mmHg < PaO2/FiO2 ≤ 300 mmHg with PEEP/CPAP ≥5cmH2O
Moderate	100 mmHg < PaO2/FiO2 ≤ 200 mmHg with PEEP ≥5cmH2O
Severe	PaO2/FiO2 ≤ 100 mmHg with PEEP ≥5cmH2O

PEEP positive end-expiratory pressure, *CPAP* continuous positive airway pressure

and treatment of infection, respiratory support including oxygenation and positive pressure ventilation, careful fluid administration which is particularly important in cases of shock, and general supportive measures, including nutritional support. The treatment focuses on lung-protective ventilation. No specific pharmacotherapies have been shown to be effective. Clinical studies have focused on using anti-inflammatory agents as a potential treatment for ARDS. However, clinical trials of glucocorticoids [17–19], granulocyte-macrophage colony-stimulating factor [20], statins [21, 22], aspirin [23], antioxidants [24], and vitamin C [25] have not demonstrated clinical utility.

2.2 *Pathophysiology of ARDS*

ARDS leads to pulmonary edema due to increased permeability of alveolar septal walls resulting from severe inflammation [14, 15]. ARDS has been considered a series of pathobiological phases, and the response of the distal airspace to an injury. These pathological processes can be divided into the exudative, proliferative, and fibrotic phases. The exudative phase is the initial response to ALI; disrupting the alveolar epithelial-endothelial barrier in which the edematous flooding of the alveolar and interstitial compartments occurs. Inflammatory cells, such as macrophages and neutrophils are activated and release inflammatory chemokines and cytokines including tumor necrosis factor alpha (TNF-α), interleukin (IL)-6, CXCL8, and arachidonic acid metabolites. Neutrophils play a central role in the inflammation and tissue injury of ARDS [26]. Activated neutrophils have reduced plasticity, making it difficult for them to pass through the pulmonary microvascular network [27]. Simultaneously, changes, such as the increased expression of adhesion molecules (e.g., intercellular adhesion molecule-1) occur on the endothelial side, thereby resulting in increased adhesion between the neutrophils and endothelial cells and the accumulation of peripheral blood neutrophils within the pulmonary vasculature [27]. Neutrophils in the pulmonary vasculature migrate from the pulmonary vessels under the influence of chemotactic factors derived from alveolar macrophages. Those that reach the pulmonary interstitium and alveolar space release neutrophil elastase and reactive oxygen species [27]. This results in severe inflammation of the lungs with cellular injury of the vascular endothelium and alveolar epithelium and the increased permeability of the pulmonary microvascular endothelium and alveolar epithelium. Increased endothelial permeability leads to the leakage and retention of fluid in the interstitium around the blood vessels and bronchioles resulting in interstitial pulmonary edema. With alveolar injury, exudate-containing plasma components fill the alveolar space, thus resulting in pulmonary edema. Secondarily, the proliferative phase begins as early as day 3 to repair the injury by re-establishing the alveolar barrier with the clearance of exudative fluid. In this phase, the M2 phenotype predominates as both resident and recruited macrophages are polarized from the M1 to M2 (anti-inflammatory) phenotype. M2 macrophages exert anti-inflammatory effects by clearing apoptotic neutrophils and cell debris, and reducing lung inflammation [28]. M2 polarization mitigates inflammatory conditions observed during ARDS [28, 29].

Notwithstanding advances in revealing the complex mechanisms underlying these initial phases of ARDS, the details of ARDS pathogenesis, in particular the fibrotic phase, remains poorly understood.

2.3 Possible Mechanisms of Action of Macrolides in ARDS

Macrolides exert beneficial effects on patients with inflammatory lung disease, in addition to their ability to inhibit the growth of pathogenic bacteria. In vitro and in vivo studies have demonstrated that macrolides suppress inflammation and modulate the immune system as discussed in several chapters of this book. Macrolides can regulate cytokine balance, inhibit chemokine production and neutrophil elastase activity, accelerate neutrophil apoptosis, alter macrophage morphology, block the activation of nuclear transcription factors, and stabilize the epithelial cell membrane [30–34]. These effects may contribute to the improved outcome of ARDS. Moreover, they decrease lung inflammation and injury, reduce inflammatory cytokines and oxidative stress, and improve survival in animal models of lung injury [35–37].

Reports on the effects of macrolides on cytokine production and neutrophil function emphasize this as a primary pathway of their beneficial effects in ARDS. However, the mechanisms by which macrolides influence the outcomes in patients with ARDS remains speculative.

3 Possible Mechanisms of Action of Macrolides in ARDS-related conditions

3.1 Ventilator-Associated Lung Injury (VALI)

Despite the application of high-flow nasal cannula and extracorporeal support, mechanical ventilation remains the mainstay of care for a patient with ARDS. Mechanical ventilation for ARDS is a double-edged sword because it is a lifesaving technique but is also associated with potentially harmful complications [38]. It adds mechanical stress to the airway [39] and may induce an additional injury called ventilator-associated lung injury (VALI). Minimizing the duration of mechanical ventilation is the best way to minimize complications and reduce mortality in patients with ARDS. Inflammation is one main driver of VALI [40]. Melatonin [41] and dexamethasone [42] have anti-inflammatory effects and reportedly decrease VALI. Researchers have reported on the pleiotropic beneficial effects of macrolides in VALI in in vivo and using in vitro models [43–46].

A recent randomized controlled trial aiming to evaluate the immunomodulatory effects of azithromycin (AZM) in preventing mechanical ventilation-induced lung injury in very low birth weight preterm neonates demonstrated that the use of AZM was significantly associated with decreased serum IL-2 and CXCL8 levels, and a lower incidence of death and oxygen dependency at 28 days in AZM-treated patients [45].

3.2 Ventilator-Associated Pneumonia (VAP)

Notwithstanding the initial lung injury, patients with ARDS may develop a secondary pulmonary infection, ventilator-associated pneumonia (VAP) [47]. VAP-complicating ARDS appears to affect between 20% and 40% of these patients [48, 49]. The incidence of VAP was 1.18 (0.86–1.60) per 100 days of invasive mechanical ventilation in a post hoc analysis of a clinical trial evaluating the prone position in ARDS [49], and VAP was associated with higher mortality, with a hazard ratio of 2.2 (95% confidence interval 1.39–3.52, $p < 0.001$) after adjusting for confounding factors. Recent data from the Center for Disease Control and Prevention suggest that VAP rates are not decreasing in the USA [50].

Giamarellos-Bourboulis et al. reported on a multicenter trial of macrolide therapy in patients with sepsis who had VAP [51]. Macrolides significantly shortened the time to the resolution of VAP (10 days in the clarithromycin group vs. 15.5 days in the placebo group, $p = 0.011$) and the time to ventilation liberation (16 days in the clarithromycin group vs. 22.5 days in the placebo group, $p = 0.049$). The macrolide group also had faster improvement in lung inflammation scores and less progression to multiple organ failure [51]. The all-cause mortality on day 90 was 60% and 43% in the placebo arm and clarithromycin arm, respectively ($P = 0.023$), and intravenous clarithromycin for 3 consecutive days as an adjunctive treatment in VAP and sepsis offered long-term survival benefits along with a considerable reduction in the hospitalization costs [52]. They also reported on serum markers, immunophenotyping characteristics of monocytes and neutrophils, and the ex vivo function of monocytes and neutrophils in patients who participated in this trial. Macrolides restored the balance between pro-inflammatory and anti-inflammatory mediators [53].

3.3 Pulmonary Fibrosis after ARDS

ARDS can also lead to pulmonary fibrosis [54–56]. Distinct from the idiopathic form of pulmonary fibrosis or progressive interstitial lung diseases, ARDS-mediated fibrosis appears to be nonprogressive and in some cases many resolve. However, some may have a persistently decreased lung function [56]. Macrolides exert an antifibrotic effect in animal models of ALI [57, 58]. Wuyts et al. reported that AZM reduced fibrosis and the restrictive lung function pattern in a bleomycin mouse model. This effect was caused by the modulation of both innate and adaptive immunity [57]. Zhang et al. reported that bleomycin-induced pulmonary fibrosis was ameliorated by macrolides, owing to the effects of macrolide-targeting senescent cells mediated by the NADPH oxidase 4 pathway [58].

4 Current Evidence for Macrolides in ALI and ARDS from Human Data

4.1 Effects of Macrolides in Patients with ARDS

The association between the administration of a macrolide antibiotic and mortality in patients with ALI was evaluated using publicly available data from the Acute Respiratory Distress Network Lisofylline and Respiratory Management of Acute Lung Injury trial, in which 235 patients were randomized in a two-by-two fashion to receive low tidal volume vs. standard tidal volume ventilation and either lisofylline (an anti-inflammatory metabolite of pentoxifyline) or placebo [10]. It was found that 47 of 235 patients received a macrolide within 24 h of study enrollment. Following adjustment for confounding variables, subjects who had received a macrolide antibiotic had a significant reduction in 180-day mortality and a shorter time to discontinuation of mechanical ventilation. By contrast, fluoroquinolone and cephalosporin antibiotics had no survival advantage [10].

We have been using AZM for ARDS and other cases of severe acute respiratory failure since 2012, based on the above report [10]. AZM administration within 24 h of septic ARDS diagnosis improved the long-term survival and reduced the time to the liberation from mechanical ventilation [11]. We performed a single-center retrospective cohort study that identified 62 patients with moderate or severe ARDS who had received AZM. Treatment with AZM significantly reduced both 90-day mortality and time to successful liberation from mechanical ventilation [12]. In a subsequent large multicenter prospective observational study, 158 of 873 patients with ARDS admitted to the ICU received macrolides (97% erythromycin), and this was associated with a decreased 30-day mortality [13].

However in a retrospective analysis of prospectively collected data from 7182 patients admitted to 20 French intensive care units with acute respiratory failure, 1295 patients received a macrolide for 3 days, and were compared with 5887 patients who did not receive a macrolide. Using the inverse probability of treatment weighting approach, showed no difference in the 28-day outcomes including the duration of mechanical ventilation [59].

Recently, researchers performed a retrospective observational study using data from the Diagnosis Procedure Combination database of Japan to compare the effects of AZM when used with β-lactam with that of β-lactam alone in mechanically ventilated patients with CAP-associated ARDS [60]. The propensity score matching analysis and the inverse probability of treatment weighting analysis revealed no significant difference between the groups with respect to the 28-day mortality and in-hospital mortality. However, this study had several limitations, such as inadequate detailed clinical data and missing information on the severity of ARDS based on the Berlin criteria [60].

4.2 Severe Pneumonia

4.2.1 Severe Community-Acquired Pneumonia

Severe pneumonia is the leading cause of ARDS. The American Thoracic Society/ Infectious Diseases Society of America (ATS/IDSA) guidelines recommend the use of macrolides in combination with beta-lactams, for the treatment of community-acquired pneumonia (CAP), including critically ill patients admitted to the ICU and beta-lactams and macrolide combination are preferred over beta-lactams and fluoroquinolone [61].

A recent large randomized controlled study assessing empiric antibiotic regimens for patients with suspected CAP demonstrated that β-lactam monotherapy was not inferior to combination therapy with a macrolide or to respiratory fluoroquinolone monotherapy [62]. There was no statistical difference in either the overall survival or complication rates between the three treatment arms. The study was pragmatic, however it was impossible to recruit only patients admitted to non-ICU wards. Thus, the results could not be generalized to either critically ill patients or those with severe CAP in ICU settings.

A multicenter, prospective observational study of intubated patients with CAP receiving guideline-concordant therapy demonstrated that the combination treatment of a β-lactam and macrolide significantly decreased 30-day mortality (hazard ratio [H.R.]: 0.48; 95% CI: 0.23–0.97; and $P = 0.04$), including in those with shock (HR: 0.44; 95% CI: 0.2–0.95; and $P = 0.03$), compared with fluoroquinolone monotherapy [63].

Sligl and colleagues performed a meta-analysis of observatiwonal studies with approximately 10,000 critically ill patients with CAP, and demonstrated that macrolide-containing therapies (often in combination with a b-lactam) were associated with a significant mortality reduction (18% relative risk, 3% absolute risk), compared with non–macrolide-containing therapies [64]. A mortality benefit from macrolides has been principally observed in cohorts of patients with severe CAP. In a systematic review, Vardakas and colleagues compared β-lactam/fluoroquinolone to the β-lactam/macrolide combination for the treatment of patients with CAP. β-lactam/fluoroquinolone combination therapy resulted in higher mortality than β-lactam/macrolide combination therapy. However, the studies had an overall low quality, and the researchers could not recommend for or against either of the regimens [65]. A prospective study demonstrated that macrolide treatment in patients with nonresponding CAP lowered IL-6 and TNF-α in the bronchoalveolar lavage fluid and IL-6, CXCL8, and IL-10 in the plasma. Patients had a shorter length of hospitalization and reached clinical stability earlier [66]. The magnitude of survival benefits appears to be independent of the antimicrobial efficacy.

4.2.2 Viral Pneumonia

Viral pneumonia is a common cause of ARDS. Macrolides have been assessed in vitro and in respiratory viral infections for their potential immunomodulatory and antiviral effects, with inconsistent results [67].

An open-label RCT conducted in patients hospitalized for influenza ($n = 107$) reported that the combination of clarithromycin, naproxen, and oseltamivir in the early stages of diagnosis significantly reduced mortality and hospital days, compared with oseltamivir alone [68]. Lee et al. conducted a multicenter trial in adults hospitalized for laboratory-confirmed influenza. The patients were randomized to receive oseltamivir-AZM or oseltamivir alone [69]. This study demonstrated a rapid reduction in plasma concentrations of pro-inflammatory cytokines and chemokines IL-6, CXCL8, IL-17, CXCL9/membrane immunoglobulin, soluble TNF receptor 1, and IL-18 and in C-reactive protein in the oseltamivir-AZM group, with a trend toward earlier symptom resolution [69].

In a randomized phase 2 clinical trial of 48 children with respiratory failure due to respiratory syncytial virus, high-dose AZM reduced matrix metalloproteinase-9 levels, TNF-α, IL-1β, and IL-10. Patients treated with high-dose AZM displayed reduced ventilator use and days on oxygen as well as shorter hospital stay. These high doses of AZM were considered safe [70]. By contrast, a multicenter observational study reported that macrolide treatment did not affect survival in severely ill patients with H1N1 influenza A [71]. Macrolides were not associated with decreased 90-day mortality and viral RNA clearance in Middle East respiratory syndrome [72].

Considering their potent immunomodulatory and antiviral potential, macrolides have been investigated for their efficacy against the pandemic of coronavirus disease 2019 (COVID-19). In the early phase of the pandemic, researchers performed various clinical trials examining the efficacy of macrolides against COVID-19. Particularly, these trials focused on the combination of AZM with hydroxychloroquine (HCQ), an antimalarial agent also used as an immunomodulator in rheumatoid arthritis and systemic lupus erythematosus. Predominantly observational studies reported that combination therapy with AZM and HCQ promoted recovery, reduced disease symptoms, viral load, and the risk of hospitalization [73–76]. However, several studies reported on no clinical benefits or no improvement in mortality of patients prescribed AZM/HCQ combination therapy, compared with controls on standard therapy [77–79], with caution about adverse events and safety risks [80].

The RECOVERY trial, a randomized, controlled, open-label, adaptive platform trial, identified no benefits of AZM on the outcomes in hospitalized patients with COVID-19 [81]. It randomized 7763 patients to AZM or standard care, thus providing strong evidence of lack of benefit in this group. Macrolides may be of no use for mild symptoms of COVID-19; nonetheless, their evaluation in-hospital settings to treat established ARDS warrants further investigation.

4.3 Acute Exacerbation of Pulmonary Fibrosis

Idiopathic pulmonary fibrosis (IPF), is a chronic and progressive disease with poor prognosis, characterized by progressive lung scarring and the destruction of the lung parenchyma. Most patients with IPF have a relatively prolonged clinical course but up to 15% experience an acute exacerbation (AE) of IPF each year [82], defined as an acute worsening or development of dyspnea and bilateral ground-glass abnormality and/or consolidation on computed tomography [83]. The definition of AE resembles the Berlin definition of ARDS. AE-fibrosing ILD may be interpreted as ARDS that develops in patients with fibrosing ILD. Furthermore, the basic mechanisms of pulmonary fibrosis are common, despite differences in the subtypes of pulmonary fibrosis following ARDS and in chronic diseases, such as IPF [84].

AE are not unique to IPF but occurs in nonspecific interstitial pneumonia, connective-tissue disease associated with interstitial lung disease, and chronic hypersensitivity pneumonitis [85]. A previous epidemiologic survey of Japanese patients with IPF demonstrated that AE-IPF was the most common cause of death [86]. AE had 50% in-hospital mortality and a major impact on the overall survival of patients with IPF [82]. Current guidelines recommend the use of steroids, despite no clear evidence of benefit. Based on the beneficial effects of macrolides on ALI [10], we investigated the efficacy of macrolides in patients with AE of chronic fibrotic interstitial pneumonia. Using a historical cohort as the control group, we investigated the efficacy of intravenous macrolides (500 mg for 5 days) in patients with AE of fibrotic interstitial pneumonia [87]. The use of intravenous AZM improved the 60 day survival compared with the historical cohort treated with a fluoroquinolone (60-day mortality: 20% in the AZM group vs. 69.6% in the fluoroquinolone group). We also reported on the efficacy of macrolides for AE in an analysis limited to patients with AE-IPF [88].

A study using a large contemporary and comprehensive Japanese clinical database assessed the efficacy of combined treatment options, including high-dose corticosteroids in patients with IPF who had severe rapid progression and required ventilator support. Treatment using the combination of macrolides with high-dose corticosteroids was associated with better prognosis [89]. Macrolide-containing regimens may improve the prognosis in patients with acute respiratory failure from interstitial lung disease requiring extracorporeal membrane oxygenation [90].

5 Summary of the Use of Macrolides in ARDS and ALI

The effect of macrolides in ARDS and AE of interstitial pneumonia is probably insufficient at conventional oral doses owing to bioavailability, suggesting that intravenous macrolides may be necessary to achieve a beneficial effect. However, the increased bioavailability may increase side effects, such as QT prolongation, so cardiac monitoring is recommended during macrolide administration. AZM may marginally increase cardiovascular events [91, 92]. However, ARDS, severe pneumonia, and AE of interstitial pneumonia can be fatal, and the benefits of macrolides probably outweigh the potential increased risk of cardiovascular events.

6 Future Research Perspectives

6.1 The Impact of ARDS Phenotypes on Therapeutic Response

ARDS is a syndrome rather than a distinct pathological entity. Therefore, patients with ARDS display substantial heterogeneity in their clinical, physiological, radiological, and biological phenotypes. A latent class analysis of clinical and biomarker data from five randomized trial cohorts of patients with ARDS identified two distinct endotypes [93]. One endotype, representing approximately 30% of the patients with ARDS, had higher plasma concentrations of inflammatory cytokines, lower plasma concentrations of the coagulation factor protein C and bicarbonate, higher prevalence of shock, and consistently worse clinical outcomes than patients with endotypes characterized by lower inflammatory markers [93]. Pulmonary ARDS is likely to respond differently than extrapulmonary ARDS [94], and the pathogenesis may differ within these broad categories.

Almost all clinical trials of ARDS therapies have focused on large patient cohorts, without considering the heterogeneous nature of this syndrome and the varying immune responses of each patient. Therefore, a precision medicine approach, identifying a potential subgroup of patients who are likely more responsive to macrolides, may be helpful.

7 Conclusion

There is limited evidence for the usefulness of macrolides for acute respiratory diseases, such as ARDS (summarized in Table 2). The pleiotropic immunomodulatory effects of macrolides may be effective in ARDS and AE of interstitial pneumonia, characterized by excessive cytokine/chemokine release and neutrophil activation. The results of several animal models of ALI and preclinical studies

Table 2 Evidence of macrolides from clinical studies involving patients with ARDS or ALI

	Disease (participants)	Study design	Intervention	Main effect attributed to macrolide	Reference
Walkey et a, 2012	ARDS ($n = 235$)	Retrospective analysis of prospective cohort	Macrolide ($n = 47$) or no macrolide ($n = 188$)	Use of macrolide was associated with lower 180-day mortality (hazard ratio [HR], 0.46; 95% CI, 0.23–0.92; P 5 0.028) and shorter time to successful discontinuation of mechanical ventilation (HR, 1.93; 95% CI, 1.18–3.17; P 5 0.009).	[10]
Kawamura et al., 2016	ARDS ($n = 125$)	Retrospective analysis of prospective cohort	AZM ($n = 29$) or no macrolide ($n = 96$)	Use of azithromycin was associated with lower 60-day mortality (adjusted hazard ratio [HR] 0.38; 95% CI 0.18–0.79; $P = 0.009$) and a shorter time to successful discontinuation of mechanical ventilation (adjusted HR for successful ventilation discontinuation: 2.22; 95% CI 1.24–3.99; $P = 0.007$.)	[11]
Kawamura et al., 2018	Sepsis-associated ARDS ($n = 191$)	Retrospective analysis of prospective cohort	AZM (i = 62) or no macrolide ($n = 129$)	Use of azithromycin was associated with improvement in 90-day survival rate (Hazard ratio [HR], 0.49; 95% confidence interval [CI], 0.27–0.87; $P = 0.015$) and a shorter time to successful discontinuation of mechanical ventilation (HR, 1.74; 95% CI, 1.07–2.81; $P = 0.026$).	[12]
Simonis et al., 2018	ARDS ($n = 873$)	Retrospective analysis of prospective cohort	Macrolide ($n = 158$) or no macrolide ($n = 715$)	Use of macrolide was associated with reduced 30-day mortality in the whole cohort [22.8% vs. 31.6%; crude odds ratio (OR), 0.64 (interquartile range, 0.43–0.96), $P = 0.03$].Subgroup analyses of propensity-matched cohort: Lower 30-day mortality remained only in ARDS of nonpulmonary origin (OR 0·50, 95% CI 0·26–0·95) and nonhyperinflammatoryphenotype 1 (0·20, 0·06–0·65)	[13]
Pons et al., 2019	ARDS ($n = 7182$)	Retrospective analysis of prospective cohort	Macrolide ($n = 1295$) or no macrolide ($n = 5887$)	The IPTW-adjusted probability of a better outcome (death and mechanical ventilation duration)	[59]

(continued)

Table 2 (continued)

	Disease (participants)	Study design	Intervention	Main effect attributed to macrolide	Reference
				within 28 days after ICU admission in the macrolides group was 49.4% (95% CI 46.8–51.6%)	
Suzuki et al., 2022	CAP-associated ARDS ($n = 1257$)	Retrospective analysis	AZM ($n = 226$) or no macrolide ($n = 1031$)	No significant difference was observed between the groups with respect to 28-day mortality (34.5% vs. 37.6%, $p = 0.556$) or in-hospital mortality (46.0% vs. 49.1%, $p = 0.569$).The inverse probability of treatment weighting analysis showed similar results.	[60]
Martin-Loeches et al., 2010	Intubated patients with CAP ($n = 218$)	Prospective analysis	Macrolide ($n = 46$) or no macrolide ($n = 172$)	Use of macrolide was associated with lower ICU mortality (hazard ratio, HR 0.48, confidence intervals, 95% CI 0.23–0.97, $P = 0.04$) when compared to the use of fluoroquinolones.	[63]
Sligel et al., 2014	Severe CAP ($n = 9850$)	Systematic review and meta-analysis	Macrolide ($n = 4036$) or no macrolide ($n = 5814$)	Use of macrolide was associated with a significant 18% relative (3% absolute) reduction in mortality compared with nonmacrolide therapies.	[64]
Kawamura et al., 2014	AE of PPF ($n = 20$)	Prospective analysis with historical controls	AZM ($n = 20$) or fluoroquinolone ($n = 56$)	Use of AZM was associated with significantly lower 60-day mortality compared with fluoroquinolone (AZM, 20% vs. control, 69.6%; $p < 0.001$).	[87]
Kawamura et al., 2017	AE of IPF ($n = 85$)	Retrospective analysis	Maclodide [38] or fluoroquinolone ($n = 47$)	Use of AZM was associated with significantly lower 60-day mortality compared with fluoroquinolone (azithromycin, 26% vs. fluoroquinolone, 70%; $p < 0.001$).	[88]

AE acute exacerbation, *ARDS* acute respiratory distress syndrome, *AZM* azithromycin, *CAP* community-acquired pneumonia, *IPF* idiopathic pulmonary fibrosis, *PPF* progressive pulmonary fibrosis

support this hypothesis. Preclinical studies have described macrolides as promising immunomodulatory agents that appear to have the potential to rectify imbalanced immune homeostasis in critically ill patients. This warrants future trials to investigate macrolides in terms of their dosing, duration, type, and side effects as well as focus on preventing antibiotic resistance. Future studies should identify the endotypes of ARDS that may respond to adjunctive macrolide treatment.

Acknowledgments This chapter did not receive funding

Conflict of interest The author has no conflict of interest to disclose.

Ethical approval Not applicable.

References

1. Sweeney RM, McAuley DF. Acute respiratory distress syndrome. Lancet. 2016;388(10058): 2416–30.
2. Force ADT, Ranieri VM, Rubenfeld GD, Thompson BT, Ferguson ND, Caldwell E, et al. Acute respiratory distress syndrome: the Berlin definition. JAMA. 2012;307(23):2526–33.
3. Bellani G, Laffey JG, Pham T, Fan E, Brochard L, Esteban A, et al. Epidemiology, patterns of care, and mortality for patients with acute respiratory distress syndrome in intensive care units in 50 countries. JAMA. 2016;315(8):788–800.
4. Matthay MA, Zemans RL, Zimmerman GA, Arabi YM, Beitler JR, Mercat A, et al. Acute respiratory distress syndrome. Nat Rev Dis Primers. 2019;5(1):18.
5. Boyle AJ, Mac Sweeney R, McAuley DF. Pharmacological treatments in ARDS; a state-of-the-art update. BMC Med. 2013;11(1):166.
6. Gibson PG, Yang IA, Upham JW, Reynolds PN, Hodge S, James AL, et al. Effect of azithromycin on asthma exacerbations and quality of life in adults with persistent uncontrolled asthma (AMAZES): a randomised, double-blind, placebo-controlled trial. Lancet. 2017;390 (10095):659–68.
7. Donath E, Chaudhry A, Hernandez-Aya LF, Lit L. A meta-analysis on the prophylactic use of macrolide antibiotics for the prevention of disease exacerbations in patients with chronic obstructive pulmonary disease. Respir Med. 2013;107(9):1385–92.
8. Uzun S, Djamin RS, Kluytmans JA, Mulder PG, van't Veer NE, Ermens AA, et al. Azithromycin maintenance treatment in patients with frequent exacerbations of chronic obstructive pulmonary disease (COLUMBUS): a randomised, double-blind, placebo-controlled trial. Lancet. Respir Med. 2014;2(5):361–8.
9. Kudoh S, Azuma A, Yamamoto M, Izumi T, Ando M. Improvement of survival in patients with diffuse panbronchiolitis treated with low-dose erythromycin. Am J Respir Crit Care Med. 1998;157(6 Pt 1):1829–32.
10. Walkey AJ, Wiener RS. Macrolide antibiotics and survival in patients with acute lung injury. Chest. 2012;141(5):1153–9.
11. Kawamura K, Ichikado K, Takaki M, Sakata Y, Yasuda Y, Shingu N, et al. Efficacy of azithromycin in sepsis-associated acute respiratory distress syndrome: a retrospective study and propensity score analysis. Springerplus. 2016;5(1):1193.
12. Kawamura K, Ichikado K, Takaki M, Eguchi Y, Anan K, Suga M. Adjunctive therapy with azithromycin for moderate and severe acute respiratory distress syndrome: a retrospective,

propensity score-matching analysis of prospectively collected data at a single center. Int J Antimicrob Agents. 2018;51(6):918–24.
13. Simonis FD, de Iudicibus G, Cremer OL, Ong DSY, van der Poll T, Bos LD, et al. Macrolide therapy is associated with reduced mortality in acute respiratory distress syndrome (ARDS) patients. Ann Transl Med. 2018;6(2):24.
14. Meyer NJ, Gattinoni L, Calfee CS. Acute respiratory distress syndrome. Lancet. 2021;398 (10300):622–37.
15. Ware LB, Matthay MA. The acute respiratory distress syndrome. N Engl J Med. 2000;342(18): 1334–49.
16. Ashbaugh DG, Bigelow DB, Petty TL, Levine BE. Acute respiratory distress in adults. Lancet. 1967;2(7511):319–23.
17. Bernard GR, Luce JM, Sprung CL, Rinaldo JE, Tate RM, Sibbald WJ, et al. High-dose corticosteroids in patients with the adult respiratory distress syndrome. N Engl J Med. 1987;317(25):1565–70.
18. Meduri GU, Headley AS, Golden E, Carson SJ, Umberger RA, Kelso T, et al. Effect of prolonged methylprednisolone therapy in unresolving acute respiratory distress syndrome: a randomized controlled trial. JAMA. 1998;280(2):159–65.
19. Steinberg KP, Hudson LD, Goodman RB, Hough CL, Lanken PN, Hyzy R, et al. Efficacy and safety of corticosteroids for persistent acute respiratory distress syndrome. N Engl J Med. 2006;354(16):1671–84.
20. Paine R 3rd, Standiford TJ, Dechert RE, Moss M, Martin GS, Rosenberg AL, et al. A randomized trial of recombinant human granulocyte-macrophage colony stimulating factor for patients with acute lung injury. Crit Care Med. 2012;40(1):90–7.
21. McAuley DF, Laffey JG, O'Kane CM, Perkins GD, Mullan B, Trinder TJ, et al. Simvastatin in the acute respiratory distress syndrome. N Engl J Med. 2014;371(18):1695–703.
22. Needham DM, Colantuoni E, Dinglas VD, Hough CL, Wozniak AW, Jackson JC, et al. Rosuvastatin versus placebo for delirium in intensive care and subsequent cognitive impairment in patients with sepsis-associated acute respiratory distress syndrome: an ancillary study to a randomised controlled trial. Lancet Respir Med. 2016;4(3):203–12.
23. Toner P, Boyle AJ, McNamee JJ, Callaghan K, Nutt C, Johnston P, et al. Aspirin as a treatment for ARDS: a randomized, placebo-controlled clinical trial. Chest. 2022;161(5):1275–84.
24. Bernard GR, Wheeler AP, Arons MM, Morris PE, Paz HL, Russell JA, et al. A trial of antioxidants N-acetylcysteine and procysteine in ARDS. The antioxidant in ARDS study group. Chest. 1997;112(1):164–72.
25. Fowler AA 3rd, Truwit JD, Hite RD, Morris PE, DeWilde C, Priday A, et al. Effect of vitamin C infusion on organ failure and biomarkers of inflammation and vascular injury in patients with sepsis and severe acute respiratory failure: the CITRIS-ALI randomized clinical trial. JAMA. 2019;322(13):1261–70.
26. Steinberg KP, Milberg JA, Martin TR, Maunder RJ, Cockrill BA, Hudson LD. Evolution of bronchoalveolar cell populations in the adult respiratory distress syndrome. Am J Respir Crit Care Med. 1994;150(1):113–22.
27. Yang SC, Tsai YF, Pan YL, Hwang TL. Understanding the role of neutrophils in acute respiratory distress syndrome. Biom J. 2021;44(4):439–46.
28. Huang X, Xiu H, Zhang S, Zhang G. The role of macrophages in the pathogenesis of ALI/ARDS. Mediat Inflamm. 2018;2018:1264913.
29. Chen X, Tang J, Shuai W, Meng J, Feng J, Han Z. Macrophage polarization and its role in the pathogenesis of acute lung injury/acute respiratory distress syndrome. Inflamm Res. 2020;69 (9):883–95.
30. Tamaoki J, Sakai N, Tagaya E, Konno K. Macrolide antibiotics protect against endotoxin-induced vascular leakage and neutrophil accumulation in rat trachea. Antimicrob Agents Chemother. 1994;38(7):1641–3.
31. Kanoh S, Rubin BK. Mechanisms of action and clinical application of macrolides as immunomodulatory medications. Clin Microbiol Rev. 2010;23(3):590–615.

32. Kricker JA, Page CP, Gardarsson FR, Baldursson O, Gudjonsson T, Parnham MJ. Nonantimicrobial actions of macrolides: overview and perspectives for future development. Pharmacol Rev. 2021;73(4):233–62.
33. Reijnders TDY, Saris A, Schultz MJ, van der Poll T. Immunomodulation by macrolides: therapeutic potential for critical care. Lancet Respir Med. 2020;8(6):619–30.
34. Haydar D, Cory TJ, Birket SE, Murphy BS, Pennypacker KR, Sinai AP, et al. Azithromycin polarizes macrophages to an M2 phenotype via inhibition of the STAT1 and NF-kappaB signaling pathways. J Immunol. 2019;203(4):1021–30.
35. Tamaoki J. The effects of macrolides on inflammatory cells. Chest. 2004;125(2 Suppl):41S–50S. quiz 1S
36. Sato K, Suga M, Akaike T, Fujii S, Muranaka H, Doi T, et al. Therapeutic effect of erythromycin on influenza virus-induced lung injury in mice. Am J Respir Crit Care Med. 1998;157(3 Pt 1):853–7.
37. Lee SJ, Yi CO, Heo RW, Song DH, Cho YJ, Jeong YY, et al. Clarithromycin attenuates radiation-induced lung injury in mice. PLoS One. 2015;10(6):e0131671.
38. Villar J, Blanco J, Anon JM, Santos-Bouza A, Blanch L, Ambros A, et al. The ALIEN study: incidence and outcome of acute respiratory distress syndrome in the era of lung protective ventilation. Intensive Care Med. 2011;37(12):1932–41.
39. Albaiceta GM, Blanch L. Beyond volutrauma in ARDS: the critical role of lung tissue deformation. Crit Care. 2011;15(2):304.
40. Santos CC, Zhang H, Liu M, Slutsky AS. Bench-to-bedside review: biotrauma and modulation of the innate immune response. Crit Care. 2005;9(3):280–6.
41. Pedreira PR, Garcia-Prieto E, Parra D, Astudillo A, Diaz E, Taboada F, et al. Effects of melatonin in an experimental model of ventilator-induced lung injury. Am J Physiol Lung Cell Mol Physiol. 2008;295(5):L820–7.
42. Nin N, Penuelas O, de Paula M, Lorente JA, Fernandez-Segoviano P, Esteban A. Ventilation-induced lung injury in rats is associated with organ injury and systemic inflammation that is attenuated by dexamethasone. Crit Care Med. 2006;34(4):1093–8.
43. Amado-Rodriguez L, Gonzalez-Lopez A, Lopez-Alonso I, Aguirre A, Astudillo A, Batalla-Solis E, et al. Anti-inflammatory effects of clarithromycin in ventilator-induced lung injury. Respir Res. 2013;14:52.
44. Lee H, Fei Q, Streicher A, Zhang W, Isabelle C, Patel P, et al. mTORC1 is a mechanosensor that regulates surfactant function and lung compliance during ventilator-induced lung injury. JCI Insight. 2021;6(14)
45. Nunes CR, Procianoy RS, Corso AL, Silveira RC. Use of azithromycin for the prevention of lung injury in mechanically ventilated preterm neonates: a randomized controlled trial. Neonatology. 2020;117(4):522–8.
46. Joelsson JP, Myszor IT, Sigurdsson S, Lehmann F, Page CP, Gudmundsson GH, et al. Azithromycin has lung barrier protective effects in a cell model mimicking ventilator-induced lung injury. ALTEX. 2020;37(4):545–60.
47. Iregui MG, Kollef MH. Ventilator-associated pneumonia complicating the acute respiratory distress syndrome. Semin Respir Crit Care Med. 2001;22(3):317–26.
48. Forel JM, Voillet F, Pulina D, Gacouin A, Perrin G, Barrau K, et al. Ventilator-associated pneumonia and ICU mortality in severe ARDS patients ventilated according to a lung-protective strategy. Crit Care. 2012;16(2):R65.
49. Ayzac L, Girard R, Baboi L, Beuret P, Rabilloud M, Richard JC, et al. Ventilator-associated pneumonia in ARDS patients: the impact of prone positioning. A secondary analysis of the PROSEVA trial. Intensive Care Med. 2016;42(5):871–8.
50. Magill SS, O'Leary E, Janelle SJ, Thompson DL, Dumyati G, Nadle J, et al. Changes in prevalence of health care-associated infections in U.S. Hospitals. N Engl J Med. 2018;379(18):1732–44.

51. Giamarellos-Bourboulis EJ, Pechere JC, Routsi C, Plachouras D, Kollias S, Raftogiannis M, et al. Effect of clarithromycin in patients with sepsis and ventilator-associated pneumonia. Clin Infect Dis. 2008;46(8):1157–64.
52. Tsaganos T, Raftogiannis M, Pratikaki M, Christodoulou S, Kotanidou A, Papadomichelakis E, et al. Clarithromycin leads to long-term survival and cost benefit in ventilator-associated pneumonia and sepsis. Antimicrob Agents Chemother. 2016;60(6):3640–6.
53. Spyridaki A, Raftogiannis M, Antonopoulou A, Tsaganos T, Routsi C, Baziaka F, et al. Effect of clarithromycin in inflammatory markers of patients with ventilator-associated pneumonia and sepsis caused by gram-negative bacteria: results from a randomized clinical study. Antimicrob Agents Chemother. 2012;56(7):3819–25.
54. Marshall R, Bellingan G, Laurent G. The acute respiratory distress syndrome: fibrosis in the fast lane. Thorax. 1998;53(10):815–7.
55. Dos Santos CC. Advances in mechanisms of repair and remodelling in acute lung injury. Intensive Care Med. 2008;34(4):619–30.
56. Burnham EL, Janssen WJ, Riches DW, Moss M, Downey GP. The fibroproliferative response in acute respiratory distress syndrome: mechanisms and clinical significance. Eur Respir J. 2014;43(1):276–85.
57. Wuyts WA, Willems S, Vos R, Vanaudenaerde BM, De Vleeschauwer SI, Rinaldi M, et al. Azithromycin reduces pulmonary fibrosis in a bleomycin mouse model. Exp Lung Res. 2010;36(10):602–14.
58. Zhang X, Dong Y, Li WC, Tang BX, Li J, Zang Y. Roxithromycin attenuates bleomycin-induced pulmonary fibrosis by targeting senescent cells. Acta Pharmacol Sin. 2021;42(12):2058–68.
59. Pons S, Timsit JF, Ruckly S, Schwebel C, Papazian L, Azoulay E, et al. Impact of macrolide therapy in critically ill patients with acute respiratory failure: a desirability of outcome ranking analysis to investigate the OUTCOMEREA database. Intensive Care Med. 2019;45(7):1043–5.
60. Suzuki J, Sasabuchi Y, Hatakeyama S, Matsui H, Sasahara T, Morisawa Y, et al. Additional effect of azithromycin over beta-lactam alone for severe community-acquired pneumonia-associated acute respiratory distress syndrome: a retrospective cohort study. Pneumonia (Nathan). 2022;14(1):1.
61. Metlay JP, Waterer GW. Update in adult community-acquired pneumonia: key points from the new American Thoracic Society/Infectious Diseases Society of America 2019 guideline. Curr Opin Pulm Med. 2020;26(3):203–7.
62. Postma DF, van Werkhoven CH, van Elden LJ, Thijsen SF, Hoepelman AI, Kluytmans JA, et al. Antibiotic treatment strategies for community-acquired pneumonia in adults. N Engl J Med. 2015;372(14):1312–23.
63. Martin-Loeches I, Lisboa T, Rodriguez A, Putensen C, Annane D, Garnacho-Montero J, et al. Combination antibiotic therapy with macrolides improves survival in intubated patients with community-acquired pneumonia. Intensive Care Med. 2010;36(4):612–20.
64. Sligl WI, Asadi L, Eurich DT, Tjosvold L, Marrie TJ, Majumdar SR. Macrolides and mortality in critically ill patients with community-acquired pneumonia: a systematic review and meta-analysis. Crit Care Med. 2014;42(2):420–32.
65. Vardakas KZ, Trigkidis KK, Falagas ME. Fluoroquinolones or macrolides in combination with beta-lactams in adult patients hospitalized with community acquired pneumonia: a systematic review and meta-analysis. Clin Microbiol Infect. 2017;23(4):234–41.
66. Lorenzo MJ, Moret I, Sarria B, Cases E, Cortijo J, Mendez R, et al. Lung inflammatory pattern and antibiotic treatment in pneumonia. Respir Res. 2015;16:15.
67. Damle B, Vourvahis M, Wang E, Leaney J, Corrigan B. Clinical pharmacology perspectives on the antiviral activity of azithromycin and use in COVID-19. Clin Pharmacol Ther. 2020;108(2):201–11.
68. Hung IFN, To KKW, Chan JFW, Cheng VCC, Liu KSH, Tam A, et al. Efficacy of clarithromycin-naproxen-oseltamivir combination in the treatment of patients hospitalized for

influenza a(H3N2) infection: an open-label randomized, controlled. Phase IIb/III Trial Chest. 2017;151(5):1069–80.
69. Lee N, Wong CK, Chan MCW, Yeung ESL, Tam WWS, Tsang OTY, et al. Anti-inflammatory effects of adjunctive macrolide treatment in adults hospitalized with influenza: a randomized controlled trial. Antivir Res. 2017;144:48–56.
70. Kong M, Zhang WW, Sewell K, Gorman G, Kuo HC, Aban I, et al. Azithromycin treatment vs placebo in children with respiratory syncytial virus-induced respiratory failure: a phase 2 randomized clinical trial. JAMA Netw Open. 2020;3(4):e203482.
71. Martin-Loeches I, Bermejo-Martin JF, Valles J, Granada R, Vidaur L, Vergara-Serrano JC, et al. Macrolide-based regimens in absence of bacterial co-infection in critically ill H1N1 patients with primary viral pneumonia. Intensive Care Med. 2013;39(4):693–702.
72. Arabi YM, Deeb AM, Al-Hameed F, Mandourah Y, Almekhlafi GA, Sindi AA, et al. Macrolides in critically ill patients with Middle East respiratory syndrome. Int J Infect Dis. 2019;81:184–90.
73. Gautret P, Lagier JC, Parola P, Hoang VT, Meddeb L, Mailhe M, et al. Hydroxychloroquine and azithromycin as a treatment of COVID-19: results of an open-label non-randomized clinical trial. Int J Antimicrob Agents. 2020;56(1):105949.
74. Sekhavati E, Jafari F, SeyedAlinaghi S, Jamalimoghadamsiahkali S, Sadr S, Tabarestani M, et al. Safety and effectiveness of azithromycin in patients with COVID-19: an open-label randomised trial. Int J Antimicrob Agents. 2020;56(4):106143.
75. Gautret P, Hoang VT, Lagier JC, Raoult D. Effect of hydroxychloroquine and azithromycin as a treatment of COVID-19: results of an open-label non-randomized clinical trial, an update with an intention-to-treat analysis and clinical outcomes. Int J Antimicrob Agents. 2021;57(1): 106239.
76. Rashad A, Nafady A, Hassan MH, Mansour H, Taya U, Bazeed SES, et al. Therapeutic efficacy of macrolides in management of patients with mild COVID-19. Sci Rep. 2021;11(1):16361.
77. Furtado RHM, Berwanger O, Fonseca HA, Correa TD, Ferraz LR, Lapa MG, et al. Azithromycin in addition to standard of care versus standard of care alone in the treatment of patients admitted to the hospital with severe COVID-19 in Brazil (COALITION II): a randomised clinical trial. Lancet. 2020;396(10256):959–67.
78. Cavalcanti AB, Zampieri FG, Rosa RG, Azevedo LCP, Veiga VC, Avezum A, et al. Hydroxychloroquine with or without azithromycin in mild-to-moderate Covid-19. N Engl J Med. 2020;383(21):2041–52.
79. Rosenberg ES, Dufort EM, Udo T, Wilberschied LA, Kumar J, Tesoriero J, et al. Association of Treatment with Hydroxychloroquine or azithromycin with in-hospital mortality in patients with COVID-19 in New York state. JAMA. 2020;323(24):2493–502.
80. Group PTC. Azithromycin for community treatment of suspected COVID-19 in people at increased risk of an adverse clinical course in the UK (PRINCIPLE): a randomised, controlled, open-label, adaptive platform trial. Lancet. 2021;397(10279):1063–74.
81. Abaleke E, Abbas M, Abbasi S, Abbott A, Abdelaziz A, Abdelbadiee S, et al. Azithromycin in patients admitted to hospital with COVID-19 (RECOVERY): a randomised, controlled, open-label, platform trial. Lancet. 2021;397(10274):605–12.
82. Song JW, Hong SB, Lim CM, Koh Y, Kim DS. Acute exacerbation of idiopathic pulmonary fibrosis: incidence, risk factors and outcome. Eur Respir J. 2011;37(2):356–63.
83. Collard HR, Ryerson CJ, Corte TJ, Jenkins G, Kondoh Y, Lederer DJ, et al. Acute exacerbation of idiopathic pulmonary fibrosis. An international working group report. Am J Respir Crit Care Med. 2016;194(3):265–75.
84. Michalski JE, Kurche JS, Schwartz DA. From ARDS to pulmonary fibrosis: the next phase of the COVID-19 pandemic? Transl Res. 2022;241:13–24.
85. Park IN, Kim DS, Shim TS, Lim CM, Lee SD, Koh Y, et al. Acute exacerbation of interstitial pneumonia other than idiopathic pulmonary fibrosis. Chest. 2007;132(1):214–20.

86. Natsuizaka M, Chiba H, Kuronuma K, Otsuka M, Kudo K, Mori M, et al. Epidemiologic survey of Japanese patients with idiopathic pulmonary fibrosis and investigation of ethnic differences. Am J Respir Crit Care Med. 2014;190(7):773–9.
87. Kawamura K, Ichikado K, Suga M, Yoshioka M. Efficacy of azithromycin for treatment of acute exacerbation of chronic fibrosing interstitial pneumonia: a prospective, open-label study with historical controls. Respiration. 2014;87(6):478–84.
88. Kawamura K, Ichikado K, Yasuda Y, Anan K, Suga M. Azithromycin for idiopathic acute exacerbation of idiopathic pulmonary fibrosis: a retrospective single-center study. BMC Pulm Med. 2017;17(1):94.
89. Oda K, Yatera K, Fujino Y, Ishimoto H, Nakao H, Hanaka T, et al. Efficacy of concurrent treatments in idiopathic pulmonary fibrosis patients with a rapid progression of respiratory failure: an analysis of a national administrative database in Japan. BMC Pulm Med. 2016;16(1):91.
90. Usagawa Y, Komiya K, Yamasue M, Fushimi K, Hiramatsu K, Kadota JI. Efficacy of extracorporeal membrane oxygenation for acute respiratory failure with interstitial lung disease: a case control nationwide dataset study in Japan. Respir Res. 2021;22(1):211.
91. Cheng YJ, Nie XY, Chen XM, Lin XX, Tang K, Zeng WT, et al. The role of macrolide antibiotics in increasing cardiovascular risk. J Am Coll Cardiol. 2015;66(20):2173–84.
92. Gorelik E, Masarwa R, Perlman A, Rotshild V, Muszkat M, Matok I. Systematic Review, Meta-analysis, and network meta-analysis of the cardiovascular safety of macrolides. Antimicrob Agents Chemother 2018;62(6).
93. Calfee CS, Delucchi K, Parsons PE, Thompson BT, Ware LB, Matthay MA, et al. Subphenotypes in acute respiratory distress syndrome: latent class analysis of data from two randomised controlled trials. Lancet Respir Med. 2014;2(8):611–20.
94. Luo L, Shaver CM, Zhao Z, Koyama T, Calfee CS, Bastarache JA, et al. Clinical predictors of hospital mortality differ between direct and indirect ARDS. Chest. 2017;151(4):755–63.

Azithromycin for Other Lung Diseases: Lung Transplantation and Sarcoidosis

Geert M. Verleden and Stijn E. Verleden

Abstract Azithromycin was introduced in lung transplantation in an attempt to improve the pulmonary function in patients with chronic allograft dysfunction (CLAD), which is defined as a progressive and usually irreversible decline in FEV_1 of at least 20% compared to the best postoperative values and is considered to be the net result of chronic rejection. In fact, in a first case series by Gerhardt et al., a response to azithromycin was observed in 30% of the patients with CLAD (Cooper et al. Am J Respir Crit Care Med 168:85, 2003). Although its mechanism of action is still unknown, it is nowadays specifically used in the treatment and in the prevention of CLAD. After the first case series, many centers have published their experience, all pointing to an increased FEV_1 and improved survival, at least in a subset of patients with the bronchiolitis obliterans (BO) phenotype of CLAD. Also, in sarcoidosis, there has been interest in azithromycin, however, mostly in combination with broad-spectrum antimycobacterial drugs (Royer et al. Sarcoidosis Vasc Diffuse Lung Dis 30:201-11, 2014).

In this chapter, we will give an overview of the possible treatment indications and effects of azithromycin in lung transplantation and sarcoidosis.

Keywords Azithromycin · Lung transplantation · CLAD · BOS · Sarcoidosis

---

G. M. Verleden (✉)
Department of Respiratory Diseases and Lung Transplantation Unit, University Hospital Gasthuisberg, Leuven, Belgium and Chrometa Department, Breathe Lab, Katholieke Universiteit Leuven, Leuven, Belgium
e-mail: geert.verleden@uzleuven.be

S. E. Verleden
ASTARC, Department of Thoracic and Vascular Surgery, University of Antwerp, Wilrijk, Belgium

B. K. Rubin, M. Shinkai (eds.), *Macrolides as Immunomodulatory Agents*, Progress in Inflammation Research 92, https://doi.org/10.1007/978-3-031-42859-3_10

1 Role of Azithromycin in Lung Transplantation

1.1 Short-Term Treatment Effects in Patients with Bronchiolitis Obliterans Syndrome (BOS)

Azithromycin was first introduced as a potential treatment for the obstructive phenotype of CLAD (BOS), which is believed to be the clinical correlate of chronic rejection [1]. The pathophysiology of BOS may be the consequence of a primary insult toward the respiratory epithelium, such as ischemia–reperfusion injury, acute rejection, infection, or aspiration, which may be either isolated (for instance one acute rejection episode, such as a respiratory syncytial virus infection) or repetitive infection of the airways with bacteria or fungi). Injury to the epithelium may locally upregulate dendritic cells, attracting more inflammatory cells (macrophages, neutrophils, T-lymphocytes, and NK cells), leading to epithelial damage and inflammation, with resulting production of chemokines and cytokines from the epithelium, the smooth muscle cells, macrophages, and neutrophils. Activated neutrophils may further increase epithelial damage via the production of reactive oxygen species and metalloproteinases [2, 3]. After an initial inflammatory phase, a fibro-proliferative phase occurs, driven by a variety of growth factors, such as platelet-derived growth factor, insulin-like growth factor, fibroblast growth factor, transforming growth factor-b and endothelin-1, leading to proliferation of smooth muscle cells and fibroblasts (myofibroblasts), epithelial to mesenchymal transition, with deposition of collagen resulting in the typical fibrous, obliterative lesions of the airways [4, 5]. On the other hand, other immunological factors such as human leukocyte antigen–antibody driven chronic rejection may also play a role in this process.

An increased bronchoalveolar lavage fluid (BAL) neutrophilia with upregulation of CXCL8 seems to be common in BOS patients [6]. Riise et al. described an increased BAL neutrophilia in patients with BOS between 1% and 96.5%, [7]. Although the mean percentage of BAL neutrophilia in most publications is increased in patients with BOS, there is also a significant proportion of patients without BAL neutrophilia, despite the fact that their progressive decrease in FEV_1 is comparable. Interestingly, there is some controversial evidence that BAL neutrophilia is a prerequisite for macrolide therapy to be effective in BOS patients as reducing this neutrophilic inflammation may be one of its main mechanisms of action [8].

Since 2003, when the first case series on azithromycin add-on treatment of BOS patients was published by Gerhardt et al. [9], different publications have corroborated these results, demonstrating that adding azithromycin (250 mg, 3 times a week) to the stable immunosuppressive treatment may improve the FEV_1 in some of the lung transplant patients at different stages of BOS [10–12]. In contrast, only one study failed to show an improvement in FEV_1 in 11 patients [13]. Taking all these publications together, 30–35% of all patients at different stages of BOS responded to azithromycin treatment by a mean increase in their FEV_1 of about 14%. A comparable effect on FEV_1 was demonstrated with clarithromycin, proving that the effects are rather class-dependent and not drug specific. Indeed, 12 of 31 patients with BOS or potential BOS responded with a mean FEV_1 increase of 732 ml, 10 of them by 3 months of treatment, 2 after 6 months [14]. These studies were open-label add-on azithromycin studies with a rather small number of patients. However, in 2015, Corris et al. published the first placebo-controlled trial with add-on azithromycin in a population of 48 patients with BOS after lung transplantation. They compared azithromycin (250 mg alternate days over 12 weeks) with placebo and their primary outcome was FEV_1 change after 12 weeks of treatment. Of the initially 48 randomized patients (25 azithromycin and 23 placebo), two were excluded because they did not have BOS. Thus, 46 patients were analyzed as intention to treat (ITT) with 33 patients completing the study. Study completers showed an estimated mean difference in FEV_1 between treatment groups (azithromycin minus placebo) of 0.278 L, ($p = <0.001$). Nine of 23 (39%) ITT patients in the azithromycin group had ≥10% gain in FEV_1 from baseline. No patients in the placebo group had ≥10% improvement in FEV_1 from baseline ($p = 0.002$) [15].

As a consequence of these publications, it became clear that different BOS phenotypes or different disease stages needed to be distinguished [16, 17]. BOS may present with neutrophilic airway inflammation, starting rather early after lung transplantation and characterized by an increase in the FEV_1 while being treated with azithromycin, whereas the other phenotype has no neutrophilic airway inflammation, starts rather late after transplantation and does not respond to azithromycin [17]. Therefore, the first phenotype could no longer be considered as classical BOS, since this is still defined as a largely irreversible and mostly progressive airways obstruction [17]. It was, therefore, proposed to rename this phenotype as neutrophilic reversible allograft dysfunction (NRAD) or azithromycin reversible allograft dysfunction (ARAD), and it was also accepted in recent guidelines that BOS can only be diagnosed after an unsuccessful azithromycin treatment trial of at least 8 weeks, to specifically exclude NRAD/ARAD [18, 19].

The possible mechanisms of action of azithromycin in BOS patients are unknown at present, although several hypotheses have been put forward, such as inhibition of the transcription of quorum-sensing genes, which may then prevent the production of tissue-damaging proteins that have been detected in clinically stable lung transplant recipients without any signs of infection [19], nevertheless leading to a neutrophilic inflammatory response. Other mechanisms include a positive effect on gastroesophageal reflux, which is accepted as a risk factor for the development of BOS, an effect involving neutrophils and CXCL8 through inhibition of IL-17 induced CXCL8 release from airway epithelial cells and smooth muscle cells [20, 21] via inhibition of different mitogen-activated protein kinases and via its anti-oxidative effect [22, 23]. This seems important as it has been shown that a BAL neutrophilia of at least 15% [8] was the best predictor to obtain an improvement of the FEV_1 with azithromycin. Different other possible mechanisms, including antibacterial and immunomodulatory, may be operative and have been previously reviewed in detail by Parnham et al. [24].

1.2 Long-Term Effects of Add-on Azithromycin in Patients with BOS

Several authors have investigated the long-term effects of adding azithromycin in patients with BOS, with specific attention to the FEV_1 improvement and survival. The first paper was published by the Hannover group and included 81 patients with at least BOS stage 0p who have been treated with azithromycin for a mean period of 1.3 years [25]. In this study, 24 out of 81 (30%) patients experienced an improvement of their FEV_1. However, 23% of the initial responders later developed a progressive decrease in FEV_1, compatible with chronic rejection, while still being treated with azithromycin. The authors also found the BAL neutrophilia (>20%) to be predictive for a positive FEV_1 response and demonstrated that most patients responded within 3 months after the addition of azithromycin [25].

In a retrospective study, including 178 patients with BOS, Jain et al. compared 78 patients who had been treated with add-on azithromycin versus 100 who were not [26]. Compared with the no-azithromycin cohort, the azithromycin cohort did not demonstrate a survival benefit; however, for those started on azithromycin before the development of BOS stage 2 ($n = 31$) there was a significant decrease in the risk of death (unadjusted hazard ratio [HR] = 0.29, 95% CI 0.11 to 0.82, $p = 0.02$). In contrast, compared with the no-azithromycin cohort, there was no difference in the risk of death for those started on azithromycin after BOS stage 2 ($n = 47$, unadjusted HR = 1.54, 95% CI 0.91 to 2.61, $p = 0.11$). This was the first study to suggest that azithromycin therapy may specifically improve survival in lung transplant recipients with BOS stage 1 and that early treatment initiation (before the development of BOS stage 2) may be important [26].

In another retrospective study, Vos et al. also demonstrated a survival benefit in 107 BOS patients treated with azithromycin during a mean of 3.1 years [27]. They showed an increase in $FEV_1 \geq 10\%$ after 3–6 months of treatment in 40% of their patients; 33% later redeveloped BOS. Pre-treatment neutrophilia was again higher in responders: 29.3% (9.3% to 69.7%) vs 11.5% (2.9% to 43.8%) ($p = 0.025$), and decreased significantly to 4.2% (1.8% to 17.6%) ($p = 0.041$) after 3 to 6 months of azithromycin therapy. Responders demonstrated better survival compared to non-responders with 6 and 21 deaths, respectively, during follow-up ($p = 0.027$). Multivariate analysis identified initial azithromycin response and earlier post-transplant initiation of azithromycin to be protective for both BOS progression and relapse (HR = 0.12 [95% CI 0.05 to 0.28], $p < 0.0001$; and HR = 0.98 [95% CI 0.97 to 0.98], $p < 0.0001$, respectively) and retransplantation and death during follow-up (HR 0.10 [95% CI 0.02 to 0.48], $p = 0.004$; and HR 0.96 [95% CI 0.95 to 0.98], $p < 0.0001$, respectively) [27].

A meta-analysis performed by Kingah et al., not only demonstrated a significant improvement in lung function in BOS patients following a mean of 7 months of additional azithromycin treatment, but also demonstrated that patients were less likely to die from BOS compared to non-treated patients [28].

1.3 Azithromycin Treatment as Prevention for the Development of BOS

Since it was shown that addition of azithromycin may improve the FEV_1 in some patients with established (neutrophilic) BOS, the question arose whether preventive treatment with azithromycin might also impact on the development of new onset BOS. To answer this question, a placebo-controlled study was performed in Leuven, including 83 lung transplant patients who were either initiated on azithromycin (250 mg, 3 times a week) from discharge after their lung transplantation ($n = 40$) or received additional placebo ($n = 43$) [29]. Primary end-points were BOS-free and overall survival 2 years after transplantation. All patients who developed BOS during the trial, were treated with open-label azithromycin to assess the change in FEV_1. The study demonstrated that BOS development was significantly decreased in patients receiving azithromycin: 12.5% versus 44.2% ($p = 0.0017$) and also that the BOS-free survival was better with azithromycin (HR 0.27, 95% CI 0.092–0.816; $p = 0.020$), while overall survival was comparable. Patients receiving azithromycin also had a better FEV_1 ($p = 0.028$) and less airway neutrophilia ($p = 0.015$) over time. Open-label azithromycin for BOS improved FEV_1 in 52.2% of the patients. No serious adverse events were noted. The authors concluded that azithromycin prophylaxis, compared to placebo, reduces BOS prevalence 2 years after lung transplantation, improves FEV_1 and attenuates neutrophilic airways inflammation [29].

In a post hoc analysis of this study, Ruttens et al. [30] evaluated the development of BOS on the long term in view of the updated classification of CLAD that was published in 2014 [31]. This study was a retrospective, ITT analysis of the previously described randomized controlled trial comparing prophylactic treatment with placebo versus azithromycin [29]. CLAD, graft loss (retransplantation and mortality) and evolution of pulmonary function were analyzed 7 years after inclusion of the last study subject. During this follow-up period, 22/43 (51%) subjects in the placebo group and 11/40 (28%) subjects in the azithromycin group eventually developed CLAD ($p = 0.043$), with the CLAD-free survival being significantly longer in the azithromycin group ($p = 0.024$). No difference was found in the prevalence of obstructive (BOS) versus restrictive (restrictive allograft syndrome, RAS) CLAD between both groups. Graft loss was similar in both groups: 23/43 (53%) versus 16/40 (40%) patients ($p = 0.27$). Long-term pulmonary function and functional exercise capacity were significantly better in the azithromycin group ($p < 0.05$). It was concluded that prophylactic azithromycin therapy reduced long-term CLAD prevalence and improved CLAD-free survival, pulmonary function, and functional exercise capacity [30].

This survival benefit with prophylactic azithromycin treatment was recently corroborated by Li et al. [32]. In their study, including 445 double lung transplant recipients, 344 received prophylactic azithromycin, starting at a median of 51 days after transplantation. Azithromycin was associated with improved survival (HR: 0.59; 95% CI: 0.42–0.82; $p = 0.002$) and a reduced risk of baseline lung allograft dysfunction (BLAD), which is defined as a lower pulmonary function than what would be expected after lung transplantation. (Odds ratio: 0.53; 95% CI: 0.33–0.85; $p = 0.046$). The time to CLAD onset was significantly longer in the azithromycin treated group compared to the non-treated group ($p = 0.02$); however, there was no clear reduction in the adjusted risk of CLAD (HR: 0.69; 95% CI: 0.47–1.03; $p = 0.07$), although there was a reduction in the severity of CLAD. The authors again concluded that prophylactic azithromycin improved the survival after lung transplantation, potentially through an improved baseline pulmonary function, which may also affect the prevalence and the severity of CLAD [32].

1.4 Other Possible Indications for Azithromycin Treatment after Lung Transplantation

Aiming to investigate the effect of azithromycin on early allograft function, Van Herck et al. performed a double-blind, placebo-controlled randomized study with azithromycin add-on versus placebo in 68 lung transplant recipients, where azithromycin (1000 mg) or placebo was initiated immediately before lung transplantation and from the first day of transplantation on (250 mg azithromycin or placebo, 3 times a week). Both groups comprised 34 subjects. There was no difference in FEV_1 at 30 and 90 days after the transplantation, but the azithromycin treated subjects demonstrated significantly less BAL neutrophilia with lower CXCL8 levels [33]. Although azithromycin had no effect on the early post-transplant FEV_1, it cannot be excluded that it might affect the best post-transplant FEV_1, in agreement with the study from Li et al. [32].

The role of azithromycin in the treatment of acute cellular rejection remains unclear, although a positive effect has also been demonstrated in lymphocytic bronchiolitis (LB), which is considered as a manifestation of acute airway rejection. Important also is that LB was proven to be rather refractory to high dose corticosteroid treatment, in contrast to classical acute cellular perivascular rejection [34]. IL-17/CD8 cells have been demonstrated to be present in LB after lung transplantation, but not in acute A-grade/rejection nor during infection [35]. Azithromycin significantly decreased the number of IL-17+ cells in the airway wall, which may further explain why it reduces BAL neutrophilia (via inhibition of the IL-17 induced CXCL8 production in the bronchial epithelium [21]) and may improve FEV_1 [35].

Since lymphocytic airway inflammation is a major risk factor for CLAD, it seemed logical to investigate whether azithromycin could control LB and improve allograft function. With this aim, Vos et al. included 15 lung transplant recipients with acute allograft dysfunction due to isolated LB. They were prospectively treated with open-label azithromycin (250 mg, 3 times a week) for at least 6 months. Spirometry was assessed before and up to 12 months after initiation of azithromycin. Radiologic features, local inflammation assessed on airway biopsy (rejection score, IL-17(+) cells/mm^2 lamina propria), and bronchoalveolar lavage fluid (total and differential cell counts, chemokine and cytokine levels) as well as systemic C-reactive (CRP) protein levels were compared between baseline and after 3 months of treatment. Azithromycin treatment significantly improved pulmonary function after 1 month. After 3 months, radiologic abnormalities, submucosal cellular inflammation, bronchoalveolar lavage protein levels of different cyto- and chemokines, number of neutrophils and eosinophils, as well as plasma CRP levels significantly decreased compared to baseline ($p < 0.05$). It was concluded that azithromycin significantly decreased LB and its associated inflammation with concomitant improvement in lung allograft function [36].

In another study, a mixed model was fitted to examine the association between daily variations in air pollution, measured as particulate matter $(PM)_{10}$ and A-grade rejection/LB on 1276 bronchoscopic biopsies in 397 patients. A difference of 10 μg/m^3 in PM_{10} 3 days before diagnosis of LB had an OR of 1.15 (95% CI 1.04–1.27; $p = 0.0044$) but not with A-grade rejection. These variations in PM_{10} also correlated with BAL neutrophilia ($p = 0.013$), lymphocytes ($p = 0.0031$) and total cell count ($p = 0.024$), however, this effect was only present in patients not taking azithromycin, again proving that azithromycin may have a protective effect in this setting [37]. Azithromycin also protected against the development of BOS and mortality risk, due to traffic air pollution, again by its immunomodulatory effect, possibly via neutrophils [38].

Despite these rather overwhelming positive effects of azithromycin, either as prophylactic treatment or as treatment for established BOS after lung transplantation, there exists great variability in the clinical use of azithromycin among lung transplant providers. Indeed, in a survey to capture azithromycin practices in 103 responders (in 15 different countries) from the International Society for Heart and Lung Transplantation community, 36% reported inconsistency even within their own center. Azithromycin was prophylactically initiated by 30 responders, 10/73 other responders waited until CLAD diagnosis was established. Most responders, however, initiated azithromycin after a CLAD risk factor and/or event, including 59 for a persistent ≥10% decline in FEV_1, 32 for LB, and 27 for BAL neutrophilia [39]. We did not identify if there are lung transplant centers who do not use azithromycin for any indication, although, as already mentioned before, the recent guidelines on treatment of CLAD do call for an 8 week course of azithromycin, before being able to establish a CLAD diagnosis [18, 19, 31]. This means that almost every lung transplant patient will benefit from azithromycin treatment at some time during the course of follow up.

2 Azithromycin in the Treatment of Sarcoidosis

Sarcoidosis is a disease of unknown origin that involves the lungs in >90% of affected patients. Not every patient needs treatment, as sarcoidosis can spontaneously resolve, at least in earlier stages. The classical treatment, when deemed necessary, involves a stepwise approach, and depends on the affected organs. At least for pulmonary sarcoidosis, the initial treatment option mostly consists of corticosteroids followed, if necessary, by antimetabolites such as azathioprine, mycophenolate, and methotrexate, or leflunomide in an attempt to taper the daily corticosteroid dose. The next treatment step may involve anti-TNF treatment in case of disease progression or toxic effects, followed by corticotropin, vasoactive intestinal peptide or CLEAR (concomitant levofloxacin, ethambutol, azithromycin, and rifabutin), in case of insufficient response [39]. Treatment with CLEAR is based on the presence of mycobacterial DNA and proteins in sarcoidosis granulomas [40].

The first evidence for CLEAR therapy (8 weeks) comes from a randomized, placebo-controlled single-masked trial in 30 subjects with symptomatic chronic cutaneous sarcoidosis lesions. In the ITT analysis, the CLEAR-treated group had a significant improvement in symptoms, along with a significant decrease in lesion dimeter, in granuloma burden and in lesion severity. In the CLEAR-treated group 4/15 subjects discontinued the treatment, whereas in the placebo group 3/15 also stopped the treatment because of side effects [41].

In an open-label trial, involving 15 subjects with chronic pulmonary sarcoidosis, Drake et al. evaluated the effect of CLEAR therapy on forced vital capacity (FVC) as a primary outcome, and on change in six-minute walking distance (6MWD) and quality of life as secondary endpoints. Of the 15 subjects included in the study, 11 completed 4 weeks of therapy and 8 completed 8 weeks of therapy. At 4 and 8 weeks, FVC significantly increased with 0.23 and 0.42 L, respectively. The 6MWD increased by 87 meters from baseline. The mean score on the St George's Respiratory Questionnaire (SGRQ) significantly improved at 8 weeks. Discontinuation of the CLEAR regimen in half of the subjects was due to adverse events such as leucopenia, arthralgia, insomnia, and rash. The authors concluded that these data were promising and needed to be validated by a placebo-controlled trial [42].

In a more recent double-blind, placebo-controlled, multicenter investigation, 97 subjects with pulmonary sarcoidosis were randomly assigned to receive 16 weeks of CLEAR ($n = 49$) or matching placebo ($n = 48$) in addition to their baseline immunosuppressive regimen. The primary outcome of this study was a comparison of the change in percentage of predicted FVC among the two patient groups. Secondary outcomes included 6MWD, SGRQ score, adverse events, and decrease in mycobacterial early secreted antigenic target of 6 kDa (ESAT-6) immune responses. The ITT analysis showed no significant differences in change in FVC between both groups, nor in 6MWD, whereas the change in SGRQ favored placebo (−8.0 for placebo vs −1.5 for CLEAR; $P = 0.028$). The per-protocol analysis also demonstrated no significant change in FVC, nor in 6MWD nor in SGRQ at 16 weeks between groups. A decline in ESAT-6 immune responses at 16 weeks was noted among CLEAR-treated group ($P = 0.0003$) but not subjects receiving placebo ($P = 0.24$). In the CLEAR group, 8 subjects stopped the treatment, due to toxicity, while only 4 in the placebo group. The number of serious adverse events was comparable in both groups. The authors concluded that a 16-week CLEAR regimen provided no benefit in FVC or 6MWD despite a significant decline in ESAT-6 immune responses [43].

In an open-label exploratory clinical trial, 21 patients with chronic cough due to sarcoidosis were treated with azithromycin, 250 mg, once daily for 3 months. Only 5/21 were on corticosteroids, none took other immunosuppressive agents. The primary outcome was number of coughs in 24 h. In the 20 subjects completing the trial, the median number of coughs significantly decreased from a mean of 228 at baseline, to 122 at 1 month and 81 at 3 months. All reported outcomes improved (cough visual analog scale, quality of life as measured by the Leicester Cough Questionnaire and King's Sarcoidosis Questionnaire [44]).

3 Conclusion

Azithromycin can be an important add-on treatment after lung transplantation, as it may improve survival and may reduce the development of CLAD, which remains the most important risk factor for mortality. When it should be initiated remains a matter of debate; either as a prophylactic add-on treatment, where it may indeed impact on survival and the development of CLAD, or as a treatment when CLAD is diagnosed, where it may (partially) reverse the decline in FEV_1 at least in some 30–35% of the patients. As a consequence, a treatment trial with azithromycin of at least 8 weeks before CLAD can be definitely diagnosed, is now implemented in the most recent guidelines. Overall, the treatment seems safe and well tolerated by most of the patients.

Whether azithromycin has any effect in pulmonary sarcoidosis is unclear. Open-label studies suggest it may improve the FVC as a part of CLEAR therapy, but a recent placebo-controlled trial was negative, suggesting that further studies may be needed. There may still be a role in the treatment of sarcoidosis-induced cough, although these data needs validation with a placebo-controlled trial [45].

COI statement The authors report no COI

Ethics compliant statement The authors confirm that this work fulfills the rules of ethics compliance.

References

1. Cooper JD, Billingham M, Egan T, Hertz MI, Higenbottam T, Lynch J, Mauer J, Paradis I, Patterson GA, Smith C, et al. A working formulation for the standardization of nomenclature and for clinical staging of chronic dysfunction in lung allografts. International Society for Heart and Lung Transplantation. J Heart Lung Transplant. 1993;12:713–6.
2. Royer PJ, Olivera-Botello G, Koutsokera A, et al. Chronic lung allograft dysfunction: a systematic review of mechanisms. Transplantation. 2016 Sep;100(9):1803–14.
3. Verleden SE, Sacreas A, Vos R, Vanaudenaerde BM. Verleden GM advances in understanding bronchiolitis obliterans after lung transplantation. Chest. 2016;150:219–25.

4. Vanstapel A, Verleden SE, Verbeken EK, et al. Beyond Bronchiolitis Obliterans: In-depth histopathologic characterization of Bronchiolitis Obliterans Syndrome after lung transplantation. J Clin Med. 2021 Dec;25(11):111.
5. Vanstapel A, Goldschmeding R, Broekhuizen R, et al. Connective Tissue Growth Factor is overexpressed in explant lung tissue and broncho-alveolar lavage in transplant-related pulmonary fibrosis. Front Immunol. 2021 May;25(12):661761.
6. DiGiovine B, Lynch JP III, Martinez FJ, et al. Bronchoalveolar lavage neutrophilia is associated with obliterative bronchiolitis after lung transplantation. J Immunol. 1996;157:4194–202.
7. Riise GC, Williams A, Kjellstrom C, et al. Bronchiolitis obliterans syndrome in lung transplant recipients is associated with increased neutrophil activity and decreased antioxidant status in the lung. Eur Respir J. 1998;12:82–8.
8. Verleden GM, Vanaudenaerde BM, Dupont LJ, Van Raemdonck DE. Azithromycin reduces airway neutrophilia and interleukin-8 in patients with bronchiolitis obliterans syndrome. Am J Respir Crit Care Med. 2006 Sep;1(174):566–70.
9. Gerhardt S, McDyer JF, Girgis RE, et al. Maintenance azithromycin therapy for bronchiolitis obliterans syndrome. Am J Respir Crit Care Med. 2003;168(121–125):85.
10. Verleden GM, Dupont LJ. Azithromycin therapy for patients with bronchiolitis obliterans syndrome after lung transplantation. Transplantation. 2004;77:1465–7.
11. Yates B, Murphy DM, Forrest IA, et al. Azithromycin reverses airflow obstruction in established bronchiolitis obliterans syndrome. Am J Respir Crit Care Med. 2005;176:772–5.
12. Porhownik NR, Batobara W, Kepron W, et al. Effect of maintenance azithromycin on established bronchiolitis obliterans syndrome in lung transplant patients. Can Respir J. 2008;15:199–202.
13. Shitrit D, Bendayan D, Gidon S, et al. Long-term azithromycin use for treatment of bronchiolitis obliterans syndrome in lung transplant recipients. J Heart Lung Transplant. 2005;24:1440–3.
14. Benden C, Boehler A. Long-term clarithromycin therapy in the management of lung transplant rejection. Transplantation. 2009;87:1538–40.
15. Corris P, Ryan VA, Small T, et al. A randomised controlled trial of azithromycin therapy in bronchiolitis obliterans syndrome (BOS) post lung transplantation. Thorax. 2015;70:442–50.
16. Verleden GM, Dupont LJ, Van Raemdonck DE. Is it bronchiolitis obliterans syndrome or is it chronic rejection: a reappraisal? Eur Respir J. 2005;25:221–4.
17. Vanaudenaerde BM, Meyts I, Vos R, et al. A dichotomy in bronchiolitis obliterans syndrome after lung transplantation revealed by azithromycin therapy. Eur Respir J. 2008;32:832–43.
18. Verleden GM, Glanville AR, Lease ED, et al. Chronic lung allograft dysfunction: Definition, diagnostic criteria, and approaches to treatment-A consensus report from the Pulmonary Council of the ISHLT. J Heart Lung Transplant. 2019;38(4):93–503.
19. Meyer KC, Raghu G, Verleden GM, Corris PA, Aurora P, Wilson KC, Brozek J, Glanville AR, ISHLT/ATS/ERS BOS Task Force Committee; ISHLT/ATS/ERS BOS Task Force Committee. An international ISHLT/ATS/ERS clinical practice guideline: diagnosis and management of bronchiolitis obliterans syndrome. Eur Respir J. 2014;44:1479–50.
20. Ward C, Camara M, Forrest I, et al. Preliminary findings of quorum signal molecules in clinically stable lung allograft recipients. Thorax. 2003;58:444–6.
21. Murphy DM, Forrest IA, Ward C, et al. Effect of azithromycin on primary bronchial epithelial cells derived from stable lung allografts. Thorax. 2007;62:834.
22. Vanaudenaerde BM, Wuyts WA, Geudens N, et al. Macrolides inhibit IL17-induced IL8 and 8-isoprostane release from human airway smooth muscle cells. Am J Transplant. 2007;7:76–82.
23. Wuyts WA, Vanaudenaerde BM, Dupont LJ, et al. Interleukin-17-induced interleukin-8 release in human airway smooth muscle cells: role for mitogen-activated kinases and nuclear factor kappa B. J Heart Lung Transplant. 2005;24:875–81.
24. Parnham MJ, Erakovic Haber V, Diamarellos-Bourboulis EJ, Perletti G, Verleden GM, Vos R. Azirhromycin: mechanisms of action and their relevance for clinical applications. Pharmacol Ther. 2014;143:225–45.

25. Gottlieb J, Szangolies J, Koehnlein T, et al. Long-term azithromycin for bronchiolitis obliterans syndrome after lung transplantation. Transplantation. 2008;85:36–41.
26. Jain R, Hachem RR, Morrell MR, et al. Azithromycin is associated with increased survival in lung transplant recipients with bronchiolitis obliterans syndrome. J Heart Lung Transplant. 2010;29:531–7.
27. Vos R, Vanaudenaerde BM, Ottevaere A, et al. Long-term azithromycin therapy for bronchiolitis obliterans syndrome: divide and conquer. J Heart Lung Transplant. 2010;29:1358–68.
28. Kingah PL, Muma G, Soubani A. Azithromycin improves lung function in patients with pos-lung transplant bronchiolitis obliterans syndrome: a meta-analysis. Clin Transpl. 2014;328:906–10.
29. Vos R, Vanaudenaerde BM, Verleden SE, et al. A randomised controlled trial of azithromycin to prevent chronic rejection after lung transplantation. Eur Respir J. 2011;37:164–72.
30. Ruttens D, Verleden SE, Vandermeulen E, et al. Prophylactic azithromycin therapy after lung transplantation: post hoc analysis of a randomized controlled trial. Am J Transplant. 2016;16:254–61.
31. Verleden GM, Raghu G, Meyer KC, Glanville AR, Corris P. A new classification system for chronic lung allograft dysfunction. J Heart Lung Transplant. 2014;33:127–33.
32. Li D, Duan Q, Weinkauf J, et al. Azithromycin prophylaxis after lung transplantation is associated with improved overall survival. J Heart Lung Transplant. 2020;39:1426–34.
33. Van Herck A, Frick AE, Schaevers V, et al. Azithromycin and early allograft function after lung transplantation: a randomize, controlled trial. J Heart Lung Transplant. 2019;38:252–9.
34. Ross DJ, Marchevsky A, Kramer M, et al. "Refractoriness" of airflow obstruction associated with isolated lymphocytic bronchiolitis/bronchitis in pulmonary allografts. J Heart Lung Transplant. 1997;16:832–8.
35. Verleden SE, Vos R, Vandermeulen E, Ruttens D, et al. Involvement of interleukin-17 during lymphocytic bronchiolitis in lung transplant patients. J Heart Lung Transplant. 2013;32:447–53.
36. Vos R, Verleden SE, Ruttens D, et al. Azithromycin and the treatment of lymphocytic airway inflammation after lung transplantation. Am J Transplant. 2014;14:2736-48.
37. Verleden SE, Scheers H, Nawrot TS, et al. Lymphocytic bronchiolitis after lung transplantation is associated with daily changes in air pollution. Am J Transplant. 2012;12:1831–8.
38. Nawrot TS, Vos R, Jacobs L, et al. The impact of traffic air pollution on bronchiolitis obliterans syndrome and mortality after lung transplantation. Thorax. 2011;66:748–54.
39. Kapnadak SG, Morrell ED, Wai TH, et al. Variability in azithromycin practices among lung transplant providers in the International Society for Heart and Lung Transplantation community. J Heart Lung Transplant. 2022;41:20–3.
40. Drake WP, Pei Z, Pride DT, Collins RD, Cover TL, Blaser MJ. Molecular analysis of sarcoidosis tissues for mycobacterium species DNA. Emerg Infect Dis. 2002;8:1334–41.
41. Drake WP, Oswald-Richter K, Richmond BW, et al. Oral antimycobacterial therapy in chronic cutaneous sarcoidosis. JAMA Dermat. 2013;149:1040–9.
42. Drake WP, Richmond BW, Oswald-Richter K, et al. Effects of broad-spectrum antimycobacterial therapy on chronic pulmonary sarcoidosis. Sarcoidosis Vasc Diffuse Lung Dis. 2014;30:201–11.
43. Drake WP, Culver DA, Baughman RP, et al. Phase II investigation of the efficacy of antimycobacterial therapy in chronic pulmonary sarcoidosis. Chest. 2021;159:1902–12.
44. Fraser SD, Thackray-Nocera S, Shepherd M, et al. Azithromycin for sarcoidosis cough: an open-label exploratory clinical trial. ERJ Open Res. 2020;6:00534–2020.
45. Baughman RP, Grutters JC. New treatment strategies for pulmonary sarcoidosis: antimetabolites, biological drugs, and other treatment approaches. Lancet Respir Med. 2015;3:813–22.

Macrolides for Rhinosinusitis and Nasal Polyps

Isao Suzaki

Abstract Low-dose and long-term administration of a 14- or 15-membered ring macrolide (macrolide therapy) is well known to be effective in the treatment of chronic airway inflammatory diseases, including diffuse panbronchiolitis, chronic rhinosinusitis (CRS), and cystic fibrosis. The mechanism of action of macrolide therapy is probably immunomodulatory rather than antibacterial. In CRS, macrolide therapy appears to be particularly effective when there is neutrophil-dominant (T17) inflammation, and where there is mucus hypersecretion with nasal discharge and posterior rhinorrhea. However, macrolide therapy is not very effective for CRS with eosinophil-dominant (T2) inflammation, characterized by serum and tissue eosinophilia.

Keywords Chronic rhinosinusitis · Macrolide therapy · Nasal polyps · Neutrophils · Immunomodulation

Abbreviations

AZM	azithromycin
CRS	chronic rhinosinusitis
CRSwNP	chronic rhinosinusitis with nasal polyps
CRSsNP	chronic rhinosinusitis without nasal polyps
CAM	clarithromycin
DPB	diffuse panbronchiolitis
ESS	endoscopic sinus surger
ECRS	eosinophilic chronic rhinosinusitis
EM	erythromycin
EPOS	European Position Paper on Rhinosinusitis and Nasal Polyps

I. Suzaki (✉)
Department of Otorhinolaryngology, Head and Neck Surgery, Showa University, School of Medicine, Tokyo, Japan
e-mail: i-suzaki@med.showa-u.ac.jp

B. K. Rubin, M. Shinkai (eds.), *Macrolides as Immunomodulatory Agents*, Progress in Inflammation Research 92, https://doi.org/10.1007/978-3-031-42859-3_11

ILC	innate lymphoid cell
IFN	interferon
IL	interleukin
RXM	roxithromycin
T1	Type 1
T2	Type 2
T17	Type 17
TNF-α	tumor necrosis factor-α

1 Introduction

Chronic rhinosinusitis (CRS) is a prolonged inflammatory condition of the nose and the paranasal sinuses characterized by two or more sinonasal symptoms, including nasal obstruction, nasal discharge, facial pain, and loss of smell for more than 12 weeks [1]. The CRS prevalence in the population has been estimated to be between 5.5% and 28% [2–4]. CRS is a multifactorial disease with no single etiology but rather is a complex interplay of factors, including genetic, nutritional, environmental, anatomic, infectious, and allergic predisposition. CRS was conventionally divided into two clinical phenotypes based on the endoscopic findings, CRSwNP or CRSsNP (chronic rhinosinusitis with or without nasal polyps). CRSwNPs generally have a greater disease burden than CRSsNPs in terms of severity, recurrence, frequent exacerbations, and less response to conventional therapy [5]. CRS endotype classification has been based on the biomarkers derived from canonical pathophysiology, such as type 1 (T1), type 2 (T2), and/or type 17 (T17) inflammation. The T1 immune response is classically observed with intracellular microbes and viruses stimulating T1 cytokines, e.g., interferon (IFN)-γ produced by T1 cells and innate lymphoid cell (ILC1). T2 inflammation is caused by adaptive and innate immune responses, and is characterized by T2 cytokines, including interleukin (IL)-4, 5, 13 secreted from T2 cells, mast cells, and ILC2 to directly and indirectly induce eosinophilic inflammation. T17 inflammation is associated with the immune reaction to the bacteria and fungi to promote neutrophilic inflammation, and is characterized by the Treg/T17 cytokines, IL-17, IL-21, and IL-22, produced from T17 cells and ILC3. Among these inflammatory pathways, it is suggested that the T2-dominant endotype is associated with the refractory CRS subtype [6], and is characterized by eosinophilia, olfactory dysfunction, and comorbidity with asthma. EPOS2020 proposed to classify primary CRS to T2 or non-T2-dominant endotypes based on biomarkers such as serum and tissue eosinophils [1]. Treatments targeting T2 inflammation in CRS include corticosteroids and biologics, such as an anti-IL-4 receptor α monoclonal antibody, dupilumab. CRS endotypes are thought to be influenced by genetics, geography, age, and environment. The primary inflammation type of CRS in Europe, the United States, and Asia is thought to differ, with a higher European proportion having T2 inflammation compared to Asians [7, 8]. The T2 mucosal inflammation presence in CRS varies from about 15%–85%, depending on geographic region and "ethnicity" [8–14]. However, it is not always possible to classify CRS endotypes in clinical practice, and some present have a mixture of endotype biomarkers [6, 15].

Macrolide antibiotics are a group of antibacterial agents with a distinctive macrocyclic lactone ring combined with sugars. They are active against many Gram-positive and some Gram-negative bacteria. In addition to antibacterial activity, these compounds exert immunomodulatory activities in vitro and in vivo through inhibiting inflammatory cell migration and inflammatory cytokine and chemokine production [16–20]. Macrolide antibiotics, especially the 14- and 15-membered ring macrolides, are used to treat chronic airway inflammatory diseases, such as diffuse panbronchiolitis (DPB), CRS, and cystic fibrosis [21, 22]. Studies have revealed that the immunomodulatory actions, not the antibacterial action of macrolides, are responsible for their clinical efficacy in CRS [16–24].

2 Progress in Macrolide Therapy for CRS

Long-term treatment with a low-dose macrolide treatment (macrolide therapy) for CRS was developed in Japan. Macrolide therapy has since been recognized in many countries as evidence-based therapy [25, 26]. Kudoh et al. first reported the clinical effectiveness of low-dose, long-term erythromycin (EM) treatment in 18 DPB patients. The introduction of macrolide therapy for DPB increased the 5-year survival rate for DPB to 91.4% between 1985 and 1990 [27].

The response to macrolide therapy suggests an immunomodulatory effect as (1) low-dose treatment is sufficient for a therapeutic response, (2) long-term (at least 1–3 months) treatment is required, and (3) treatment is also effective against macrolide-resistant bacteria, such as *Pseudomonas aeruginosa*. Many investigators have demonstrated that macrolides exhibit immunomodulatory activities [20], including inhibiting mucus hypersecretion [28] affecting ion transport [29]; improving mucociliary clearance [30]; inhibiting inflammatory cytokine/chemokine production [31]; transcription factor suppression and inflammatory cytokine/chemokine gene expression [32]; effects on inflammatory cells, fibroblasts, and epithelial cells [33–35]; and decreasing bacterial quorum-sensing, twitching motility, and biofilm formation [36, 37].

DPB is a sinobronchial syndrome often associated with refractory CRS. Suzaki et al. investigated the effects of low-dose, long-term EM treatment for CRS complicated by DPB in 38 patients aged 17–79 years (mean 50.7 years). All patients were treated with EM at 600 mg/day for 6–66 months (mean 20.8 months). The lower airway symptom improvement rate was 84.2% and that of sinonasal symptoms in CRS associated with DPB was 71% [38]. Subsequently, this group reported the clinical efficacy of low-dose, long-term administration of EM (400–600 mg/day for 3–19 months) in a study of 26 patients with intractable CRS without DPB, who did not benefit from surgery or standard therapies [39] and the same group also

Table 1 Macrolide therapy recommendations for chronic rhinosinusitis in Japan [43]

1.	Macrolides:	14-membered macrolides; erythromycin (EM), clarithromycin (CAM), roxithromycin (RXM)
2.	Indication:	(1) Cases with hypersecretory symptoms such as nasal discharge and/or postnasal drip(2) Postoperative cases
3.	Daily dosage:	As a rule, one-half of the usual dose.Adult: EM (400–600 mg/day), CAM (200 mg/day), RXM (150 mg/day) Child: EM (10 mg/kg/day), CAM (5 mg/kg/day) Except for the following cases: a. In cases with severe clinical symptoms, macrolides should be administered at the usual dosage initially. b. In cases of acute exacerbation, macrolides should be increased to the usual dosage, or switched to other antibiotics.
4.	Duration of therapy:	As a rule, macrolide therapy is administered for 3 months. (1) Responders If adequate response has been obtained, the therapy should be suspended. (2) Non-responders If the patients failed to improve clinical condition, the drug should be switched to other antibiotics or alternative therapies including surgery.
5.	Clinical assessment:	Assessment of clinical efficacy should be based primarily on improvements in subjective symptoms. Radiological findings are informative, but they are not suitable for clinical assessment.
6.	Relapse of symptoms:	About half of patients experience relapse of symptoms after discontinuation of the therapy. Such patients often respond to readministration of macrolide therapy. Patients with multicycles of relapse and remission, at short intervals, may require alternative therapies, including surgery.
7.	Poor responders:	(1) Type I allergic inflammation(2) Acute exacerbation(3) Large nasal polyps and severe obstruction of the middle nasal meatus(4) Type 2 predominant chronic rhinosinusitis characterized by serum and tissue eosinophilia, high serum IgE levels, and asthma co-existence
8.	Combination therapies:	Macrolide therapy could be more effective in combination with endoscopic sinus surgery and nasal irrigation.
9.	Clinical precautions:	Pay sufficient attention to cross-reaction, which may occur with some anti-allergic drug.

demonstrated benefit with the low-dose, long-term administration efficacy of EM (400–600 mg/day for adults and 200–300 mg/day for children for 3–27 months) in 130 refractory CRS patients including 21 children [40]. Long-term treatment of CRS with low-dose roxithromycin (RXM) and clarithromycin (CAM) had good efficacy in most reports [41, 42]. In 2007, the Japan Rhinologic Society proposed guidelines for the treatment of CRS with a strong recommendation to use macrolide therapy (Table 1) [43].

The 15-membered ring macrolide/azalide azithromycin (AZM) has immunomodulatory effects similar to those of EM, CAM, and RXM, and good clinical response has been demonstrated with low-dose, long-term AZM administration for CF in the United States and Europe [44]. A multinational randomized controlled trial showed the clinical efficacy of low-dose, long-term AZM administration (250 mg or 500 mg three times a week for 6 months) for primary ciliary dyskinesia in Europe. However, the study showed no significant improvement in sinonasal symptoms as measured by QOL-PCD questionnaire. The reason for the lack of improvement might be that patients included in the study had more severe symptoms, making it difficult to achieve significant improvement [45]. The 16-membered ring macrolides, including josamycin, do not exhibit immunomodulatory effects [26, 28].

Cervin et al. [46] from Sweden reported that 1-year EM administration improved symptoms, mucociliary transport, and endoscopic findings in patients with persistent CRS after surgery. In the first double-blind, randomized, placebo-controlled study of macrolide CRS therapy, subjects were given RXM 150 mg/day for 3 months to treat CRSsNP. This treatment resulted in improved Sinonasal Outcome Test-20 (SNOT-20) scores, saccharin transit time, and nasal endoscopic findings in the RXM group compared to the placebo group [47]. The pathophysiological CRS background is that most CRSwNP cases are accompanied by high IgE levels and severe eosinophilic inflammation; however, the benefit of macrolides was best seen in patients with low serum IgE levels.

The evidence-based guideline for CRS established by the European Position Paper on Rhinosinusitis and Nasal Polyps (EPOS) 2007 and separately, the British Society for Allergy and Clinical Immunology designated low-dose, long-term macrolide therapy as a strong grade-A recommendation for CRSsNP treatment based on the results of this placebo-controlled study [48, 49]. Macrolide therapy, local corticosteroid treatment, and nasal irrigation are recommended for moderate/severe CRSsNP.

However, in EPOS 2012 [50], the grade-A designation for macrolide therapy was reduced to grade C based on a randomized clinical trial of AZM 500 mg/week for 3 months) [51]. However, this study included patients with high IgE levels, nasal polyposis, and asthma, against which macrolide therapy is ineffective. It has been reported that macrolide therapy is most effective against neutrophilic inflammation, including non-T2-dominant inflammation; however, its effect on eosinophilic inflammation is limited.

A systematic review and meta-analysis of macrolide therapy in CRS assessed the prognostic factors that predict favorable outcomes: CRS phenotypes; specifically, CRSwNP or CRSsNP, serum IgE, size of the macrolide lactone ring, concurrent endoscopic sinus surgery (ESS), and macrolide dosage and duration. Subgroup analysis revealed that low-dose macrolide administration was clinically effective in CRSsNP, and macrolide therapy for at least 24 weeks was more effective than shorter duration therapy [52]. They also concluded that macrolide therapy success was not associated with serum IgE, size of the lactone ring, concurrent ESS, and dosage of macrolides. The EPOS 2020 Steering Group using the Grading of Recommendations Assessment, Development and Evaluation (GRADE) system gave the overall recommendation for long-term systemic antibiotics as "uncertain" due to the relatively low quality of available evidence [1] and this included macrolide therapy. The International Consensus Statement on Allergy and Rhinology: rhinosinusitis 2021 positions macrolide therapy as a treatment option for CRSsNP and CRSwNP, especially in persons with nasal polyps and

Table 2 Evidence of macrolide therapy on adult patients with CRS

Study	Year	Method	Participants	Macrolides	Main results
Suzaki et al. [38]	1990	Prospective open study	38 CRS Complicated by DPB	EM	Lower airway symptoms improved 84.2% and sinonasal symptoms improved 71.0%
Kikuchi et al. [39]	1991	Prospective open study	26 CRS	EM	Improvement in sinonasal symptoms and endoscopic findings.
Kikuchi et al. [40]	1992	Prospective open study	109 CRS	EM	Improvement in sinonasal symptoms and endoscopic findings.
Hashiba et al. [54]	1997	Single-blind study	59 CRS	CAM vs. EM	CAM was significantly more effective when compared to EM.
Cervin et al. [46]	2002	Prospective open study	17 CRS	EM	Significant improvement on symptom VAS scale, endoscopic finding and saccharin transit time. Trend toward an increase in nasal nitric oxide.No significant effect on ciliary beat frequency.
Wallwork et al. [47]	2006	Double-blind placebo control study	64 CRSsNP	RXM vs. placebo	Significant improvement on SNOT-20, endoscopic finding, and saccharin transit time. Subgroup analysis on low vs high IgE levels found a 93% improvement in the low IgE group.
Videler et al. [51]	2011	Double-blind placebo control study	60 CRSwNP and CRSsNP	AZM vs. placebo	No significant effects.

AZM azithromycin; *CAM* clarithromycin; *CRS* chronic rhinosinusitis; *CRSwNP* chronic rhinosinusitis with nasal polyps; *CRSsNP* chronic rhinosinusitis without nasal polyps; *DPB* diffuse panbronchiolitis; *EM* erythromycin; *PNIF* peak nasal inspiratory flow; roxythromycin; *SNOT* Sinonasal Outcome Test; *VAS* visual analog scale

neutrophil-dominant inflammation with poor response to corticosteroids [53]. Appropriate patient selection for CRS macrolide therapy is thought to be important for good therapeutic efficacy, and future pathogenesis and identification analysis of biomarkers useful for predicting therapeutic efficacy in CRS is expected. The progress and evidence of macrolide therapy on adult CRS are summarized in Table 2.

3 The Therapeutic Mechanism of Macrolides on CRS

EM, CAM, and RXM are used to treat CRS in Japan [25, 26], as previously described. There is a better clinical response to CRS with CAM (400 mg/day) compared to EM (600 mg/day) based on a single-blind study [54]. However, clinical efficacy comparisons among macrolides to treat CRS have rarely been reported, and thus which agent is most effective is uncertain. Macrolides have been shown to inhibit viral attachment, infection, reproduction, and accentuate the host's antiviral defenses [55–58]. The sites of action of CRS macrolide therapy are shown in Fig. 1. As discussed in other chapters, macrolides have immunomodulatory properties to suppress proinflammatory cytokines and chemokines [23, 31, 59–61].

Macrolide therapy decreases CXCL8 in CRS nasal lavage ameliorating neutrophil inflammation [47, 60, 62] by inhibiting neutrophil chemotaxis and recruitment [28, 63, 64]. Macrolides are also reported to block airway epithelial nasal gland cells Cl^- channels, which can decrease water and mucin secretion and enhance ciliary clearance [20, 28, 65–68]. Macrolide therapy appears to be most effective in persons with CRS who have neutrophilic predominant inflammation, mucus hypersecretion, and a history of sinus surgery [69–73]. However, macrolide therapy is less effective for patients with CRS who have large nasal polyps and T2 inflammation marked by asthma, aspirin intolerance, and eosinophilia; also known as Samter's triad [74–76]. CRS with predominant T2 inflammation is usually treated with topical and/or systemic corticosteroids, sinus surgery, and occasionally biologic agents targeting T2 inflammation.

Reactive oxygen species and free radicals contribute to local tissue damage. Macrolides inhibit reactive oxygen species production by neutrophils and fibroblasts [77–79]. Inflammatory cytokine production, e.g., IL-1β and TNF-α production, is modulated by circadian rhythms, and this is modulated in part, by plasma corticosteroid concentration. Macrolides may act on the hypothalamus–pituitary system to enhance endogenous corticosterone production in the adrenal cortex [80]. Immunologically, the effects of macrolides on CRS may be expected to modulate inflammatory immune responses and tissue damage factor production, resulting in improvement of the condition and suppression of prolonged disease.

4 Macrolide Therapy in Children

CRS is less common in children at 2.1–4% [1, 81–84], but the negative impact on quality of life is similar to that in adults [81, 85]. The primary causes of CRS in children and adults are thought to differ, with environmental tobacco smoke and

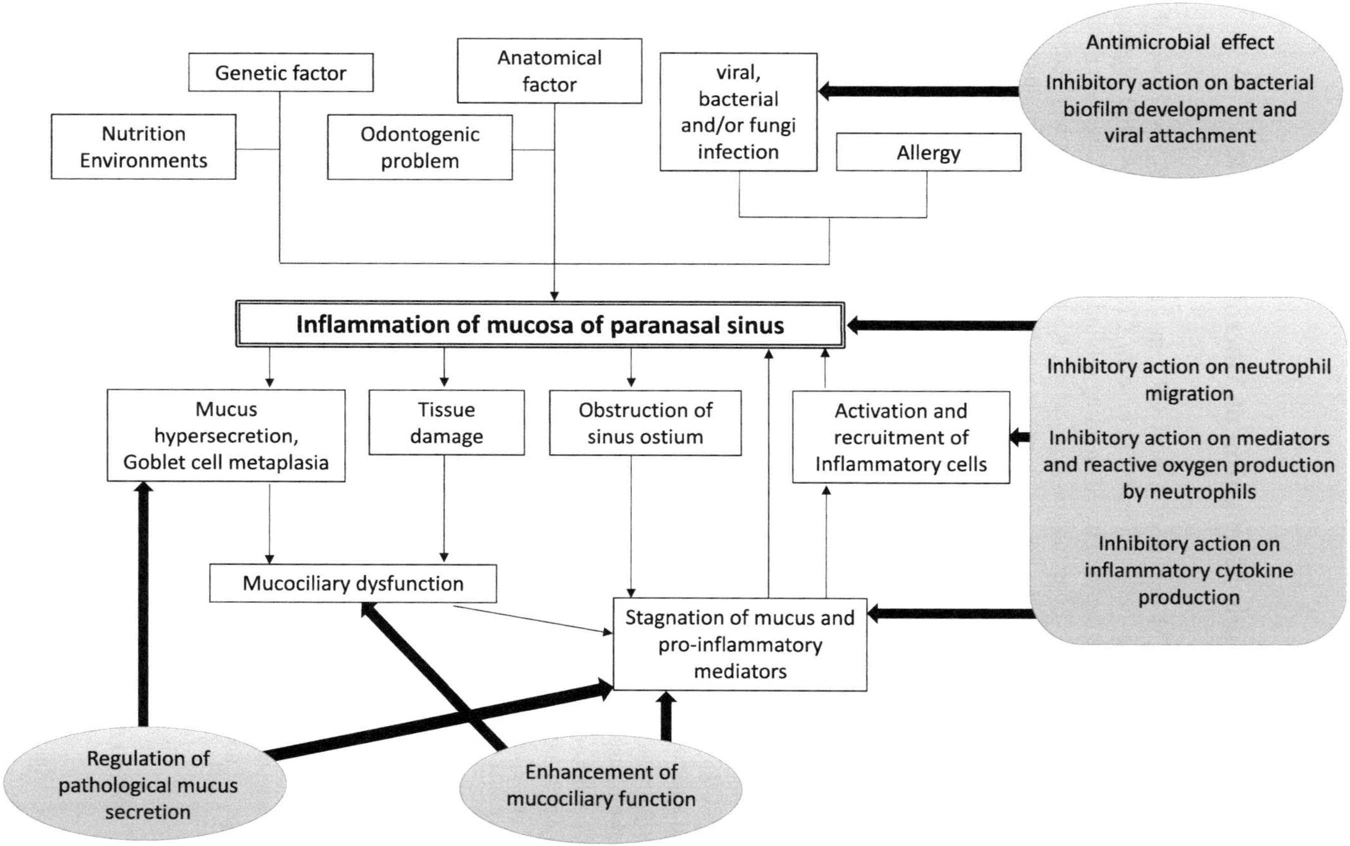

Fig. 1 Proposed mechanisms for macrolide therapy of chronic rhinosinusitis

adenoid hypertrophy as a reservoir of pathogenic bacteria and/or a cause of nasal obstruction being more important in children [1]. Macrolide therapy appears to be effective in treating CRS in children although studies in children are limited [26]. The benefit of adding macrolide therapy to intranasal corticosteroids and saline irrigation was shown in a retrospective study of a small number of children with CRS who have failed conventional therapy [86]. The macrolide dose for children is half the usual EM dose at 10 mg/kg and CAM at 6 mg/kg. In children, acute exacerbations due to bacterial infection can occur during therapy and thus there may be a benefit to add an antibiotic directed against the etiologic bacterial pathogen. The duration of macrolide administration should be as short as possible since pediatric CRS may resolve spontaneously. ESS is performed less frequently in children because of concerns about the effect on facial bone development. EPOS2020 proposed that saline irrigation and nasal corticosteroid therapy are acceptable conventional treatments for pediatric CRS patients, but there was a lack of evidence to support macrolide adjunctive therapy [1].

5 Conclusion

Macrolide therapy is useful in non-eosinophilic (non-T2) CRS treatment due, in part, to immunomodulation. Macrolide therapy should be initiated for the treatment of CRS patients with mucopurulent rhinorrhea lasting more than 1 month, and the drug should be discontinued if efficacy is not observed 2 months after administration. Care should be taken to avoid unnecessary prolonged macrolide use since macrolide therapy is not uniformly effective in CRS. Attempts should be made to identify the endotype of each patient and consider macrolide therapy in combination with other drugs and surgical treatment as indicated.

Declarations None.

Conflict of Interest The authors declare no conflicts of interest in association with the present study.

Funding This research was funded, in part, by a grant from the Denny Hamlin Foundation.

Authors' contributions I.S. collected data and prepared the article.

Acknowledgments Not applicable.

Ethical Approval This chapter does not contain any studies with human participants performed by any of the authors.

References

1. Fokkens WJ, Lund VJ, Hopkins C, Hellings PW, Kern R, Reitsma S, et al. European position paper on rhinosinusitis and nasal polyps 2020. Rhinology. 2020;58:1–464. https://doi.org/10.4193/Rhin20.600.
2. Hastan D, Fokkens WJ, Bachert C, Newson RB, Bislimovska J, Bockelbrink A, et al. Chronic rhinosinusitis in Europe–an underestimated disease. A GA^{2}LEN study. Allergy. 2011;66:1216–23. https://doi.org/10.1111/j.1398-9995.2011.02646.x.
3. Hirsch AG, Stewart WF, Sundaresan AS, Young AJ, Kennedy TL, Scott Greene J, et al. Nasal and sinus symptoms and chronic rhinosinusitis in a population-based sample. Allergy. 2017;72:274–81. https://doi.org/10.1111/all.13042.
4. Pilan RR, Pinna FR, Bezerra TF, Mori RL, Padua FG, Bento RF, et al. Prevalence of chronic rhinosinusitis in Sao Paulo. Rhinology. 2015;70:533–9. https://doi.org/10.1111/all.12577.
5. Akdis CA, Bachert C, Cingi C, Dykewicz MS, Hellings PW, Naclerio RM, et al. Endotypes and phenotypes of chronic rhinosinusitis: a PRACTALL document of the European academy of allergy and clinical immunology and the american academy of allergy, asthma & immunology. J Allergy Clin Immunol. 2013;131:1479–90. https://doi.org/10.1016/j.jaci.2013.02.036.
6. Kato A, Peters AT, Stevens WW, Schleimer RP, Tan BK, Kern RC. Endotypes of chronic rhinosinusitis: relationships to disease phenotypes, pathogenesis, clinical findings, and treatment approaches. Allergy. 2022;77:812–26. https://doi.org/10.1111/all.15074.
7. Staudacher AG, Peters AT, Kato A, Stevens WW. Use of endotypes, phenotypes, and inflammatory markers to guide treatment decisions in chronic rhinosinusitis. Ann Allergy Asthma Immunol. 2020;124:318–25. https://doi.org/10.1016/j.anai.2020.01.013.
8. Wang X, Zhang N, Bo M, Holtappels G, Zheng M, Lou H, et al. Diversity of T(H) cytokine profiles in patients with chronic rhinosinusitis: a multicenter study in Europe, Asia, and Oceania. J Allergy Clin Immunol. 2016;138:1344–53. https://doi.org/10.1016/j.jaci.2016.05.041.
9. Tomassen P, Vandeplas G, Van Zele T, Cardell LO, Arebro J, Olze H, et al. Inflammatory endotypes of chronic rhinosinusitis based on cluster analysis of biomarkers. J Allergy Clin Immunol. 2016;137:1449–56.e4. https://doi.org/10.1016/j.jaci.2015.12.1324.
10. Zhang Y, Gevaert E, Lou H, Wang X, Zhang L, Bachert C, et al. Chronic rhinosinusitis in Asia. J Allergy Clin Immunol. 2017;140:1230–9. https://doi.org/10.1016/j.jaci.2017.09.009.
11. Wang ET, Zheng Y, Liu PF, Guo LJ. Eosinophilic chronic rhinosinusitis in east Asians. World J Clin Cases. 2014;2:873–82. https://doi.org/10.12998/wjcc.v2.i12.873.
12. Cao PP, Li HB, Wang BF, Wang SB, You XJ, Cui YH, et al. Distinct immunopathologic characteristics of various types of chronic rhinosinusitis in adult Chinese. J Allergy Clin Immunol. 2009;124:478–84.
13. Zhang N, Van Zele T, Perez-Novo C, Van Bruaene N, Holtappels G, DeRuyck N, et al. Different types of T-effector cells orchestrate mucosal inflammation in chronic sinus disease. J Allergy Clin Immunol. 2008;122:961–8. https://doi.org/10.1016/j.jaci.2008.07.008.
14. Tokunaga T, Sakashita M, Haruna T, Asaka D, Takeno S, Ikeda H, et al. Novel scoring system and algorithm for classifying chronic rhinosinusitis: the JESREC study. Allergy. 2015;70:995–1003. https://doi.org/10.1111/all.12644.
15. Stevens WW, Peters AT, Tan BK, Klingler AI, Poposki JA, Hulse KE, et al. Associations between inflammatory endotypes and clinical presentations in chronic rhinosinusitis. J Allergy Clin Immunol Pract. 2019;7:2812–20.e3. https://doi.org/10.1016/j.jaip.2019.05.009.
16. Asano K, Suzuki M, Shimane T, Suzaki H. Suppression of co-stimulatory molecule expressions on splenic B lymphocytes by a macrolide antibiotic, roxithromycin in vitro. Int Immunopharmacol. 2001;1:1385–92. https://doi.org/10.1016/s1567-5769(01)00070-4.
17. Suzaki H, Asano K, Yu M, Hisamitsu T. Influence of roxithromycin on inflammatory cytokine production from nasal polyp fibroblasts in vitro. Acta Otolaryngol. 2003;123:637–42. https://doi.org/10.1080/0001648021000028132.

18. Furuya A, Asano K, Shoji N, Hirano K, Hamasaki T, Suzaki H. Suppression of nitric oxide production from nasal fibroblasts by metabolized clarithromycin in vitro. J Inflamm. 2010;7:56. https://doi.org/10.1186/1476-9255-7-56.
19. Suzaki I, Asano K, Kanei A, Suzaki H. Enhancement of thioredoxin production from nasal epithelial cells by the macrolide antibiotic, clarithromycin in vitro. In Vivo. 2013;27:351–6.
20. Kanoh S, Rubin BK. Mechanisms of action and clinical application of macrolides as immunomodulatory medications. Clin Microbiol Rev. 2010;23:590–615. https://doi.org/10.1128/cmr.00078-09.
21. Keicho N, Kudoh S. Diffuse panbronchiolitis: role of macrolides in therapy. Am J Respir Med. 2002;1:119–31. https://doi.org/10.1007/bf03256601.
22. Rubin BK, Henke MO. Immunomodulatory activity and effectiveness of macrolides in chronic airway disease. Chest. 2004;125:70s–8s. https://doi.org/10.1378/chest.125.2_suppl.70s.
23. Culić O, Eraković V, Parnham MJ. Anti-inflammatory effects of macrolide antibiotics. Eur J Pharmacol. 2001;429:209–29. https://doi.org/10.1016/s0014-2999(01)01321-8.
24. Kwiatkowska B, Maślińska M. Macrolide therapy in chronic inflammatory diseases. Med Inf. 2012;2012:636157. https://doi.org/10.1155/2012/636157.
25. Suzaki H. Clinical study and action mechanisms of macrolide therapy for chronic rhinosinusitis. Asian Rhinol J. 2013;1:14–20.
26. Shimizu T, Suzaki H. Past, present and future of macrolide therapy for chronic rhinosinusitis in Japan. Auris Nasus Larynx. 2016;43:131–6. https://doi.org/10.1016/j.anl.2015.08.014.
27. Kudoh S, Azuma A, Yamamoto M, Izumi T, Ando M. Improvement of survival in patients with diffuse panbronchiolitis treated with low-dose erythromycin. Am J Respir Crit Care Med. 1998;157:1829–32. https://doi.org/10.1164/ajrccm.157.6.9710075.
28. Shimizu T, Shimizu S, Hattori R, Gabazza EC, Majima Y. In vivo and in vitro effects of macrolide antibiotics on mucus secretion in airway epithelial cells. Am J Respir Crit Care Med. 2003;168:581–7. https://doi.org/10.1164/rccm.200212-1437OC.
29. Tamaoki J, Isono K, Sakai N, Kanemura T, Konno K. Erythromycin inhibits cl secretion across canine tracheal epithelial cells. Eur Respir J. 1992;5:234–8.
30. Tamaoki J, Chiyotani A, Sakai N, Takeyama K, Takizawa T. Effect of erythromycin on ciliary motility in rabbit airway epithelium in vitro. J Antimicrob Chemother. 1992;29:173–8. https://doi.org/10.1093/jac/29.2.173.
31. Takizawa H, Desaki M, Ohtoshi T, Kawasaki S, Kohyama T, Sato M, et al. Erythromycin modulates IL-8 expression in normal and inflamed human bronchial epithelial cells. Am J Respir Crit Care Med. 1997;156:266–71.
32. Desaki M, Takizawa H, Ohtoshi T, Kasama T, Kobayashi K, Sunazuka T, et al. Erythromycin suppresses nuclear factor-kappaB and activator protein-1 activation in human bronchial epithelial cells. Biochem Biophys Res Commun. 2000;267:124–8. https://doi.org/10.1006/bbrc.1999.1917.
33. Kanai K, Asano K, Hisamitsu T, Suzaki H. Suppression of matrix metalloproteinase production from nasal fibroblasts by macrolide antibiotics in vitro. Eur Respir J. 2004;23:671–8. https://doi.org/10.1183/09031936.04.00057104.
34. Ichikawa Y, Ninomiya H, Koga H, Tanaka M, Kinoshita M, Tokunaga N, et al. Erythromycin reduces neutrophils and neutrophil-derived elastolytic-like activity in the lower respiratory tract of bronchiolitis patients. Am Rev Respir Dis. 1992;146:196–203. https://doi.org/10.1164/ajrccm/146.1.196.
35. Kikuchi T, Hagiwara K, Honda Y, Gomi K, Kobayashi T, Takahashi H, et al. Clarithromycin suppresses lipopolysaccharide-induced interleukin-8 production by human monocytes through AP-1 and NF-kappa B transcription factors. J Antimicrob Chemother. 2002;49:745–55. https://doi.org/10.1093/jac/dkf008.
36. Tateda K, Comte R, Pechere JC, Köhler T, Yamaguchi K, Van Delden C. Azithromycin inhibits quorum sensing in Pseudomonas aeruginosa. Antimicrob Agents Chemother. 2001;45:1930–3. https://doi.org/10.1128/aac.45.6.1930-1933.2001.

37. Yanagihara K, Tomono K, Imamura Y, Kaneko Y, Kuroki M, Sawai T, et al. Effect of clarithromycin on chronic respiratory infection caused by Pseudomonas aeruginosa with biofilm formation in an experimental murine model. J Antimicrob Chemother. 2002;49:867–70. https://doi.org/10.1093/jac/dkf013.
38. Suzaki H, Kudoh S, Oritsu S, Kurashima A, Nagai H. The effects of low-dose long-term erythromycin administration treatment on chronic rhinosinusitis complicated by diffuse panbronchiolitis. Ther Res. 1990;11:29–31. [in Japanese]
39. Kikuchi S, Suzaki H, Aoki A, Ito O, Nomura Y. Clinical effect of long-term low-dose erythromycin therapy for chronic sinusitis. Pract Otorhinolaryngol. 1991;84:41–7. [in Japanese]. https://doi.org/10.5631/jibirin.84.41.
40. Kikuchi S, Yamasoba T, Suzaki H, Aoki A, Hara M, Nomura Y. Long-term low-dose erythromycin therapy for chronic sinusitis practica oto-rhino-laryngologica 1992;85:1245–1252. [in Japanese] doi:https://doi.org/10.5631/jibirin.85.1245.
41. Ohyama M, Ueno K, Matsune S, Hanamure Y, Tsurumaru H. Current status on macrolide therapy in chronic sinusitis. Pract Otorhinolaryngol. 1999;92:571–82. [in Japanese]. https://doi.org/10.5631/jibirin.92.571.
42. Majima Y. Clinical implications of the immunomodulatory effects of macrolides on sinusitis. Am J Med. 2004;117:20–5. https://doi.org/10.1016/j.amjmed.2004.07.025.
43. Japan Rhinologic Society. Macrolide therapy. In: The handbook of management of chronic rhinosinusitis. Tokyo: Kanehara Press; 2007. p. 49–51. [in Japanese].
44. Southern KW, Barker PM. Azithromycin for cystic fibrosis. Eur Respir J. 2004;24(5):834–8. https://doi.org/10.1183/09031936.04.00084304.
45. Kobbernagel HE, Buchvald FF, Haarman EG, Casaulta C, Collins SA, Hogg C, et al. Efficacy and safety of azithromycin maintenance therapy in primary ciliary dyskinesia (BESTCILIA): a multicentre, double-blind, randomised, placebo-controlled phase 3 trial. Lancet Respir Med. 2020;8:493–505. https://doi.org/10.1016/s2213-2600(20)30058-8.
46. Cervin A, Kalm O, Sandkull P, Lindberg S. One-year low-dose erythromycin treatment of persistent chronic sinusitis after sinus surgery: clinical outcome and effects on mucociliary parameters and nasal nitric oxide. Otolaryngol Head Neck Surg. 2002;126:481–9. https://doi.org/10.1067/mhn.2002.124849.
47. Wallwork B, Coman W, Mackay-Sim A, Greiff L, Cervin A. A double-blind, randomized, placebo-controlled trial of macrolide in the treatment of chronic rhinosinusitis. Laryngoscope. 2006;116:189–93. https://doi.org/10.1097/01.mlg.0000191560.53555.08.
48. Fokkens W, Lund V, Mullol J. EP3OS 2007: European position paper on rhinosinusitis and nasal polyps 2007. A summary for otorhinolaryngologists. Rhinology. 2007;45:97–101.
49. Scadding GK, Durham SR, Mirakian R, Jones NS, Drake-Lee AB, Ryan D, et al. BSACI guidelines for the management of rhinosinusitis and nasal polyposis. Clin Exp Allergy. 2008;38:260–75. https://doi.org/10.1111/j.1365-2222.2007.02889.x.
50. Fokkens WJ, Lund VJ, Mullol J, Bachert C, Alobid I, Baroody F, et al. EPOS 2012: European position paper on rhinosinusitis and nasal polyps 2012. A summary for otorhinolaryngologists. Rhinology. 2012;50(1):1–12. https://doi.org/10.4193/Rhino12.000.
51. Videler WJ, Badia L, Harvey RJ, Gane S, Georgalas C, van der Meulen FW, et al. Lack of efficacy of long-term, low-dose azithromycin in chronic rhinosinusitis: a randomized controlled trial. Allergy. 2011;66:1457–68. https://doi.org/10.1111/j.1398-9995.2011.02693.x.
52. Seresirikachorn K, Suwanparin N, Srisunthornphanich C, Chitsuthipakorn W, Kanjanawasee D, Snidvongs K. Factors of success of low-dose macrolides in chronic sinusitis: systematic review and meta-analysis. Laryngoscope. 2019;129:1510–9. https://doi.org/10.1002/lary.27865.
53. Orlandi RR, Kingdom TT, Smith TL, Bleier B, DeConde A, Luong AU, et al. International consensus statement on allergy and rhinology: rhinosinusitis 2021. I Int Forum Allergy Rhinol. 2021;11:213–739. https://doi.org/10.1002/alr.22741.

54. Hashiba M. Clinical efficacy of long-term macrolides therapy for chronic sinusitis-comparison between erythromycin and clarithromycin. Pract Otorhinolaryngol. 1997;90:717–27. [in Japanese]. https://doi.org/10.5631/jibirin.90.717.
55. Sato K, Suga M, Akaike T, Fujii S, Muranaka H, Doi T, et al. Therapeutic effect of erythromycin on influenza virus-induced lung injury in mice. Am J Respir Crit Care Med. 1998;157:853–7. https://doi.org/10.1164/ajrccm.157.3.9703098.
56. Yamaya M, Shinya K, Hatachi Y, Kubo H, Asada M, Yasuda H, et al. Clarithromycin inhibits type a seasonal influenza virus infection in human airway epithelial cells. J Pharmacol Exp Ther. 2010;333:81–90. https://doi.org/10.1124/jpet.109.162149.
57. Asada M, Yoshida M, Suzuki T, Hatachi Y, Sasaki T, Yasuda H, et al. Macrolide antibiotics inhibit respiratory syncytial virus infection in human airway epithelial cells. Antivir Res. 2009;83:191–200. https://doi.org/10.1016/j.antiviral.2009.05.003.
58. Suzuki T, Yamaya M, Sekizawa K, Hosoda M, Yamada N, Ishizuka S, et al. Erythromycin inhibits rhinovirus infection in cultured human tracheal epithelial cells. Am J Respir Crit Care Med. 2002;165:1113–8. https://doi.org/10.1164/ajrccm.165.8.2103094.
59. Khan AA, Slifer TR, Araujo FG, Remington JS. Effect of clarithromycin and azithromycin on production of cytokines by human monocytes. Int J Antimicrob Agents. 1999;11:121–32. https://doi.org/10.1016/s0924-8579(98)00091-0.
60. Suzuki H, Shimomura A, Ikeda K, Furukawa M, Oshima T, Takasaka T. Inhibitory effect of macrolides on interleukin-8 secretion from cultured human nasal epithelial cells. Laryngoscope. 1997;107:1661–6. https://doi.org/10.1097/00005537-199712000-00016.
61. Tamaoki J, Kadota J, Takizawa H. Clinical implications of the immunomodulatory effects of macrolides. Am J Med. 2004;117:5s–11s. https://doi.org/10.1016/j.amjmed.2004.07.023.
62. Yamada T, Fujieda S, Mori S, Yamamoto H, Saito H. Macrolide treatment decreased the size of nasal polyps and IL-8 levels in nasal lavage. Am J Rhinol. 2000;14:143–8. https://doi.org/10.2500/105065800782102717.
63. Kadota J, Sakito O, Kohno S, Sawa H, Mukae H, Oda H, et al. A mechanism of erythromycin treatment in patients with diffuse panbronchiolitis. Am Rev Respir Dis. 1993;147:153–9. https://doi.org/10.1164/ajrccm/147.1.153.
64. Tamaoki J, Takeyama K, Yamawaki I, Kondo M, Konno K. Lipopolysaccharide-induced goblet cell hypersecretion in the Guinea pig trachea: inhibition by macrolides. Am J Phys. 1997;272:15–9. https://doi.org/10.1152/ajplung.1997.272.1.L15.
65. Ikeda K, Wu D, Takasaka T. Inhibition of acetylcholine-evoked cl- currents by 14-membered macrolide antibiotics in isolated acinar cells of the Guinea pig nasal gland. Am J Respir Cell Mol Biol. 1995;13:449–54. https://doi.org/10.1165/ajrcmb.13.4.7546775.
66. Goswami SK, Kivity S, Marom Z. Erythromycin inhibits respiratory glycoconjugate secretion from human airways in vitro. Am Rev Respir Dis. 1990;141:72–8. https://doi.org/10.1164/ajrccm/141.1.72.
67. Mori S, Saito H, Kimura Y, Takahashi N, Yamada T. Effect of macrolides on nasal ciliary activity. Jibi Inkoka Tembo. 1995;38:220–7. [in Japanese]. https://doi.org/10.11453/orltokyo1958.38.Supplement3_220.
68. Yen TT, Jiang RS, Chang CY, Wu CY, Liang KL. Erythromycin reduces nasal inflammation by inhibiting immunoglobulin production, attenuating mucus secretion, and modulating cytokine expression. Sci Rep. 2021;11:21737. https://doi.org/10.1038/s41598-021-01192-8.
69. Moriyama H, Yanagi K, Ohtori N, Fukami M. Evaluation of endoscopic sinus surgery for chronic sinusitis: post-operative erythromycin therapy. Rhinology. 1995;33:166–70.
70. Nakamura Y, Suzuki M, Yokota M, Ozaki S, Ohno N, Hamajima Y, et al. Optimal duration of macrolide treatment for chronic sinusitis after endoscopic sinus surgery. Auris Nasus Larynx. 2013;40:366–72. https://doi.org/10.1016/j.anl.2012.09.009.
71. Varvyanskaya A, Lopatin A. Efficacy of long-term low-dose macrolide therapy in preventing early recurrence of nasal polyps after endoscopic sinus surgery. Int Forum Allergy Rhinol. 2014;4:533–41. https://doi.org/10.1002/alr.21318.

72. Lin CF, Wang MC, Merton AT, Ho NH, Wu PS, Hsu AT, et al. Add-on effect of clarithromycin to oral steroids as post- operative therapy for chronic rhinosinusitis with nasal polyps: a randomised controlled trial. Rhinology. 2020;58:550–8. https://doi.org/10.4193/Rhin19.325.
73. Perić A, Baletić N, Milojević M, Sotirović J, Živić L, Perić AV, et al. Effects of preoperative clarithromycin Administration in Patients with nasal polyposis. West Indian Med J. 2014;63: 721–7. https://doi.org/10.7727/wimj.2013.313.
74. Haruna S, Shimada C, Ozawa M, Fukami S, Moriyama H. A study of poor responders for long-term, low-dose macrolide administration for chronic sinusitis. Rhinology. 2009;47:66–71.
75. Suzuki H, Ikeda K, Honma R, Gotoh S, Oshima T, Furukawa M, et al. Prognostic factors of chronic rhinosinusitis under long-term low-dose macrolide therapy. ORL. 2000;62:121–7. https://doi.org/10.1159/000027731.
76. Kim SD, Cho KS. Samter's triad: state of the art. Clin Exp Otorhinolaryngol. 2018;11:71–80. https://doi.org/10.21053/ceo.2017.01606.
77. Terao H, Asano K, Kanai K, Kyo Y, Watanabe S, Hisamitsu T, et al. Suppressive activity of macrolide antibiotics on nitric oxide production by lipopolysaccharide stimulation in mice. Mediators of Inflamm. 2003;12:195–202.
78. Park HH, Park IH, Cho JS, Lee YM, Lee HM. The effect of macrolides on myofibroblast differentiation and collagen production in nasal polyp-derived fibroblasts. Am J Rhinol Allergy. 2010;24:348–53. https://doi.org/10.2500/ajra.2010.24.3520.
79. Nozoe K, Aida Y, Fukuda T, Sanui T, Nishimura F. Mechanisms of the macrolide-induced inhibition of superoxide generation by neutrophils. Inflammation. 2016;39:1039–48. https://doi.org/10.1007/s10753-016-0333-3.
80. Yamamoto S, Asano K, Shimane T, Hisamitsu T, Suzaki H. Enhancement of endogenous corticosterone levels by a macrolide antibiotic, roxithromycin in mice. Life Sci. 2001;69:1115–21. https://doi.org/10.1016/S0024-3205(01)01199-7.
81. Cunningham MJ, Chiu EJ, Landgraf JM, Gliklich RE. The health impact of chronic recurrent rhinosinusitis in children. Arch Otolaryngol Head Neck Surg. 2000;126:1363–8. https://doi.org/10.1001/archotol.126.11.1363.
82. Adams PF, Hendershot GE, Marano MA. Current estimates from the national health interview survey, 1996. Vital Health Stat. 1999;10:1–203.
83. Sidell D, Shapiro NL, Bhattacharyya N. Obesity and the risk of chronic rhinosinusitis, allergic rhinitis, and acute otitis media in school-age children. Laryngoscope. 2013;123:2360–3. https://doi.org/10.1002/lary.24038.
84. Gilani S, Shin JJ. The burden and visit prevalence of pediatric chronic rhinosinusitis. Otolaryngol Head Neck Surg. 2017;157:1048–52. https://doi.org/10.1177/0194599817721177.
85. Sami AS, Scadding GK. Rhinosinusitis in secondary school children-part 2: main project analysis of MSNOT-20 Young persons questionnaire (MSYPQ). Rhinology. 2014;52:225–30. https://doi.org/10.4193/Rhin12-011-2.
86. Seresirikachorn K, Chetthanon T, Suwansirisuk T, Aeumjaturapat S, Chusakul S, Kanjanaumporn J, et al. Low-dose macrolides for treating pediatric rhinosinusitis: a retrospective study and literature review. SAGE Open Med. 2020;8:2050312120933642. https://doi.org/10.1177/2050312120933642.

Part III
Clinical Use for Other Diseases

Macrolides for Cancer

Masahiro Shinoda

Abstract Macrolides exert their antitumor effects through various mechanisms. Clarithromycin markedly reduced the incidence of mucosa-associated lymphoid tissue (MALT) lymphoma with *Helicobacter pylori* eradication. For cancer growth signals, clarithromycin and roxithromycin exhibit their antitumor effects by inhibiting the Raf to mitogen-activated protein-kinase pathway by acting on extracellular signal-regulated kinase and exhibit antitumor effects. Rapamycin, a mammalian target of rapamycin (mTOR) inhibitor, is effective against cancer by inhibiting the phosphatidylinositol-3 kinase/Akt/mTOR signaling pathway. Ivermectin has been shown to inhibit the Wnt/β-catenin signaling pathway and the Hippo signaling pathway. Regarding growth suppressor evasion, clarithromycin can have an antitumor effect by suppressing TGF-β in combination with other drugs. Regarding resisting cell death, clarithromycin, azithromycin, and ivermectin can induce apoptosis. Clarithromycin and azithromycin can have antitumor effects by acting on autophagy in combination with anticancer drugs. Ivermectin has been reported to induce pyroptosis. Clarithromycin, azithromycin, and ivermectin can have antiangiogenic effects. Ivermectin is expected to inhibit epithelial–mesenchymal transition. Ivermectin and clarithromycin have been reported effective in their action on reactive oxygen species. Erythromycin is effective in overcoming resistance to anticancer drugs and has synergistic effects with other drugs. In clinical trials, the efficacy of clarithromycin has been established as an eradication therapy for MALT lymphoma. Also, clarithromycin, in combination with lenalidomide and dexamethasone, is effective in multiple myeloma. Rapamycin is effective in renal cell carcinoma, neuroendocrine tumors, breast cancer, etc., and has been approved by the FDA. Macrolides, which have various antitumor effects, will be the subject of future research, especially in combination with other drugs.

Keywords Erythromycin · Clarithromycin · Azithromycin · Roxithromycin · Rapamycin · Ivermectin · Anticancer

M. Shinoda (✉)
Department of Respiratory Medicine, Tokyo Shinagawa Hospital, Tokyo, Japan

B. K. Rubin, M. Shinkai (eds.), *Macrolides as Immunomodulatory Agents*, Progress in Inflammation Research 92, https://doi.org/10.1007/978-3-031-42859-3_12

Abbreviations

CI	confidence interval
CR	complete response (remission)
HR	hazard ratio
ORR	objective response rate
OS	overall survival;
PD	progressive disease
PFS	progression-free survival
PR	partial response
SD	stable disease

1 Introduction

Cancer is a large group of diseases that occur in almost every organ or tissue of the body, in which abnormal cells grow uncontrollably, cross normal boundaries to invade adjacent parts of the body, and spread to other organs. The latter process, called metastasis, is an important cause of cancer deaths. Nearly ten million people died from cancer in 2020. The leading causes of cancer death in 2020 were lung (1.80 million deaths), colon and rectum (916,000 deaths), liver (830,000 deaths), stomach (769,000 deaths), and breast (685,000 deaths) [1].

It is recognized that 5–10% of all cancers are hereditary. The remaining 90–95% of cancers are believed to be caused by genetic mutations occurred by toxins (e.g., tobacco), lifestyle factors such as unhealthy diet and excessive alcohol consumption, infections (*Helicobacter pylori*, human papillomavirus, etc.), environmental factors (ultraviolet light, radon, asbestos, ionizing radiation, etc.). Many additional factors increase the risk of developing cancer. Accumulation of genetic mutations causes tumors to develop, grow, progress, and metastasize through various mechanisms [1, 2]. In 2011, Hanahan and Weinberg proposed 11 cancer hallmarks (sustaining proliferative signaling, evading growth suppressors, resisting cell death, enabling replicative immortality, inducing angiogenesis, activating invasion and metastasis, activating invasion and metastasis, deregulating cellular energetics, genome instability and mutation, avoiding immune destruction, and tumor promoting inflammation) and the tumor microenvironment to guide the exploration of new research areas and the devising of new treatments. In addition, resistance to anticancer drugs is an important problem for cancer chemotherapy [3].

In this chapter, we describe the expected effects of macrolides on these cancer characteristics, summarize clinical studies' results, and remark on prospects.

2 Carcinogenic Mechanisms and Macrolide Effects on Them

2.1 *Infection*

2.1.1 *Helicobacter pylori* (*H. pylori*) Infection

H. pylori is a spiral-shaped Gram-negative, microaerophilic bacterium found in the human stomach. Chronic gastric infection by *H. pylori* is strongly associated with the development of distal gastric carcinoma and gastric mucosal lymphoma in humans [4].

Mucosa-associated lymphoid tissue (MALT) lymphoma is a low-grade lymphoma originating from marginal zone B cells [5]. The stomach is the most common site of MALT lymphoma, 90% of which are caused by chronic gastritis caused by *H. pylori* infection. In total, 50%–90% of gastric MALT lymphomas achieve complete remission※ with *H. pylori* eradication treatment, including clarithromycin [6].

While tumor-shrinking effects on lymphoma may be due to the antibacterial effects of clarithromycin on *H. pylori*, some reports attribute such findings to direct antitumor or immunomodulatory effects of clarithromycin [7–10]. As for gastric cancer, eradication is known to suppress the development of gastric cancer [11].

2.2 *Sustaining Proliferative Signaling*

2.2.1 Raf to Mitogen-Activated Protein (MAP)-Kinase Pathway

Activation of Ras proteins, small guanosine triphosphatases (GTPases) related to signaling pathways involved in cell cycle progression, cell migration, apoptosis, and senescence, trigger MAPK cascade activation such as Raf/MEK/extracellular signal-regulated kinase (ERK). RAS proteins have three isotypes: HRAS, KRAS, and NRAS [12, 13]. Ras mutations have been identified in both hematological and solid tumors, with NRAS prevalent in hematological and melanomas and KRAS prevalent in pancreas, colon, and lung cancers [14].

Nodes of MAPK signaling transmit and regulate extracellular stimuli to control and fine-tune vital cellular functions, including proliferation, cell division, metabolism, motility, innate immunity, cellular stress response, apoptosis, and survival functions in eukaryotes from yeast to humans. The MAPK pathway is known to have four major branch pathways and more than a dozen MAPK enzymes, which are classified into at least seven different groups. [15, 16] The ERK pathway is induced by proliferative factors involved in proliferative signaling and is critical for cell proliferation, differentiation, and survival. MEK1 and MEK2 selectively phosphorylate ERK1 and ERK2 on serine and threonine residues, and ERK1/2 directly regulates cell cycle mediators, promotes protein and nucleotide synthesis, and regulates mammalian target of rapamycin (mTOR) signaling through interactions with proteins such as TSC2 [17]. While the upstream RAS and RAF kinases are frequently mutated in MAPK-driven cancers, mutations in MEK and ERK are less common, accounting for <1% of all observed MAPK oncogenic genomic alterations. However, despite the low frequency of MEK/ERK-activating mutations, this pathway is important because of the problem of acquired resistance to RAF inhibitor therapy and the dependence of multiple tumor types on the MAPK pathway [18].

Clarithromycin at physiological concentrations is known to suppress ERK, delay progression of bronchial epithelial cells into the S phase of the cell cycle, and delay cell growth [19]. ERK1/2 is activated and associated with more advanced tumors in non-small cell lung cancer. Antitumor effects may be partly mediated through macrolide regulation of ERK [20].

A combination of the histone deacetylase inhibitor FK228 and roxithromycin had synergistic inhibitory effects on cell survival in the HUT-78, Ki-JK, and EL-4 lymphoma cells, and inhibited the phosphorylation of Akt and extracellular signal-regulated kinase (ERK) in EL-4 cells in a dose-dependent manner [21].

2.2.2 Phosphatidylinositol-3 Kinase (PI3K)/Akt/mTOR Signal Pathway

Somatic mutations caused by PI3K/Akt/mTOR-related genes induce constitutive activation of various cancer growth pathways, leading to tumor cell proliferation, growth, differentiation, metabolism, and apoptosis, and other functional dysregulation that support tumor cell survival [22]. PI3K is activated through multiple upstream signals such as cytokines, integrins, B cell receptor (BCR) activation, or G protein-coupled receptor (GPCR) ligands. After PI3K binds to the ligand, receptor tyrosine kinases or G protein-coupled receptor (GPCR)-induced PI3K activation occurs at the cell membrane. Activated PI3K phosphorylates PIP2 to generate PIP3. Accumulating PIP3 and recruitment of proteins with pleckstrin homology domains, such as Akt and phosphoinositide-dependent kinase-1 (PDK1), subsequently trigger signaling cascades that affect cell growth, survival, calcium mobilization, cell motility, vesicle trafficking, cell proliferation, apoptosis, etc. [23] Three classes have been identified in PI3K. Class I PI3K has been reported to be associated with various malignancies [22]. Tumor types with PIK3CA mutations include breast, endometrium, urinary tract, cervix, skin, and ovary. Tumor types with PIK3R1 mutations include endometrium, colorectal, cervix, upper respiratory tract, and central nervous system [22].

The tumor suppressor PTEN inhibits Akt by suppressing the activity of signaling through PI3K and acts as a negative regulator of the PI3K/Akt/mTOR signaling cascade [24]. Somatic mutations, including PTEN homozygous deletion, truncation mutation, point mutation, and other abnormalities, have been identified in many cancers [22]. Akt is a member of the AGC family and its activation functions as a master switch for various signaling pathways, triggering many intracellular responses through downstream targets and interacting partners. These signaling abnormalities affect a wide range of diseases, including cancer, diabetes, and neurodegeneration [25]. Akt binds to PIP3 through its pleckstrin homology (PH) domain and translocates to the cell membrane. PDK1 is also translocates to the membrane via its PH domain, and threonine 308 of Akt is phosphorylated. The second phosphorylation of Akt at serine 473 by the mTOR-Rictor complex (mTORC2) results in full Akt activation [25–28]. Tumors with Akt mutations have been reported in the meninges, breast, endometrium, urinary tract, thyroid, skin, lung, ovary, hematopoietic/lymphatic system, and kidney [22]. A downstream effector of the PI3K/Akt pathway, mTOR forms complexes with different regulatory protein subunits that control various aspects of signal transduction and is activated by multiple mechanisms. mTOR comprises two protein complexes, mTORC1 and mTORC2 core catalytic unit [29]. The mTORC1 complex, composed of mTOR, Raptor, and mLST8, regulates cell growth and proliferation by phosphorylating the eukaryotic translation initiation factor 4E-binding protein 1 (4E-BP1) and the ribosomal protein S6 kinase (S6K). mTORC1 regulates various tumor cell-specific processes such as translation, ribosome biogenesis, autophagy, glucose metabolism, cellular responses to hypoxia, and metastasis [29]. The mTORC2 complex consists of mTOR, Rictor, mLST8, and mSin1 and phosphorylates multiple proteins (Akt, serum glucocorticoid-regulated kinase 1 (SGK1), and protein kinase Cα (PKCα)). mTORC2 functions to control cell survival and proliferation [30]. Tumors with mTOR mutations have been reported in the endometrium, kidney, colorectal, lung, skin, esophagus, upper respiratory tract, urinary tract, breast, ovary, hematopoietic/lymphatic system, liver, pancreas, and brain [22].

Rapamycin (sirolimus), a macrolide derived from *Streptomyces hygroscopicus* [31], has been used to prevent transplant rejection and to treat lymphangioleiomyomatosis. Rapamycin is an inhibitor of mTOR1 and has antitumor effects on head and neck cancer, ovarian cancer, glioblastoma, prostate cancer, breast cancer, endometrial cancer, renal cancer, testicular cancer, colon cancer, bladder cancer, lung cancer, and melanoma [32].

2.2.3 Wnt/β-Catenin Signal Pathway

Activation of the Wnt pathway is initiated by the interaction of Wnt/Frizzled (FZD) with low-density lipoprotein receptor-related proteins 5 and 6 (LRPS5/6). It is subsequently signaled via Dishevelled (Dvl) to downstream mediators of the Wnt signaling cascade. Accumulating β-catenin and its nuclear translocation promotes interactions with T-cell factor/lymphoid enhancer factor (TCF/LEF) family members required to transcribe target genes. The cytoplasmic protein β-catenin regulates the activity of multiple transcription factors that regulate genes involved in the development, cell cycle control, and carcinogenesis. Dvl signal propagates to planar cell polarity (PCP) and PCP signaling ultimately induces actin polymerization and microtubule stabilization required for cell polarity and migration. Dvl is also involved in Ca^{2+}-dependent regulation of calcineurin, the transcription factors nuclear factor of activated T cells (NFAT) family controls the expression of genes associated with cell fate determination and migration [33]. Ivermectin suppresses the

Wnt/β-catenin/TCF transcriptional response. This effect is rescued by continuous and direct activation of TCF transcriptional activity and is related to repression of the levels of C-terminally phosphorylated β-catenin phosphoforms and cyclin D1 [34].

2.2.4 Hippo Signaling Pathway

Hippo signaling controls organ size by regulating cell proliferation, apoptosis, and stem cell self-renewal. Dysregulation of the Hippo pathway contributes to cancer development. A kinase cascade is a core to the Hippo pathway, wherein Mst1/2 kinases and SAV1 form a complex to phosphorylate and activate large tumor suppressors 1 and 2 (LATS1/2). LATS1/2 kinases phosphorylate and inhibit the transcription co-activators YAP and TAZ, two major downstream effectors of the Hippo pathway. When dephosphorylated, YAP/TAZ translocate into the nucleus and interact with TEAD1–4 and other transcription factors to induce the expression of genes that promote cell proliferation and inhibit apoptosis [35]. Many studies have associated increased accumulation of YAP1 in the nucleus with poor prognosis in patients with intrahepatic cholangiocellular carcinoma and combined hepatocellular and cholangiocarcinoma, colorectal cancer, ovarian cancer, and gastric cancer [36]. Ivermectin can inhibit the proliferation of gastric cancer cells by inhibiting YAP1 in vivo and in vitro [37].

2.3 *Evading Growth Suppressors*

2.3.1 Corruption of the Transforming Growth Factor (TGF)-β Pathway Promotes Malignancy

TGF-β signaling is tumor-suppressive in epithelial cells but can promote invasion and metastasis during the late stage of cancer progression. During tumor progression, tumor cells often lose the antiproliferative response to TGFβ, which is associated with increased TGF-β expression in the microenvironment. TGF-β-mediated regulation in the tumor microenvironment can be attributed to many factors, including cell-autonomous signaling, stromal–epithelial interactions, inflammation, immune evasion, and angiogenesis. Cell-autonomous TGF-β signaling triggers epithelial–mesenchymal transition (EMT) in cancer cells, increasing invasion and metastasis. Conversely, abrogation of autonomous TGF-β signaling in cancer cells can increase metastasis in the apparent absence of EMT. Together, cell-type-dependent and context-dependent effects of TGF-β signaling contribute to the regulation of tumor initiation, progression, and metastasis [38]. A study using 13762NF mammary adenocarcinoma in the F-344 rat system did not observe any significant reduction in mortality with clarithromycin alone, but a significant decrease in mortality was obtained when either carboplatin or clarithromycin was administered in combination with cyclophosphamide. Clarithromycin showed no direct cytotoxicity against this tumor in vitro, although expressions of matrix metalloproteinase-9 (MMP-9), TGF-β, and tumor necrosis factor (TNF)-α were decreased. Spleen cells from clarithromycin-treated tumor-bearing rats expressed lower levels of TGF-β and IL-6 genes and stronger tumor-neutralizing activity than those obtained from rats not treated with clarithromycin [39].

2.4 *Resisting Cell Death*

2.4.1 Apoptosis

Apoptosis, the programmed autonomous cell death controlled by genes to maintain the stability of the internal environment of multicellular organisms, is generally unregulated in many types of cancer [40].The intrinsic pathway can be activated by endogenous stresses such as oncogenes, direct DNA damage, hypoxia, and survival factor deficiency. A sensor of cellular stress, p53 is a key activator of the intrinsic pathway. This pathway is tightly regulated by the balance of activities of Bcl-2 family proteins, including proteins promoting apoptosis (Bax, Bak, Bad, Bid, Puma, Bim, and Noxa) and proteins inhibiting apoptosis (Bcl-2, Bcl-xL, Bcl-w, and Mcl-1). [41, 42] There are at least two pathways in the extrinsic pathway: the receptor-mediated pathway and the cytotoxic stress-mediated pathway. Receptor-mediated pathways include those activated by death ligands. Death Receptors (DR) are cell surface receptors that transmit specific ligand-initiated apoptotic signals and play a central role in induced apoptosis. These receptors activate des-caspase (DC) within seconds of ligand binding, leading to apoptotic cell death within hours [43]. Both intrinsic and extrinsic pathways ultimately depend on the protease activity of specific caspase family members. These caspases fall into two major categories. Initiator caspases such as caspase-2, -8, -9, -10, and -12 are coupled with upstream proapoptotic signals and cleave executioner caspases such as caspase-3, -6, and -7 and ultimately modify proteins involved in cell demolition [44].

In a BALB/c murine B-cell lymphoma cell line, clarithromycin induced apoptosis through the appearance of apoptotic bodies, DNA fragmentation, degeneration, and detachment of cells, which may be induced through the TNF system [45]. Most DLBCL and gastric MALT lymphoma cases show bcl-2 expression, and NF-κB-mediated downregulation of antiapoptotic genes following clarithromycin administration. This may partially explain the suppression of tumor growth after the eradication or in the absence of *H. pylori* infection. [46, 47] Mouse studies have shown that Bcl-xL may be involved in the pathogenesis of B-cell MALT lymphoma arising from chronic infection with *Helicobacter* species. [48, 49] In activated lymphocytes, downregulation of Bcl-xL has been reported as the mechanism by which clarithromycin induces apoptosis [50]. Azithromycin inhibited cell proliferation more effectively in the HeLa cervical adenocarcinoma cells and SGC-7901 gastric cancer cells than in the transformed BHK-21 hamster fibroblast cell line. Azithromycin-induced apoptosis is partially mediated by a caspase-dependent mechanism involving upregulation of apoptotic protein-cleaved PARP and caspase-3 products and downregulation of the anti-apoptotic proteins, Mcl-1, bcl-2, and bcl-X1. Moreover, the combination of azithromycin and the common anticancer chemotherapeutic agent vincristine selectively synergized against apoptosis in HeLa and SGC-7901 cells [51]. Azithromycin enhanced tumor necrosis factor-related apoptosis-inducing ligand (TRAIL)-induced apoptosis in colon adenocarcinoma cells, mainly through the upregulation of DR4 and DR5 [52]. Azithromycin has been shown to enhance caspase 3/7 activity and induce apoptosis in chronic myelogenous leukemia cell lines. Combined administration of imatinib and azithromycin significantly induced apoptosis compared to single administration in imatinib-resistant cell lines [53].

Ivermectin has been reported to induce caspase-dependent apoptosis in HeLa cells [54], breast cancer cells [55], glioblastoma [56], chronic myelogenous leukemia cells [57], OCI-AML2 leukemia cells [58], and epithelial ovarian cancer cells [59].

2.4.2 Autophagy

Autophagy is a lysosomal degradation pathway for the breakdown of intracellular proteins and organelles. Although constitutive autophagy is a homeostatic mechanism for intracellular recycling and metabolic regulation, it is also stress-responsive and is important for removing damaged proteins and organelles. Autophagy confers stress tolerance, limits damage, and sustains viability under adverse conditions. Autophagy is a tumor-suppression mechanism, yet it enables tumor cell survival under stress (nutrient starvation, radiotherapy, and certain cytotoxic drugs) [60].

A study in myeloma and chronic myelogenous leukemia cells suggested that clarithromycin might halt the autophagic process after the fusion of autophagosomes and lysosomes. Clarithromycin may, therefore, represent a potential adjuvant for therapies in which tumors use autophagy as an escape mechanism [61]. Treatment of chronic myeloid leukemia cells with dasatinib, a tyrosine kinase inhibitor, induces autophagy [62]. The combination of clarithromycin and dasatinib inhibits late autophagy, resulting in a reduced percentage of living cells compared with dasatinib alone. Cell lines with clinically known dasatinib-resistance mutations also became more sensitive to dasatinib when clarithromycin was co-administered. Although clinically relevant dasatinib concentrations alone did not affect cell death, combination with clarithromycin achieved a cell death rate of 32% in these mutant cells [62]. The effects of combination therapy with DNA-damaging drugs (doxorubicin, etoposide, carboplatin, etc.) and azithromycin in non-small cell lung cancer cell lines, the cytotoxic activity of the DNA-damaging drugs was enhanced in the presence of azithromycin. Concomitant use of azithromycin has been reported to block autophagy and lead to the accumulation of lysosomes and autolysosomes [63]. In myeloma cell lines [64], metastatic breast cancer cell lines [65], and head and neck squamous cell carcinoma cell lines [66], macrolides have been suggested to induce cell death by inhibiting autophagy via the proapoptotic transcription factor C/EBP homologous protein (CHOP).

PAK proteins are critical modulators of nuclear signaling and cytoskeletal reorganization. Among the PAK proteins, p21 (RAC1)-activated kinase 1 (PAK1) modulates a wide range of signals involved in numerous biological activities. Blockade of PAK1 signaling contributes to tumor cell death [67]. PAK1 is associated with the development of most human cancers and functions as an Akt-binding protein that stimulates Akt phosphorylation and activation [68]. The Akt/mTOR signaling pathway was shown to play an important inhibitory role in autophagy [69]. Several studies have shown that the PAK1 inhibitor ivermectin inhibits the growth of breast [70], ovarian [71], glioblastoma [67], and NF2 tumors [71] by inducing cytostatic autophagy in vitro and in vivo.

2.4.3 Pyroptosis

Pyroptosis is a type of inflammatory cell death induced by inflammasomes. Inflammasomes initiate the conversion of pro-caspase-1 via self-shearing into activated caspase-1. Activated caspase-1 can cause pro-IL-1β and pro-IL-18 to mature and be secreted [72].

It was reported that activated caspase-1 was significantly increased in breast cancer cells after ivermectin intervention, and characteristic pyroptosis phenomena such as cell swelling and rupturing were observed [55].

2.5 *Inducing Angiogenesis*

Tumors require sustenance in the form of nutrients and oxygen as well as an ability to evacuate metabolic wastes and carbon dioxide. The tumor-associated neovasculature generated by angiogenesis addresses these needs. During tumor progression, an angiogenic switch is almost always activated and remains on, causing normally quiescent vasculature to sprout new vessels that help sustain expanding neoplastic growths continually [73].

Vascular endothelial growth factor (VEGF) is a heparin-binding homodimeric glycoprotein that acts via endothelial-specific receptor tyrosine kinases/VEGFRs (vascular endothelial growth factor receptors; VEGFR1 (FLT1), VEGFR2 (KDR/Flk1), and VEGFR3 (FLT4)) and the signaling is critical to the processes of angiogenesis and tumor growth [74–76]. The binding of VEGF-A to VEGFR-2 activates the Ras/Raf/MAPK/ERK pathway and PI3K/Akt/mTOR pathway, leading to endothelial cell proliferation [77].

Endothelial tube formation is inhibited by clarithromycin in a dose-dependent manner in vitro, and clarithromycin can inhibit tumor-induced angiogenesis [78]. In vivo and in vitro studies with mouse B16BL6 melanoma cells have also shown that clarithromycin and roxithromycin potentiate the inhibition of tumor growth by cyclophosphamide, cisplatin, doxorubicin, or vindesine, possibly via antiangiogenic effects [79].

Azithromycin inhibited capillary network formation in human lung tumor-associated endothelial cells (HLT-ECs) both in vitro and in vivo and can target VEGFR2-mediated focal adhesions and PI3K/Akt signaling pathways and may suppress angiogenesis and lung tumor growth [80].

A study investigating the effect of roxithromycin on tumor angiogenesis in the HepG2 human liver cancer cell line suggested that roxithromycin inhibits tumor angiogenesis and that changes in VEGF expression are involved in the mechanism underlying this inhibitory effect [81].

In vitro capillary network formation experiments using human brain microvascular endothelial cells (HBMECs) revealed that ivermectin eliminated the ability of HBMECs to form tubular structures, confirming the effect of ivermectin against angiogenesis, which indicated that ivermectin is a potent angiogenesis inhibitor [56].

2.6 *Activating Invasion and Metastasis*

2.6.1 Epithelial–Mesenchymal Transition

Epithelial–mesenchymal transition (EMT) is an important biological process for the migration and invasion of malignant tumor cells derived from epithelial cells and involved in angiogenesis, tumor growth, and the generation of cancer stem cells (CSCs) that might influence tumor recurrence and resistance to conventional therapies [82, 83]. The multidomain adapter proteins SIN3A and SIN3B are essential facilitators of epigenetic deregulators with no intrinsic DNA-binding activity that act as molecular scaffolds that drive interactions between sequence-specific DNA-binding transcription factors and chromatin regulators [84]. The blockage of interactions between the PAH2 domain of the chromatin regulatory factor SIN3A and SIN3 interaction domain (SID)-containing proteins via the SID peptide leads to EMT reversal and the expression of silenced genes encoding proteins involved in cell differentiation and growth [85].

It was reported that ivermectin, as a small mimetic of the SID peptide, inhibits the interaction between SIN3-PAH2 and MAD [86].

2.7 *Deregulating Cellular Energetics*

Reactive oxygen species (ROS), produced in the body primarily by the mitochondria, serve as cell signaling molecules generated in oxidative metabolism and are associated with several human diseases. The reprogramming of redox metabolism induces abnormal accumulation of ROS in cancer cells. It has been widely accepted that ROS plays opposite roles in tumor growth, metastasis, and apoptosis according to their different distributions, concentrations, and durations in specific subcellular structures. These double-edged roles in cancer progression include the

ROS-dependent malignant transformation and the oxidative stress-induced cell death [87].

In ovarian cancer cells in vitro and in vivo, clarithromycin and cisplatin decreased expression of endogenous antioxidant enzymes and increased levels of ROS [88]. Clarithromycin has been suggested to potentiate the cytotoxic effects of cisplatin. Some recent data demonstrate that ivermectin exhibits selective toxicity in inducing mitochondrial dysfunction and oxidative stress and enhances the role of BCR-ABL TKIs in CD34 chronic myeloid leukemia cells [57].

2.8 Cancer Stem Cells (CSCs)

CSCs are a cell population like stem cells with characteristics of self-renewal and differentiation potential in tumor tissue. Their robust proliferation and multidirectional differentiation abilities are unrestricted because they lack a negative feedback regulation mechanism for stem cell self-renewal. CSCs are identified in most types of liquid and solid cancers and contribute to tumor onset, expansion, resistance, recurrence, and metastasis after therapy. [89, 90]

It was reported that ivermectin would preferentially target and inhibit CSCs-rich cell populations compared with other cell populations in MDA-MB-231 breast cancer cells and the expression of the homeobox protein NANOG, octamer-binding protein 4 (OCT-4) and SRY-box 2 (SOX-2), which are closely related to the self-renewal and differentiation ability of stem cells in CSCs [91].

2.9 Drug Resistance/Synergistic Effect with Other Drugs

P-glycoprotein (P-Gp) encoded by the mdr1 gene in cells is an active efflux pump for hydrophobic, cationic anticancer drugs, such as vinca alkaloids and anthracycline antibiotics. This glycoprotein may play a vital role in the antitumor activity of these agents against anticancer drug-resistant cells through the overexpression of P-Gp [92]. In a study by Wang et al., erythromycin and clarithromycin increased the accumulation of vinblastine and cyclosporine A in anticancer drug-resistant (P388/ADR) cells without affecting sensitive mouse leukemia P388 cells, prolonging the survival of P388/ADR-bearing mic [92].

In a study evaluating the therapeutic effects of imatinib and azithromycin combination therapy in imatinib-resistant chronic myelogenous leukemia, azithromycin alone and the azithromycin/imatinib combination reduced P-Gp function in both K562S cells and high MDR-1 (P-Gp)-expressing K562R cells [53].Also, several studies have confirmed that ivermectin could reverse drug resistance by inhibiting P-Gp. [93–95]. Alpha 1 acid glycoprotein (AGP), also known as orosomucoid, is an acute-phase protein that influences the free plasma concentrations of drugs and AGP alters the distribution and metabolism of some drugs [96]. Serum concentrations of

AGP increase several-fold in response to local inflammatory stimuli, and were increased in both plasma and ascites in cancer patients. [97, 98] Erythromycin can reactivate the cell growth-inhibitory effects of paclitaxel after suppression by AGP. In an OCUM-2MD3 peritoneal carcinomatosis xenograft mouse model, administration of paclitaxel alone did not diminish peritoneal carcinoma, but co-administration of erythromycin and paclitaxel reduced peritoneal carcinomatosis [99].

Erythromycin has also been reported to modulate chemosensitivity associated with human ether-a-go-go related gene (hERG) K+ channel expression in cancer cells. The hERG encodes the pore-forming subunit of the rapidly activating delayed rectifier potassium channel (IKr) in cardiomyocytes and has been identified as a gene involved in chromosome 7-associated long QT syndrome [100]. Several studies have shown that hERG is expressed in some cancer cell lines and is absent in the healthy cells from which the respective cancers are derived. [101–103] An in vitro study using HT-29 and T84 human colon carcinoma cells, MCF-7 and SK-BR-3 human mammary adenocarcinoma cells, PG highly metastatic human lung giant-cell carcinoma cells, and A549 human lung adenocarcinoma cells found correlations between hERG expression levels and chemosensitivity to vincristine, paclitaxel, and hydroxy-camptothecin. Erythromycin suppressed the proliferation of cancer cells, with its antitumor efficacy correlating with hERG expression. Synergistic effects were identified between erythromycin and vincristine, paclitaxel, and hydroxy-camptothecin [104].

3 Clinical Data※

3.1 Clarithromycin (Table 1)

Although some studies have failed to confirm efficacy with clarithromycin monotherapy [116–118], it has been reported that clarithromycin plus dexamethasone and low-dose thalidomide have efficacy for patients with multiple myeloma and Waldenström's macroglobulinemia [105]. The addition of clarithromycin to treatment with low-dose dexamethasone and lenalidomide, in a regimen known as BiRd, has been shown efficacy in a phase II trial [106, 107] and a case-matched study [108] in treatment-naïve multiple myeloma patients. However, in a phase III trial of treatment-naïve, transplant-ineligible multiple myeloma patients, addition of clarithromycin to Rd. resulted in more toxic deaths and did not improve progression-free survival (PFS) despite increases in the complete response rate. This was attributed to side effects associated with overexposure to corticosteroids resulting from the delayed clearance induced by clarithromycin in this elderly population [109].

Eradication of *H. pylori* has shown high efficacy in several phase II trials for *H. pylori*-associated MALT lymphoma. [112, 113] As for extranodal marginal zone B-cell lymphoma relapsed/refractory stage IE and IV, in a single-center phase II trial, it was reported that clarithromycin monotherapy was effective [9].

Table 1 Clinical trials in patients with hematological malignancies and solid tumors with clarithromycin

Cancer type	Year	Design	Subject	Regimen	Outcome[a]	
Multiple myeloma (MM) / Waldenström's macroglobulinemia (WM)						
MM/WM Naïve / previously treated	2002	Phase 2 Single arm	$N = 50$	Clarithromycin (Biaxin), low-dose thalidomide and dexamethasone	CR 13% Near CR 40% Major response 13% PR 27%	[105]
MM Chemotherapy- Naïve	2008 2013	Phase 2 Single arm	$N = 72$	Clarithromycin (Biaxin)-lenalidomide-low-dose dexamethasone (BiRd)	ORR 6.6-year follow-up CR 43%, very good PR 25%, PR 25% Median PFS 49 months Median EFS 47 months 5-year OS 75.2%	[106, 107]
MM Chemotherapy-Naïve	2010	Phase 2 Retrospective Case matched study	$N = 72$	BiRd vs. lenalidomide-low-dose dexamethasone (Rd)	BiRd vs. Rd. CR 45.8 vs. 13.9%, $P < 0.001$ Very good PR or better 73.6 vs. 33.3%, $p < 0.001$ Median PFS 48.3 vs. 27.5 months, $p = 0.044$ 3-year OS 89.7 vs. 73.0%, $p = 0.218$	[108]
MM Chemotherapy- Naïve	2021	Phase 3 Randomized Open-label Two arms	$N = 286$	Rd or Rd. and clarithromycin (C-Rd)	Median PFS C-Rd vs. Rd. 23 vs. 29 months, $p = 0.14$ Rate of CR or better C-Rd vs. Rd. 22.6 vs 14.4%, $p = 0.048$	[109]

(continued)

Table 1 (continued)

Cancer type	Year	Design	Subject	Regimen	Outcome[a]	
Lymphoma: Mucosa associated lymphoid tissue (MALT), diffuse large B-cell lymphoma (DLBCL)						
Gastric MALT lymphoma Stage I or II N1	1999	Phase 2 Single arm	$N = 34$ 28 *H. pylori* positive	Amoxicillin and clarithromycin / tetracycline and clarithromycin / tetracycline and metronidazole	*H. pylori*-positive patients: CR 50%, PR 29%[b] *H. pylori*-negative patients: No response 100%[b]	[110]
Low-grade gastric MALT lymphoma stage IE	2001	Phase 2 Single arm	$N = 97$	Clarithromycin, omeprazole, and metronidazole	Complete endoscopic and histological remission 79%	[111]
Low-grade gastric MALT lymphoma Stage IE and IIE	2001	Phase 2 Single arm	$N = 44$ 34 *H. pylori* positive	Clarithromycin, amoxicillin, lansoprazole	43% complete histological regression (56% within *H. pylori*-positive patients)	[112]
Gastric marginal zone B-cell lymphoma of MALT stage I	2004	Phase 2 Single arm	$N = 95$ 90 evaluable	Clarithromycin, omeprazole, and metronidazole/amoxicillin	CR 62%[c] Minimal residual disease 18%[c] PR 12%[c] SD 4%[c]	[113]
Extranodal marginal zone B-cell lymphoma Relapsed/ refractory Stage IE and IV	2010	Phase 2 Single arm	$N = 13$	Clarithromycin	CR 15%† PR 23%† SD 31%† PD 31%†	[9]
H. pylori-positive gastric DLBCL (de novo and MALT) Stage I	2012	Phase 2 Single arm	$N = 16$	Clarithromycin, omeprazole, tinidazole/metronidazole	CR 50%†† PR 19%†† PD 31%††	[114]

Lung cancer: Non-small cell lung cancer (NSCLC), small cell lung cancer (SCLC)						
NSCLC and SCLC Stage IIIa, IIIb, IV Prior chemo and/or radiation therapy	1997	Phase 2 Randomized Two arms	$N = 49$ 42 NSCLC 7 SCLC	Clarithromycin or none	NSCLC: Increased median survival time Clarithromycin vs. control 535 vs. 277 days SCLC: No significant difference in median Survival time	[115]

[a] In multiple myeloma, response criteria were adopted from the International Myeloma Working Group criteria

Solid tumor response was assessed by Response Evaluation Criteria in solid tumor.

[b] Complete remission was defined as the absence of histopathological evidence of lymphoma on endoscopic biopsy. Partial remission was defined as a reduction in endoscopic tumor stage or 50% reduction in the size of large tumors

[c] Complete remission was defined as total disappearance of lymphoma and absence of histopathological evidence of lymphoma on endoscopic biopsy. Partial remission was assumed in cases of tumor reduction of at least 50%. Patients revealing normalization of macroscopic findings but with persistent residual lymphoma infiltrates on histological examination were classified as minimal residual disease

† Response was defined according to the National Cancer Institute standardized criteria (Cheson et al. 1999)

†† Residual macroscopic abnormalities at endoscopic examination or residual perigastric lymph nodes measuring <1 cm in diameter or gastric wall alterations at ultrasonography were considered as complete response (remission) if histopathological examination did not show lymphomatous infiltration. Persistence of areas of MALT and/or DLBCL in histopathological specimens in patients with normal/improved gastric aspect at endoscopy and ultrasonography were considered as PR

For chronic myelogenous leukemia, a clinical study, although it included a small number of 4 cases, reported that combination therapy with tyrosine kinase inhibitor (TKI) showed 25% complete hematological remission and all patients had Bcr-abl/abl transcript level reduction [119].

Regarding solid cancer, in a randomized trial with advanced lung cancer, clarithromycin maintenance therapy showed significantly longer median survival than the control group, especially in non-small cell lung cancer, which was more effective, nearly doubling median survival [115]. These findings were thought to be due to decreased serum IL-6 levels after treatment with clarithromycin [120].

3.2 Azithromycin

In a phase II trial of long-term oral azithromycin for MALT lymphoma, only 4 of 16 patients (25%) responded, with 2 complete responses and 2 partial responses, while stable disease was seen in 9 patients (56%) and progressive disease in 3 patients (19%). Administration of azithromycin showed some antilymphoma activity, but overall response rate (ORR) fell below predefined thresholds of interest and the study was discontinued [121].

In a study of low-dose azithromycin combined with paclitaxel and cisplatin for advanced non-small cell lung cancer, patients taking azithromycin displayed modest but clear advantages in both progression-free and overall survival [122].

3.3 Rapamycin (Everolimus (Table 2), Temsirolimus (Table 3), Ridaforolimus (Table 4))

In a double-blind, randomized, placebo-controlled phase III trial that investigated the efficacy of everolimus for advanced renal cell carcinoma that had progressed after VEGFR-TKI therapy, the median PFS was significantly longer in the everolimus group (4.9 months) compared with in the placebo group (1.9 months) [123]. Everolimus has shown antitumor activity in patients with advanced neuroendocrine tumors in many trials. [126, 127] In a randomized, placebo-controlled, phase III study for nonfunctional neuroendocrine tumors of the lung or gastrointestinal tract, the median PFS was significantly longer in the everolimus group compared with the placebo group [126]. In a phase III trial for hormone receptor-positive, human epidermal growth factor receptor 2 (HER2)-negative, metastatic/recurrent breast cancer, everolimus, and exemestane were compared with exemestane monotherapy as endocrine therapy after second-line treatment in patients previously treated with nonsteroidal aromatase inhibitors. The combination group significantly prolonged PFS of the overall population [124]. By these findings, the FDA approved everolimus as advanced renal cell carcinoma, pancreatic neuroendocrine tumors, and

Table 2 Clinical trials in patients with hematological malignancies and solid tumors with everolimus

Cancer type	Year	Design	Subject	Regimen	Outcome[a]	Ref
Renal cell carcinoma						
Metastatic renal cell carcinoma Progressing on vascular endothelial growth factor receptor tyrosine kinase inhibitors	2010	Phase 3 Randomized Double-blind Two arms	$N = 416$	Everolimus or placebo	Median PFS Everolimus vs. placebo 4.9 vs. 1.9 months (HR 0.33; $p < 0.001$)	[123]
Breast cancer						
Advanced breast cancer Postmenopausal hormone-receptor-positive	2012	Phase 3 Randomized	$N = 724$	Everolimus and exemestane or exemestane and placebo	Median PFS Everolimus and exemestane vs. exemestane and placebo 6.9 vs. 2.8 months (HR 0.43; 95%CI 0.35–0.54; $p < 0.001$)	[124]
Advanced breast cancer HER2-positive, trastuzumab-resistant Previously received taxane therapy.	2014	Phase 3 Randomized Double-blind Two arms	$N = 569$	Everolimus, trastuzumab and vinorelbine or Placebo, trastuzumab and vinorelbine	Median PFS Everolimus group vs. placebo group 7.00 vs. 5.78 months (HR 0.78; 95%CI 0.65–0.95; $p = 0.0067$)	[125]
Neuroendocrine tumor						
Advanced, progressive neuroendocrine tumors Lung or gastrointestinal tract	2016	Phase 3 Randomized Double-blind Two arms	$N = 302$	Everolimus or placebo	Median PFS Everolimus vs. placebo 11.0 vs. 3.9 months (HR 0·48; 95%CI 0.35–0.67; $p < 0{\cdot}00001$)	[126]

(continued)

Table 2 (continued)

Cancer type	Year	Design	Subject	Regimen	Outcome[a]	Ref
Advanced neuroendocrine tumors associated with carcinoid syndrome	2011	Phase 3 Randomized Double-blind Two arms	$N = 429$	Everolimus plus octreotide long-acting repeatable(LAR) Or placebo plus octreotide LAR	Median PFS Everolimus plus octreotide LAR vs. Placebo plus octreotide LAR 16·4 vs. 11.3 months (HR 0·77; 95%CI 0.59–1.00; $p = 0.026$)	[127]
Subependymal giant cell astrocytomas						
Subependymal giant cell astrocytomas associated with tuberous sclerosis complex	2013	Phase 3 Randomized Double-blind Two arms	$N = 117$	Everolimus or placebo	At least 50% reduction in the volume of tumor Everolimus vs. placebo 35% patients vs. none (difference 35%, 95%CI 15–52, $p < 0.0001$)	[128]

Abbreviations: *CI* confidence interval; *CR* complete response (remission); *HR* hazard ratio; *ORR* objective response rate; *OS* overall survival; *PD* progressive disease; *PFS* progression-free survival; *PR* partial response; *SD* stable disease

[a] Solid tumor response was assessed by Response Evaluation Criteria in solid tumor

Table 3 Clinical trials in patients with hematological malignancies and solid tumors with temsirolimus

Cancer type	Year	Design	Subject	Regimen	Outcome[a]	Ref
Renal-cell carcinoma (RCC)						
Advanced RCC Previously untreated, poor-prognosis metastatic	2007	Phase 3 Randomized Three arms	$N = 626$	Temsirolimus or Interferon alfa-2a or Temsirolimus and interferon alfa-2a	Median OS Temsirolimus vs. interferon 10.9 vs. 7.3 months (HR 0.73; 95%CI 0.58–0.92; $p = 0.008$) Temsirolimus and interferon vs. interferon 8.4 vs. 7.3 months (HR 0.96; 95%CI, 0.76–1.20; $p = 0.70$)	[129]
RCC	2012	Phase 2 Non-randomized	$N = 82$	Temsirolimus	Clinical benefit rate 48% (95%CI 36–59) ORR 11% (95%CI 5–20)	[130]
Head and neck squamous cell carcinoma (HNSCC)						
Recurrent and/or metastatic HNSCC Platinum and cetuximab refractory	2015	Phase 2 Single arm	$N = 40$	Temsirolimus	PFR at 12 weeks 40% Median PFS 56 days (95%CI 36–113) Median OS 152 days (95%CI 76–256)	[131]
Recurrent and/or metastatic head and neck squamous cell carcinoma	2017	Phase 2 Single arm	$N = 39$ 36 evaluable	Temsirolimus, carboplatin, and paclitaxel	ORR after two cycles of treatment PR 41.7% SD 52.3%	[132]
Melanoma						
Melanoma Unresectable stage III to IV	2013	Phase 2 Single arm	$N = 17$	Temsirolimus and bevacizumab	ORR 17.7% PR 17.7%, SD 53%	[133]

(continued)

Table 3 (continued)

Cancer type	Year	Design	Subject	Regimen	Outcome[a]	Ref
Sarcoma						
Bone and soft tissue sarcoma Allocated based on IGF-1R expression by immunohistochemistry to one of three treatment groups	2013	Phase 2 Single arm	$N = 54$	Temsirolimus and cixutumumab	PFS at 12 weeks IGF-1R-positive soft-tissue sarcoma 31% IGF-1R-positive bone sarcoma 35% IGF-1R-negative group 39%	[134]
Soft tissue sarcoma 2 and over prior chemotherapeutics	2015	Phase 2 Randomized Two arms	$N = 71$	Selumetinib or Selumetinib and temsirolimus	In the overall cohort, PFS no difference between the two arms In the leiomyosarcoma cohort, four-month PFS rate was 50% with the combination vs 0% with selumetinib alone	[135]
First relapse rhabdomyosarcoma	2019	Phase 2 Randomized Two arms	$N = 87$	Bevacizumab or temsirolimus together with vinorelbine and cyclophosphamide	6-month EFS Bevacizumab vs. temsirolimus 54.6% (95%CI 39.8–69.3%) Vs. 69.1% (95%CI 55.1–83%)	[136]
Mantle cell lymphoma						
Mantle cell lymphoma Relapsed or refractory	2009	Phase 3 Randomized Open-label Three arms	$N = 162$	Temsirolimus 175 mg weekly for 3 weeks followed by either 75 mg (175/75-mg) Or 25 mg (175/25-mg) weekly, or investigator's choice therapy (invest)	Median PFS 175/75-mg vs invest 4.8 vs. 1.9 months (HR 0.44; $p = 0.0009$) 175/25-mg vs invest 3.4 vs. 1.9 months (HR 0.65; $p = 0.0618$) ORR 175/75-mg group vs invest 22 vs. 2% ($p = 0.0019$)	[137]

Mantle cell lymphoma Relapsed or refractory	2011	Phase 2 Single arm	$N = 71$ 69 evaluable	Temsirolimus and rituximab	ORR 59% CR 19%, PR 41%	[138]

Abbreviations: *C*, confidence interval; *CR* complete response (remission); *HR* hazard ratio; *ORR* objective response rate; *OS* overall survival; *PD* progressive disease; *PFR* progression-free survival rate; *PFS* progression-free survival; *PR* partial response; *SD* stable disease

[a] Solid tumor response was assessed by Response Evaluation Criteria in solid tumor

Table 4 Clinical trials in patients with solid tumors with ridaforolimus

Cancer type	Year	Design	Subject	Regimen	Outcome[a]	Ref
Endometrial cancer						
Advanced endometrial cancer	2013	Phase 2 Single arm	$N = 45$	Ridaforolimus	PR 11% SD 18%	[139]
Advanced endometrial cancer One or two lines of chemotherapy and no hormonal therapy	2015	Phase 2 Open-label Randomized Two arms	$N = 130$ 64 Ridaforolimus	Ridaforolimus or Investigator choice chemotherapy	Ridaforolimus 3.6 months The comparator 1.9 months (HR 0.53; 95% CI, 0.31–0.90; $p = 0.008$)	[140]
Breast cancer						
Metastatic breast cancer HER2-positive trastuzumab-refractory	2015	Phase 2b	$N = 34$	Ridaforolimus	PR 15%	[141]
Soft tissue or bone sarcomas						
Metastatic soft tissue or bone sarcomas Achieved objective response or stable disease with prior chemotherapy	2013	Phase 3 Randomized Double-blind Two arms	$N = 711$ 702 evaluable	Ridaforolimus or placebo	Median PFS Ridaforolimus 17.7 vs. placebo 14.6 weeks (HR 0.72; 95%CI, 0.61–0.85; $p = 0.001$)	[142]

Abbreviations: *CI* confidence interval; *CR* complete response (remission); *HR* hazard ratio; *ORR* objective response rate; *OS* overall survival; *PD* progressive disease; *PFS* progression-free survival; *PR* partial response; *SD* stable disease

[a] Solid tumor response was assessed by Response Evaluation Criteria in solid tumor

breast cancer. In addition, phase II trials have shown everolimus could be effective in advanced/persistent/recurrent endometrial cancer [141], peripheral T-cell lymphoma [142], and refractory Hodgkin's lymphoma [143].

In a randomized controlled trial conducted in patients with previously untreated, poor-prognosis metastatic renal-cell carcinoma, patients who received temsirolimus alone significantly had a more prolonged overall survival and PFS than those who received interferon alfa alone [129]. Temsirolimus has been approved as first-line drug for advanced renal cell carcinoma. In a phase III trial, temsirolimus improved PFS and ORR compared with standard therapy in patients with relapsed or refractory mantle cell lymphoma [144].

In a phase III trial of patients with metastatic soft tissue sarcoma or osteosarcoma who had achieved objective response or stable disease on prior chemotherapy, ridaforolimus improved PFS compared to placebo and induced a mean 1.3% reduction in target lesion size [140] Additionally, phase II trials have shown efficacy in advanced endometrial cancer [145] and HER2-positive trastuzumab-refractory metastatic breast cancer [139].

4 Future Outlook and Conclusion

Macrolides modulate diverse targets and signaling pathways in cancer cells, regulate the tumor microenvironment by inhibiting CSCs activity, reduce tumor angiogenesis and metastasis, and exert antitumor effects. They have also been shown to induce cell death, including apoptosis, autophagy, and pyroptosis. They are also effective against drug-resistant cancer. Combined therapy may be expected to improve cancer patient prognosis, as evidenced by the combination of currently used anticancer agents with different mechanisms of action. Which anticancer drug and when to combinate will be the subject of future research.

In the RAS–RAF–MEK–ERK pathway, which is critical for cell proliferation, differentiation, and survival, extensive studies have been conducted to elucidate the activation mechanisms and structural components of the upstream MAPK components, but these kinases have been elusive. Relatively little attention had been directed to MEK and ERK due to the low frequency of oncogenic activating mutations. MEK inhibitors cobimetinib, trametinib, binimetinib, and selumetinib are FDA-approved, and trametinib is approved in combination with BRAF inhibitors for lung cancer and melanoma. No ERK inhibitors have been approved and are under development [18]. ERK-inhibiting clarithromycin and other macrolides are considered the subject of future research in combination therapy.

The previously widely used macrolide repurposing strategy avoids the high cost and lengthy time associated with traditional drug discovery strategies, as toxicity and pharmacokinetic profiles are already established. Therefore, repurposing approved non-anticancer macrolides for cancer treatment is an attractive strategy for anticancer drug discovery.

We believe that macrolides could be further developed and clinically introduced as a bridge role in cancer therapy in the near future.

※ For MALT lymphoma, complete remission was defined as total disappearance of lymphoma and absence of histopathological evidence of lymphoma on endoscopic biopsy. Partial remission was assumed in cases of tumor reduction of at least 50%. Patients revealing normalization of macroscopic findings but with persistent residual lymphoma infiltrates on histological examination were classified as minimal residual disease.

For extranodal marginal zone B-cell lymphoma, response was defined according to the National Cancer Institute standardized criteria (Cheson et al. 1999).

In multiple myeloma, response criteria were adopted from the International Myeloma Working Group criteria.

Solid tumor response was assessed by Response Evaluation Criteria in solid tumor.

Overall response rate is the sum of complete remission (response) and partial remission (response).

Conflict of Interest All authors declare they have no conflict of interest.

Ethics compliance statement This chapter does not contain any studies with human participants or animals performed by any of the authors.

References

1. World Health Organization. https://www.who.int/news-room/fact-sheets/detail/cancer. Accessed 9 Jan 2023.
2. National Cancer Institute. https://www.cancer.gov/about-cancer/causes-prevention/genetics. Accessed 9 Jan 2023.
3. Hanahan D, Weinberg RA. Hallmarks of cancer: the next generation. Cell. 2011;144(5): 646–74.
4. Kim SS, Ruiz VE, Carroll JD, Moss SF. Helicobacter pylori in the pathogenesis of gastric cancer and gastric lymphoma. Cancer Lett. 2011;305(2):228–38.
5. Isaacson PG, Chott A, Nakamura S, Müller-Hermelink HK, Harris NL, Swerdlow SH. Extranodal marginal zone lymphoma of mucosa associated lymphoid tissue (MALT lymphoma). WHO classification of Tumours of Haematopoietic and lymphoid tissues. In: Swerdlow SH, Campo E, Harris NL, et al., editors. IARC press. 4th ed. Lyon; 2008. p. 214–7.
6. Ruskoné-Fourmestraux A, Fischbach W, Aleman BM, Boot H, Du MQ, Megraud F, et al. EGILS consensus report. Gastric extranodal marginal zone B-cell lymphoma of MALT. Gut. 2011;60(6):747–58.
7. Arima N, Tsudo M. Extragastric mucosa-associated lymphoid tissue lymphoma showing the regression by helicobacter pylori eradication therapy. Brit J Haematol. 2003;120(5):790–2.
8. Ochi M, Tominaga K, Okazaki H, Yamamori K, Wada T, Shiba M, et al. Regression of primary low-grade mucosa-associated lymphoid tissue lymphoma of duodenum after long term treatment with clarithromycin. Scand J Gastroenterol. 2006;41(3):365–9.
9. Govi S, Dognini GP, Licata G, Crocchiolo R, Resti AG, Ponzoni M, et al. Six-month oral clarithromycin regimen is safe and active in extranodal marginal zone B-cell lymphomas:final results of a single-Centre phase II trial. Br J Haematol. 2010;150(2):226–9.

10. Ishimatsu Y, Mukae H, Matsumoto K, Harada T, Hara A, Hara S, et al. Two cases with pulmonary mucosa-associated lymphoid tissue lymphoma successfully treated with clarithromycin. Chest. 2010;138(3):730–3.
11. Fukase K, Kato M, Kikuchi S, Inoue K, Uemura N, Okamoto S, et al. Effect of eradication of helicobacter pylori on incidence of metachronous gastric carcinoma after endoscopic resection of early gastric cancer: an open-label, randomised controlled trial. Lancet. 2008;372(9636): 392–7.
12. Kolch W. Meaningful relationships: the regulation of the Ras/Raf/MEK/ERK pathway by protein interactions. Biochem J. 2000;351(Pt 2):289–305.
13. Santarpia L, Lippman SM, El-Naggar AK. Targeting the MAPK-RAS-RAF signaling pathway in cancer therapy. Expert Opin Ther Targets. 2012;16(1):103–19.
14. National Cancer Institute. https://www.cancer.gov/research/key-initiatives/ras/ras-central/blog/2014/ras-proteins-created-equal. Accessed 9 Jan 2023.
15. Morrison DK. MAP kinase pathways. Cold Spring Harb Perspect Biol. 2012;4(11):a011254.
16. Cargnello M, Roux PP. Activation and function of the MAPKs and their substrates, the MAPK-activated protein kinases. Microbiol Mol Biol Rev. 2011;75(1):50–83.
17. Frémin C, Meloche S. From basic research to clinical development of MEK1/2 inhibitors for cancer therapy. J Hematol Oncol. 2010;3:8.
18. Barbosa R, Acevedo LA, Marmorstein R. The MEK/ERK network as a therapeutic target in human cancer. Mol Cancer Res. 2021;19(3):361–74.
19. Shinkai M, Tamaoki J, Kobayashi H, Kanoh S, Motoyoshi K, Kute T, et al. Clarithromycin delays progression of bronchial epithelial cells from G1 phase to S phase and delays cell growth via extracellular signal-regulated protein kinase suppression. Antimicrob Agents Chemother. 2006;50(5):1738–44.
20. Vicent S, Lopez-Picazo JM, Toledo G, Lozano MD, Torre W, Garcia-Corchon C, et al. ERK1/2 is activated in non-small-cell lung cancer and associated with advanced tumours. Br J Cancer. 2004;90(5):1047–52.
21. Morimura S, Sugaya M, Kai H, Miyagaki T, Asano Y, Tada Y, et al. Depsipeptide and roxithromycin induce apoptosis of lymphoma cells by blocking extracellular signal-regulated kinase activation. J Dermatol. 2014;41(1):57–62.
22. Polivka J Jr, Janku F. Molecular targets for cancer therapy in the PI3K/AKT/mTOR pathway. Pharmacol Ther. 2014;142(2):164–75.
23. Vanhaesebroeck B, Stephens L, Hawkins P. PI3K signalling: the path to discovery and understanding. Nat Rev Mol Cell Biol. 13(3):195–203.
24. Song MS, Salmena L, Pandolfi PP. The functions and regulation of the PTEN tumour suppressor. Nat Rev Mol Cell Biol. 2012;13(5):283–96.
25. Arencibia JM, Pastor-Flores D, Bauer AF, Schulze JO, Biondi RM. AGC protein kinases: from structural mechanism of regulation to allosteric drug development for the treatment of human diseases. Biochim Biophys Acta. 2013;1834(7):1302–21.
26. Davies MA. Regulation, role, and targeting of Akt in cancer. J Clin Oncol. 2011;29(35): 4715–7.
27. Song G, Ouyang G, Bao S. The activation of Akt/PKB signaling pathway and cell survival. J Cell Mol Med. 2005;9(1):59–71.
28. Riaz A, Zeller KS, Johansson S. Receptor-specific mechanisms regulate phosphorylation of AKT at Ser473: role of RICTOR in 1 integrin-mediated cell survival. PLoS One. 2012;7(2): e32081.
29. Lu M, Wang J, Ives HE, Pearce D. mSIN1 protein mediates SGK1 protein interaction with mTORC2 protein complex and is required for selective activation of the epithelial sodium channel. J Biol Chem. 2011;286(35):30647–54.
30. Ballou LM, Lin RZ. Rapamycin and mTOR kinase inhibitors. J Chem Biol. 2008;1(1–4): 27–36.

31. Vezina C, Kudelski A, Sehgal SN. Rapamycin (AY-22,989), a new antifungal antibiotic. I. Taxonomy of the producing streptomycete and isolation of the active principle. J Antibiot (Tokyo). 1975;28:721–6.
32. Dowling RJO, Pollak M, Sonenberg N. Current status and challenges associated with targeting mTOR for cancer therapy. BioDrugs. 2009;23(2):77–91.
33. Niehrs C. The complex world of WNT receptor signalling. Nat Rev Mol Cell Biol. 2012;13 (12):767–79.
34. Melotti A, Mas C, Kuciak M, Lorente-Trigos A, Borges I, Ari A. The river blindness drug Ivermectin and related macrocyclic lactones inhibit WNT-TCF pathway responses in human cancer. EMBO Mol Med. 2014;6(10):1263–78.
35. Pan D. The hippo signaling pathway in development and cancer. Dev Cell. 2010;19(4): 491–505.
36. Liu J, Zhang K, Cheng L, Zhu H, Xu T. Progress in understanding the molecular mechanisms underlying the antitumour effects of Ivermectin. Drug Des Devel Ther. 2020;14:285–96.
37. Nambara S, Masuda T, Nishio M, Kuramitsu S, Tobo T, Ogawa Y, et al. Antitumor effects of the antiparasitic agent ivermectin via inhibition of yes-associated protein 1 expression in gastric cancer. Oncotarget. 2017;8(64):107666–77.
38. Bierie B, Moses HL. Tumour microenvironment: TGFbeta: the molecular Jekyll and Hyde of cancer. Nat Rev Cancer. 2006;6(7):506–20.
39. Sassa K, Mizushima Y, Fujishita T, Oosaki R, Kobayashi M. Therapeutic effect of clarithromycin on a transplanted tumor in rats. Antimicrobial Agents Chemother. 1999;43 (1):67–72.
40. Bai L, Wang S. Targeting apoptosis pathways for new cancer therapeutics. Annu Rev Med. 2014;65:139–55.
41. Cheng Q, Chen J. Mechanism of p53 stabilization by ATM after DNA damage. Cell Cycle. 2010;9(3):472–8.
42. Lahav G. Oscillations by the p53-Mdm2 feedback loop. Adv Exp Med Biol. 2008;641:28–38.
43. Muntané J. Harnessing tumor necrosis factor receptors to enhance antitumor activities of drugs. Chem Res Toxicol. 2011;24(10):1610–6.
44. McIlwain DR, Berger T, Mak TW. Caspase functions in cell death and disease. Cold Spring Harb Perspect Biol. 2013;5(4):a008656.
45. Ohara T, Morishita T, Suzuki H, Masaoka T, Ishii H, Hibi T. Antibiotics directly induce apoptosis in B cell lymphoma cells derived from BALB/c mice. Anticancer Res. 2004;24(6): 3723–30.
46. Chen Y, Han T, Iqbal J, Irons R, Chan WC, Zhu X, et al. Diffuse large B-cell lymphoma in Chinese patients: immunophenotypic and cytogenetic analyses of 124 cases. Am J Clin Pathol. 2010;133(2):305–13.
47. Ohashi S, Segawa K, Okamura S, Urano H, Kanamori S, Ishikawa H, et al. A clinicopathologic study of gastric mucosa-associated lymphoid tissue lymphoma. Cancer. 2000;88(10): 2210–9.
48. Fukui T, Okazaki K, Tamaki H, Kawasaki K, Matsuura M, Asada M, et al. Immunogenetic analysis of gastric MALT lymphoma-like lesions induced by helicobacter pylori infection in neonatally thymectomized mice. Lab Investig. 2004;84(4):485–92.
49. Morgner A, Sutton P, O'Rourke JL, Enno A, Dixon MF, Lee A. Helicobacter-induced expression of Bcl-X(L) in B lymphocytes in the mouse model: a possible step in the development of gastric mucosa-associated lymphoid tissue (MALT) lymphoma. Int J Cancer. 2001;92(5):634–40.
50. Mizunoe S, Kadota J, Tokimatsu I, Kishi K, Nagai H, Nasu M. Clarithromycin and azithromycin induce apoptosis of activated lymphocytes via down-regulation of Bcl-xL. Int Immunopharmacol. 2004;4(9):1201–7.
51. Zhou X, Zhang Y, Li Y, Hao X, Liu X, Wang Y. Azithromycin synergistically enhances anti-proliferative activity of vincristine in cervical and gastric cancer cells. Cancers (Basel). 2012;4 (4):1318–32.

52. Qiao X, Wang X, Shang Y, Li Y, Chen SZ. Azithromycin enhances anticancer activity of TRAIL by inhibiting autophagy and up-regulating the protein levels of DR4/5 in colon cancer cells in vitro and in vivo. Cancer Commun (Lond). 2018;38(1):43.
53. Ozkan T, Hekmatshoar Y, Karabay AZ, Koc A, Gunes BA, Gurel AK, et al. Assessment of azithromycin as an anticancer agent for treatment of imatinib sensitive and resistant CML cells. Leuk Res. 2021;102:106523.
54. Zhang P, Zhang Y, Liu K, Liu B, Xu W, Gao J, et al. Ivermectin induces cell cycle arrest and apoptosis of HeLa cells via mitochondrial pathway. Cell Prolif. 2019;52(2):e12543.
55. Draganov D, Gopalakrishna-Pillai S, Chen YR, Zuckerman N, Moeller S, Wang C, et al. Modulation of P2X4/P2X7/Pannexin-1 sensitivity to extracellular ATP via Ivermectin induces a non-apoptotic and inflammatory form of cancer cell death. Sci Rep. 2015;5:16222.
56. Liu Y, Fang S, Sun Q, Liu B. Anthelmintic drug ivermectin inhibits angiogenesis, growth and survival of glioblastoma through inducing mitochondrial dysfunction and oxidative stress. Biochem Biophys Res Commun. 2016;480(3):415–21.
57. Wang J, Xu Y, Wan H, Hu J. Antibiotic ivermectin selectively induces apoptosis in chronic myeloid leukemia through inducing mitochondrial dysfunction and oxidative stress. Biochem Biophys Res Commun. 2018;497(1):241–7.
58. Sharmeen S, Skrtic M, Sukhai MA, Hurren R, Gronda M, Wang X, et al. The antiparasitic agent ivermectin induces chloride-dependent membrane hyperpolarization and cell death in leukemia cells. Blood. 2010;116(18):3593–603.
59. Kodama M, Kodama T, Newberg JY, Katayama H, Kobayashi M, Hanash SM, et al. In vivo loss-of-function screens identify KPNB1 as a new druggable oncogene in epithelial ovarian cancer. Proc Natl Acad Sci U S A. 2017;114(35):E7301–10.
60. White E, DiPaola RS. The double-edged sword of autophagy modulation in cancer. Clin Cancer Res. 2009;15(17):5308–16.
61. Nakamura M, Kikukawa Y, Takeya M, Mitsuya H, Hata H. Clarithromycin attenuates autophagy in myeloma cells. Int J Oncol. 2010;37(4):815–20.
62. Schafranek L, Leclercq TM, White DL, Hughes TP. Clarithromycin enhances dasatinib-induced cell death in chronic myeloid leukemia cells, by inhibition of late stage autophagy. Leuk Lymphoma. 2013;54(1):198–201.
63. Toriyama K, Takano N, Kokuba H, Kazama H, Moriya S, Hiramoto M, et al. Azithromycin enhances the cytotoxicity of DNA-damaging drugs via lysosomal membrane permeabilization in lung cancer cells. Cancer Sci. 2021;112(8):3324–37.
64. Moriya S, Che XF, Komatsu S, Abe A, Kawaguchi T, Gotoh A, et al. Macrolide antibiotics block autophagy flux and sensitize to bortezomib via endoplasmic reticulum stress-mediated CHOP induction in myeloma cells. Int J Oncol. 2013;42(5):1541–50.
65. Komatsu S, Miyazawa K, Moriya S, Takase A, Naito M, Inazu M, et al. Clarithromycin enhances bortezomib-induced cytotoxicity via endoplasmic reticulum stress-mediated CHOP (GADD153) induction and autophagy in breast cancer cells. Int J Oncol. 2012;40(4):1029–39.
66. Hirasawa K, Moriya S, Miyahara K, Kazama H, Hirota A, Takemura J, et al. Macrolide antibiotics exhibit cytotoxic effect under amino acid-depleted culture condition by blocking autophagy flux in head and neck squamous cell carcinoma cell lines. PLoS One. 2016;11(12):e0164529.
67. Crump A. Ivermectin: enigmatic multifaceted 'wonder' drug continues to surprise and exceed expectations. J Antibiot (Tokyo). 2017;70(5):495–505.
68. Hashimoto H, Sudo T, Maruta H, Nishimura R. The direct PAK1 inhibitor, TAT-PAK18, blocks preferentially the growth of human ovarian cancer cell lines in which PAK1 is abnormally activated by autophosphorylation at Thr 423. Drug Discov Ther. 2010;4(1):1–4.
69. Shinojima N, Yokoyama T, Kondo Y, Kondo S. Roles of the Akt/mTOR/p70S6K and ERK1/2 signaling pathways in curcumin-induced autophagy. Autophagy. 2014;3(6):635–7.
70. Dou Q, Chen HN, Wang K, et al. Ivermectin induces cytostatic autophagy by blocking the PAK1/Akt axis in breast cancer. Cancer Res. 2016;76(15):4457–69.

71. Hashimoto HMS, Sudo T, Maruta H. Ivermectin inactivates the kinase PAK1 and blocks the PAK1dependent growth of human ovarian cancer and NF2 tumor cell lines. Drug Discov Ther. 2009;3(6):3.
72. Fang Y, Tian S, Pan Y, Li W, Wang Q, Tang Y, et al. Pyroptosis: a new frontier in cancer. Biomed Pharmacother. 2020;121:109595.
73. Hanahan D, Folkman J. Patterns and emerging mechanisms of the angiogenic switch during tumorigenesis. Cell. 1996;86(3):353–64.
74. Lohela M, Bry M, Tammela T, Alitalo K. VEGFs and receptors involved in angiogenesis versus lymphangiogenesis. Curr Opin Cell Biol. 2009;21(2):154–65.
75. Hicklin DJ, Ellis LM. Role of the vascular endothelial growth factor pathway in tumor growth and angiogenesis. J Clin Oncol. 2005;23(5):1011–27.
76. Tammela T, Enholm B, Alitalo K, Paavonen K. The biology of vascular endothelial growth factors. Cardiovasc Res. 2005;65(3):550–63.
77. Grothey A, Galanis E. Targeting angiogenesis: progress with anti-VEGF treatment with large molecules. Nat Rev Clin Oncol. 2009;6(9):507–18.
78. Yatsunami J, Turuta N, Wakamatsu K, Hara N, Hayashi S. Clarithromycin is a potent inhibitor of tumor-induced angiogenesis. Res Exp Med (Berl). 1997;197(4):189–97.
79. Yatsunami J, Fukuno Y, Nagata M, Tsuruta N, Aoki S, Tominaga M, et al. Roxithromycin and clarithromycin, 14-membered ring macrolides, potentiate the antitumor activity of cytotoxic agents against mouse B16 melanoma cells. Cancer Lett. 1999;147(1–2):17–24.
80. Li F, Huang J, Ji D, Meng Q, Wang C, Chen S, et al. Azithromycin effectively inhibits tumor angiogenesis by suppressing vascular endothelial growth factor receptor 2-mediated signaling pathways in lung cancer. Oncol Lett. 2017;14(1):89–96.
81. Aoki D, Ueno S, Kubo F, Oyama T, Sakuta T, Matsushita K, et al. Roxithromycin inhibits angiogenesis of human hepatoma cells in vivo by suppressing VEGF production. Anticancer Res. 2005;25(1A):133–8.
82. Lee JY, Kong G. Roles and epigenetic regulation of epithelial-mesenchymal transition and its transcription factors in cancer initiation and progression. Cell Mol Life Sci. 2016;73(24):4643–60.
83. Tam WL, Weinberg RA. The epigenetics of epithelial-mesenchymal plasticity in cancer. Nat Med. 2013;19(11):1438–49.
84. Silverstein RA, Ekwall K. Sin3: a flexible regulator of global gene expression and genome stability. Curr Genet. 2005;47(1):1–17.
85. Farias EF, Petrie K, Leibovitch B, Murtagh J, Chornet MB, Schenk T, et al. Interference with Sin3 function induces epigenetic reprogramming and differentiation in breast cancer cells. Proc Natl Acad Sci U S A. 2010;107(26):11811–6.
86. Kwon YJ, Petrie K, Leibovitch BA, Zeng L, Mezei M, Howell L, et al. Selective inhibition of SIN3 corepressor with avermectins as a novel therapeutic strategy in triple-negative breast cancer. Mol Cancer Ther. 2015;14(8):1824–36.
87. Wang Y, Qi H, Liu Y, Duan C, Liu X, Xia T, et al. The double-edged roles of ROS in cancer prevention and therapy. Theranostics. 2021;11(10):4839–57.
88. Zhou B, Xia M, Wang B, Thapa N, Gan L, Sun C, et al. Clarithromycin synergizes with cisplatin to inhibit ovarian cancer growth in vitro and in vivo. J Ovarian Res. 2019;12(1):107.
89. Huang Z, Wu T, Liu AY, Ouyang G. Differentiation and transdifferentiation potentials of cancer stem cells. Oncotarget. 2015;6(37):39550–63.
90. Najafi M, Farhood B, Mortezaee K. Cancer stem cells (CSCs) in cancer progression and therapy. J Cell Physiol. 2019;234(6):8381–95.
91. Dominguez-Gomez G, Chavez-Blanco A, Medina-Franco JL, Saldivar-Gonzalez F, Flores-Torrontegui Y, Juarez M, Diaz-Chavez J, Gonzalez-Fierro A, Duenas-Gonzalez A. Ivermectin as an inhibitor of cancer stemlike cells. Mol Med Rep. 2018;17(2):3397–403.
92. Wang L, Kitaichi K, Hui CS, Takagi K, Takagi K, Sakai M, et al. Reversal of anticancer drug resistance by macrolide antibiotics in vitro and in vivo. Clin Exp Pharmacol Physiol. 2000;27(8):587–93.

93. Lespine A, Dupuy J, Orlowski S, Nagy T, Glavinas H, Krajcsi P, et al. Interaction of ivermectin with multidrug resistance proteins (MRP1, 2 and 3). Chem Biol Interact. 2006;159(3):169–79.
94. Pouliot JF, L'Heureux F, Liu Z, Prichard RK, Georges E. Reversal of Pglycoprotein-associated multidrug resistance by ivermectin. Biochem Pharmacol. 1997;53(1):17–25.
95. Lespine A, Martin S, Dupuy J, Roulet A, Pineau T, Orlowski S, et al. Interaction of macrocyclic lactones with P-glycoprotein: structure-affinity relationship. Eur J Pharm Sci. 2007;30(1):84–94.
96. Routledge PA. The plasma protein binding of basic drugs. Br J Clin Pharmacol. 1986;22(5): 499–506.
97. Piver MS, Moyer M, Diakun K, Lele SB, Chu TM. Serum alpha1-acid glycoprotein in epithelial ovarian cancer. Gynecol Oncol. 1988;29(3):305–8.
98. Elg SA, Mayer AR, Carson LF, Twiggs LB, Hill RB, Ramakrishnan S. Alpha-1 acid glycoprotein is an immunosuppressive factor found in ascites from ovaria carcinoma. Cancer. 1997;80(8):1448–56.
99. Ohbatake Y, Fushida S, Tsukada T, Kinoshita J, Oyama K, Hayashi H, et al. Elevated alpha1-acid glycoprotein in gastric cancer patients inhibits the anticancer effects of paclitaxel, effects restored by co-administration of erythromycin. Clin Exp Med. 2016;16(4):585–92.
100. Jiang M, Dun W, Tseng GN. Mechanism for the effects of extracellular acidification on HERG-channel function. Am J Phys. 1999;277(4):H1283–92.
101. Cherubini A, Taddei GL, Crociani O, Paglierani M, Buccoliero AM, Fontana L, et al. HERG potassium channels are more frequently expressed in human endometrial cancer as compared to non-cancerous endometrium. Br J Cancer. 2000;83(12):1722–9.
102. Bianchi L, Wible B, Arcangeli A, Taglialatela M, Morra F, Castaldo P, et al. Herg encodes a K + current highly conserved in tumors of different histogenesis: a selective advantage for cancer cells? Cancer Res. 1998;58(4):815–22.
103. Pillozzi S, Brizzi MF, Balzi M, Crociani O, Cherubini A, Guasti L, et al. HERG potassium channels are constitutively expressed in primary human acute myeloid leukemias and regulate cell proliferation of normal and leukemic hemopoietic progenitors. Leukemia. 2002;16(9): 1791–8.
104. Chen SZ, Jiang M, Zhen YS. HERG K+ channel expression-related chemosensitivity in cancer cells and its modulation by erythromycin. Cancer Chemother Pharmacol. 2005;56(2):212–20.
105. Coleman M, Leonard J, Lyons L, Pekle K, Nahum K, Pearse R, et al. BLT-D (clarithromycin [Biaxin], low-dose thalidomide, and dexamethasone) for the treatment of myeloma and Waldenström's macroglobulinemia. Leuk Lymphoma. 2002;43(9):1777–82.
106. Niesvizky R, Jayabalan DS, Christos PJ, Furst JR, Naib T, Ely S, et al. BiRD (Biaxin [clarithromycin]/Revlimid [lenalidomide]/dexamethasone) combination therapy results in high complete- and overall-response rates in treatment-naive symptomatic multiple myeloma. Blood. 2008;111(3):1101–9.
107. Rossi A, Mark T, Jayabalan D, Christos P, Zafar F, Pekle K, et al. BiRd (clarithromycin, lenalidomide, dexamethasone): an update on long-term lenalidomide therapy in previously untreated patients with multiple myeloma. Blood. 2013;121(11):1982–5.
108. Gay F, Rajkumar SV, Coleman M, Kumar S, Mark T, Dispenzieri A, et al. Clarithromycin (Biaxin)-lenalidomide-low-dose dexamethasone (BiRd) versus lenalidomide-low-dose dexamethasone (Rd) for newly diagnosed myeloma. Am J Hematol. 2010;85(9):664–9.
109. Puig N, Hernandez MT, Rosinol L, Gonzalez E, Arriba F, Oriol A, et al. Lenalidomide and dexamethasone with or without clarithromycin in patients with multiple myeloma ineligible for autologous transplant: a randomized trial. Blood Cancer J. 2021;11(5):101.
110. Steinbach G, Ford R, Glober G, Sample D, Hagemeister FB, Lynch PM, et al. Antibiotic treatment of gastric lymphoma of mucosa-associated lymphoid tissue. An uncontrolled trial Ann Intern Med. 1999;131(2):88–95.
111. Thiede C, Wündisch T, Alpen B, Neubauer B, Morgner A, Schmitz M, et al. Long-term persistence of monoclonal B cells after cure of helicobacter pylori infection and complete

histologic remission in gastric mucosa-associated lymphoid tissue B-cell lymphoma. J Clin Oncol. 2001;19(6):1600–9.
112. Ruskone-Fourmestraux A, Lavergne A, Aegerter PH, Megraud F, Palazzo L, Mascarel AD, et al. Predictive factors for regression of gastric MALT lymphoma after anti-helicobacter pylori treatment. Gut. 2001;48(3):297–303.
113. Fischbach W, Goebeler-Kolve ME, Dragosics B, Greiner A, Stolte M. Long term outcome of patients with gastric marginal zone B cell lymphoma of mucosa associated lymphoid tissue (MALT) following exclusive helicobacter pylori eradication therapy: experience from a large prospective series. Gut. 2004;53(1):34–7.
114. Ferreri AJ, Govi S, Raderer M, Mulè A, Andriani A, Caracciolo D, et al. Helicobacter pylori eradication as exclusive treatment for limited-stage gastric diffuse large B-cell lymphoma: results of a multicenter phase 2 trial. Blood. 2012;120(18):3858–60.
115. Mikasa K, Sawaki M, Kita E, Hamada K, Teramoto S, Sakamoto M, et al. Significant survival benefit to patients with advanced non-small-cell lung cancer from treatment with clarithromycin. Chemotherapy. 1997;43(4):288–96.
116. Musto P, Falcone A, Sanpaolo G, Bodenizza C, Carotenuto M, Carella AM. Inefficacy of clarithromycin in advanced multiple myeloma: a definitive report. Haematologica. 2002;87(6): 658–9.
117. Stewart AK, Trudel S, Al-Berouti BM, Sutton DM, Meharchand J. Lack of response to short-term use of clarithromycin (BIAXIN) in multiple myeloma. Blood. 1999;93(12):4441.
118. Moreau P, Huynh A, Facon T, Bouilly I, Sotto JJ, Legros L, et al. Lack of efficacy of clarithromycin in advanced multiple myeloma. Intergroupe Français du Myélome(IFM). Leukemia. 1999;13(3):490–1.
119. Carella AM, Beltrami G, Pica G, Carella A, Catania G. Clarithromycin potentiates tyrosine kinase inhibitor treatment in patients with resistant chronic myeloid leukemia. Leuk Lymphoma. 2012;53(7):1409–11.
120. Sakamoto M, Mikasa K, Majima T, Hamada K, Konishi M, Maeda K, et al. Anti-cachectic effect of clarithromycin for patients with unresectable non-small cell lung cancer. Chemotherapy. 2001;47(6):444–51.
121. Lagler H, Kiesewetter B, Dolak W, Obermueller M, Simonitsch-Klupp I, Lukas J, et al. Treatment of mucosa associated lymphoid tissue lymphoma with a long-term once-weekly regimen of oral azithromycin: results from the phase II MALT-A trial. Hematol Oncol. 2019;37(1):22–6.
122. Chu DJ, Yao DE, Zhuang YF, Hong Y, Zhu XC, Fang ZR, et al. Azithromycin enhances the favorable results of paclitaxel and cisplatin in patients with advanced non-small cell lung cancer. Genet Mol Res. 2014;13(2):2796–805.
123. Motzer RJ, Escudier B, Oudard S, Hutson TE, Porta C, Bracarda S, et al. Phase 3 trial of everolimus for metastatic renal cell carcinoma: final results and analysis of prognostic factors. Cancer. 2010;116(18):4256–65.
124. Baselga J, Campone M, Piccart M, Burris HA 3rd, Rugo HS, Sahmoud T, et al. Everolimus in postmenopausal hormone-receptor-positive advanced breast cancer. N Engl J Med. 2012;366 (6):520–9.
125. André F, O'Regan R, Ozguroglu M, Toi M, Xu B, Jerusalem G, et al. Everolimus for women with trastuzumab-resistant, HER2-positive, advanced breast cancer (BOLERO-3): a randomised, double-blind, placebo-controlled phase 3 trial. Lancet Oncol. 2014;15(6):580–91.
126. Yao JC, Fazio N, Singh S, Buzzoni R, Carnaghi C, Wolin E, et al. Everolimus for the treatment of advanced, non-functional neuroendocrine tumours of the lung or gastrointestinal tract (RADIANT-4): a randomised, placebo-controlled, phase 3 study. Lancet. 2016;387(10022): 968–77.
127. Pavel ME, Hainsworth JD, Baudin E, Peeters M, Hörsch D, Winkler RE, et al. Everolimus plus octreotide long-acting repeatable for the treatment of advanced neuroendocrine tumours associated with carcinoid syndrome (RADIANT-2): a randomised, placebo-controlled, phase 3 study. Lancet. 2011;378(9808):2005–12.

128. Franz DN, Belousova E, Sparagana S, Bebin EB, Frost M, Kuperman R, et al. Efficacy and safety of everolimus for subependymal giant cell astrocytomas associated with tuberous sclerosis complex (EXIST-1): a multicentre, randomised, placebo-controlled phase 3 trial. Lancet. 2013;381(9861):125–32.
129. Hudes G, Carducci M, Tomczak P, Dutcher J, Figlin R, Kapoor A, et al. Temsirolimus, interferon alfa, or both for advanced renal-cell carcinoma. N Engl J Med. 2007;356(22): 2271–81.
130. Sun Y, Rha S, Lee SH, Guo J, Ueda T, Qin S, et al. Phase II study of the safety and efficacy of temsirolimus in east Asian patients with advanced renal cell carcinoma. Jpn J Clin Oncol. 2012;42(9):836–44.
131. Grünwald V, Keilholz U, Boehm A, Guntinas-Lichius O, Hennemann B, Schmoll HJ, et al. TEMHEAD: a single-arm multicentre phase II study of temsirolimus in platin- and cetuximab refractory recurrent and/or metastatic squamous cell carcinoma of the head and neck (SCCHN) of the German SCCHN group (AIO). Ann Oncol. 2015;26(3):561–7.
132. Dunn LA, Fury MG, Xiao H, Baxi SS, Sherman EJ, Korte S, et al. A phase II study of temsirolimus added to low-dose weekly carboplatin and paclitaxel for patients with recurrent and/or metastatic (R/M) head and neck squamous cell carcinoma (HNSCC). Ann Oncol. 2017;28(10):2533–8.
133. Slingluff CL Jr, Petroni GR, Molhoek KR, Brautigan DL, Chianese-Bullock KA, Shada AL, et al. Clinical activity and safety of combination therapy with temsirolimus and bevacizumab for advanced melanoma: a phase II trial (CTEP 7190/Mel47). Clin Cancer Res. 2013;19(13): 3611–20.
134. Schwartz GK, Tap WD, Qin LX, Livingston MB, Undevia SD, Chmielowski B, et al. Cixutumumab and temsirolimus for patients with bone and soft-tissue sarcoma: a multicentre, open-label, phase 2 trial. Lancet Oncol. 2013;14(4):371–82.
135. Eroglu Z, Tawbi HA, Hu J, Guan M, Frankel PH, Ruel NH, et al. A randomised phase II trial of selumetinib vs selumetinib plus temsirolimus for soft-tissue sarcomas. Br J Cancer. 2015;112(10):1644–51.
136. Mascarenhas L, Chi YY, Hingorani P, Anderson JR, Lyden ER, Rodeberg DA, et al. Randomized phase II trial of bevacizumab or Temsirolimus in combination with chemotherapy for first relapse rhabdomyosarcoma: a report from the Children's oncology group. J Clin Oncol. 2019;37(31):2866–74.
137. Ansell SM, Tang H, Kurtin PJ, Koenig PA, Inwards DJ, Shah K, et al. Temsirolimus and rituximab in patients with relapsed or refractory mantle cell lymphoma: a phase 2 study. Lancet Oncol. 2011;12(4):361–8.
138. Colombo N, McMeekin DS, Schwartz PE, Sessa C, Gehrig PA, Holloway R, et al. Ridaforolimus as a single agent in advanced endometrial cancer: results of a single-arm, phase 2 trial. Br J Cancer. 2013;108(5):1021–6.
139. Seiler M, Ray-Coquard I, Melichar B, Yardley DA, Wang RX, Dodion PF, et al. Oral ridaforolimus plus trastuzumab for patients with HER2+ trastuzumab-refractory metastatic breast cancer. Clin Breast Cancer. 2015;15(1):60–5.
140. Demetri GD, Chawla SP, Ray-Coquard I, Le Cesne A, Staddon AP, Milhem MM, et al. Results of an international randomized phase III trial of the mammalian target of rapamycin inhibitor ridaforolimus versus placebo to control metastatic sarcomas in patients after benefit from prior chemotherapy. J Clin Oncol. 2013;31(19):2485–92.
141. Slomovitz BM, Filiaci VL, Walker JL, Taub MC, Finkelstein KA, Moroney JW, et al. A randomized phase II trial of everolimus and letrozole or hormonal therapy in women with advanced, persistent or recurrent endometrial carcinoma: a GOG foundation study. Gynecol Oncol. 2022;164(3):481–91.
142. Kim SJ, Shin DY, Kim JS, Yoon DH, Lee WS, Lee H, et al. A phase II study of everolimus (RAD001), an mTOR inhibitor plus CHOP for newly diagnosed peripheral T-cell lymphomas. Ann Oncol. 2016;27(4):712–8.

143. Janku F, Park H, Call SG, Madwani K, Oki Y, Subbiah V, et al. Safety and efficacy of Vorinostat plus Sirolimus or Everolimus in patients with relapsed refractory Hodgkin lymphoma. Clin Cancer Res. 2020;26(21):5579–87.
144. Hess G, Herbrecht R, Romaguera J, Verhoef G, Crump M, Gisselbrecht C, et al. Phase III study to evaluate temsirolimus compared with investigator's choice therapy for the treatment of relapsed or refractory mantle cell lymphoma. J Clin Oncol. 2009;27(23):3822–9.
145. Oza AM, Pignata S, Poveda A, McCormack M, Clamp A, Schwartz B, et al. Randomized phase II trial of Ridaforolimus in advanced endometrial carcinoma. J Clin Oncol. 2015;33(31): 3576–82.

Macrolides in Chronic Skin Disorders

Yozo Ishiuji

Abstract Macrolide antibiotics are widely used to treat infections of soft tissues and the respiratory tract due to their efficacy against Gram-negative and Gram-positive bacteria. In addition to being antimicrobials, in the late 1980s long-term therapy with the macrolide antibiotic erythromycin was shown to alter the clinical course of diffuse panbronchiolitis. Since that time, macrolides have been found to have immunomodulatory properties. These effects provided the rationale for studies performed to assess the usefulness of macrolides in other inflammatory diseases including skin and hair disorders, including rosacea, palmoplantar pustulosis, psoriasis, pityriasis rosea, bullous pemphigoid, pityriasis lichenoides, alopecia areata, cutaneous adverse reactions specific to epidermal growth factor receptor inhibitors, and atopic dermatitis. This review summarizes these clinical studies, case reports, and animal studies dealing with the potential benefits of macrolides antibiotics in the treatment of selected dermatoses which have primarily been classified as noninfectious.

Keywords Macrolides · Chronic Skin Disorders · Immunomodulatory effects · rosacea · CXCL8 · tumor necrosis factor (TNF)-α · interferons (IFNs)γ

1 Introduction

Erythromycin A, the prototype macrolide antibiotic was isolated from a Philippine soil sample in the 1940s and was first marketed in 1952. During the 1990s clarithromycin, roxithromycin (RXM), and azithromycin were introduced. Macrolides inhibit RNA-dependent protein synthesis by reversibly binding to the 50S ribosomal subunit of a susceptible microorganism [1].

Macrolides are widely used to treat infections of soft tissues and the respiratory tract due to their efficacy against Gram-negative and Gram-positive bacteria, including intracellular organisms such as Chlamydia and Legionella [2, 3]. In addition to

Y. Ishiuji (✉)
Department of Dermatology, Jikei University School of Medicine, Tokyo, Japan

B. K. Rubin, M. Shinkai (eds.), *Macrolides as Immunomodulatory Agents*, Progress in Inflammation Research 92, https://doi.org/10.1007/978-3-031-42859-3_13

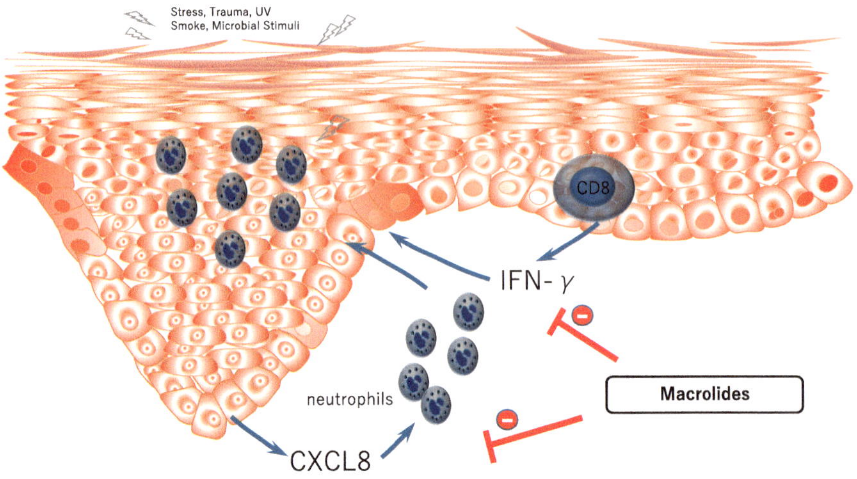

Fig. 1 The mechanisms of action for the anti-inflammatory properties of the macrolides are clearly multifactorial. Macrolides inhibit the production of many proinflammatory chemokines and cytokines, such as CXCL8, and IFNγ

being antimicrobials, macrolides antibiotics have immunomodulatory properties and are thus beneficial in treating chronic pulmonary diseases. It must be pointed out that immune modulation is the suppression of inflammation and immune hyperactivation without causing immunosuppression [4]. Macrolides may directly influence phagocyte and lymphocyte function and chemotaxis. Effects on the generation and release of chemokines and cytokines involved in the inflammatory process have been studied both in vivo and in vitro [5]. The immunomodulatory properties have been studied most thoroughly in chronic inflammatory airway diseases, particularly diffuse panbronchiolitis (DPB) and cystic fibrosis (CF). The immunomodulatory activity of macrolides has been a source of mechanistic and clinical research in non-DPB inflammatory airway disease. Erythromycin (EM), azithromycin, clarithromycin, and roxithromycin (RXM) inhibit chemotaxis and infiltration of neutrophils into the airway and, subsequently, decrease mucus secretion. The mechanisms of action for these properties are clearly multifactorial. Macrolides inhibit the production of many proinflammatory chemokines and cytokines, such as interleukin (IL)-1, IL-6, CXCL8, and tumor necrosis factor (TNF)-α and increase production of IL-10 and, possibly, IL-4 (Fig. 1). Macrolides also inhibit leukotriene B4 and the release of superoxide anion by neutrophils. In addition, macrolides block formation of adhesion molecules necessary for neutrophil migration. EM and its derivatives inhibit T-lymphocyte proliferation and induce T-lymphocyte apoptosis [6, 7]. In this chapter, I summarize clinical studies, case reports and animal studies dealing with the potential benefits of macrolides in the treatment of selected noninfectious dermatoses (Table 1).

Table 1 The summary of the potential benefits of macrolides antibiotics in the treatment of selected dermatoses which have primarily been classified as noninfectious

Diseases	The clinical evidence	Ref.
Rosacea	Ten patients who were intolerant of or had persistent symptoms of rosacea despite conventional treatment, improved with the oral use of azithromycin.	[8]
	A 67-year-old man who had photosensitivity to doxycycline and hyperpigmented dyschromia to minocycline with oral azithromycin in a dose of 250 mg 3 times weekly.	[9]
	Azithromycin decreased the number of lesions by 75% and the number of inflammatory lesions 89% after therapy.	[10]
	Azithromycin is as effective as doxycycline and improves the quality of life of patients.	[11]
	52-year-old woman with 2 weeks of oral azithromycin who had intractable rosacea not responding to conventional treatments including topical benzoyl peroxide and metronidazole, as well as oral metronidazole, isotretinoin, and doxycycline.	[12]
Palmoplantar pustulosis and SAPHO syndrome	Low-dose and long-term oral macrolide therapy significantly improves refractory PPP which was unresponsive to topical corticosteroids in more than 75% of patients treated.	[13]
	Several authors have also reported successful control of SAPHO syndrome with azithromycin.	[14–16]
	Five patients with SAPHO syndrome, ages 27 to 44 years, with a beneficial response to macrolide, clindamycin, and the nonsteroidal anti-inflammatory drug, lornoxicam.	[17]
Psoriasis	Some studies have shown the efficacy of macrolides in psoriasis.	[18]
	Ten subjects with chronic plaque psoriasis to take 150 mg RXM orally twice daily for 1 to 7 weeks. Six out of the ten patients had a decreased psoriasis area and severity index (PASI) score.	[19]
	Oral azithromycin in a single blind randomized case-control trial of 50 subjects with moderate-to-severe chronic plaque psoriasis. Of these, 30 subjects received azithromycin for 48 weeks as a single oral 500 mg daily dose for 4 days with a gap of 10 days. A significant improvement in PASI score was noted from 12 weeks most of the subjects in the azithromycin group.	[20]
Adult-onset Still's disease (AOSD)	Remarkable improvement followed rechallenges with clarithromycin for subsequent AOSD flares.	[21]
	Therapeutic responses using clarithromycin in some patients with AOSD.	[22]

(continued)

Table 1 (continued)

Diseases	The clinical evidence	Ref.
Chronic Urticaria	Antibiotics for HP eradication suppressed CSU (chronic spontaneous Urticaria) symptoms and improved remission with or without HP eradication. Some antibiotics, such as clarithromycin, attenuate proinflammatory cytokine production during the innate immune response by inhibiting T2 cytokine secretion.	[23, 24]
Pityriasis Rosea	EM is probably more beneficial in reducing the severity of itching than placebo.	[25]
Pityriasis Lichenoides	Oral EM showed clearance rates ranging between 66% and 83%.	[26]
Bullous pemphigoid	Tetracyclines and macrolides have been used as third-line options due to their immunomodulatory activity, and have shown efficacy as both monotherapy and adjuvant therapy.	[27]
Idiopathic thrombocytopenic purpura	HP-positive ITP patients can be successfully treated by using a proton pump inhibitor, amoxicillin, and clarithromycin.	[28, 29]
Alopecia Areata	RXM increased the percentage of HFs in the anagen phase.	[30]
Targeted therapy and chemotherapy associated skin toxicities	Oral tetracyclines are effective in the treatment of dverse skin reactions induced by targeted therapies. There is insufficient evidence for the usefulness of macrolide antibiotics. However, considering their immunomodulatory effects, they may be an alternative to tetracyclines in patients with tetracycline side effects. Macrolide antibiotics may be an alternative to tetracyclines in patients with tetracycline side effects.	[31]
Atopic dermatitis (itch)	Seventeen subjects participated in an open trial of macrolides for treatment of psoriasis. Mean PASI scores dropped significantly, and itch was reduced in 11 subjects after therapy.	[32]
	Six subjects with severe pruritus and six with moderate pruritus in the study group reported that itch disappeared completely after the treatment.	[33]
	Topical application of josamycin to AD lesions colonized by *S. aureus* may help control AD.	[34]

2 Rosacea

Rosacea is a chronic cutaneous disorder affecting primarily the face and characterized by erythema, transient or persistent, telangiectasia, and inflammatory lesions including papulo-pustules and swelling [35]. Topical medications, systemic drugs, lasers, and light-based therapies have been used for the management of rosacea with variable results. Tetracyclines and their derivatives, including minocycline and doxycycline, have anti-inflammatory properties that correlate with certain aspects of the pathophysiology and are commonly used to treat rosacea [36]. However, long-term treatment with tetracycline is not well tolerated due to requiring frequent administration, poor adherence and side effects including gastrointestinal intolerance, photosensitivity, and candidiasis [10]. Moreover, given the chronic nature of the disease, bacterial resistance will develop. Azithromycin is also effective in treating rosacea as confirmed by several clinical studies. Fernandez-Obregon reported that 10 patients who were intolerant of or had persistent symptoms of rosacea despite conventional treatment, improved with the oral use of azithromycin [8]. Modi et al. treated a 67-year-old man who had photosensitivity to doxycycline and hyperpigmented dyschromia to minocycline with oral azithromycin in a dose of 250 mg 3 times weekly [9]. Bakar et al. reported that treatment with oral azithromycin decreased the number of lesions by 75% and the number of inflammatory lesions 89% after therapy [10]. An open-label study showed that azithromycin is as effective as doxycycline and improves the quality of life of patients [11]. Kim et al. treated a 52-year-old woman with 2 weeks of oral azithromycin who had intractable rosacea not responding to conventional treatments including topical benzoyl peroxide and metronidazole, as well as oral metronidazole, isotretinoin, and doxycycline [12]. The authors reported that the lesions had markedly improved, and no side effects related to azithromycin were noted. Rosacea patients have more skin reactive oxygen species levels than healthy controls. A significant decrease in chemiluminescence, a measurement of the generation of reactive oxygen species, was shown after treatment with azithromycin 500 mg on three days each week for 4 weeks [10].

3 Palmoplantar Pustulosis and SAPHO Syndrome

Palmoplantar pustulosis or pustulosis palmaris et plantaris (PPP) is a refractory pustular eruption of the palms and soles with unknown etiology. In addition to skin lesions, PPP patients may present with severe joint pain and pustulotic arthro-osteitis (PAO), especially of the sternoclavicular joint. PAO is sometimes regarded as a variant of synovitis, acne, pustulosis, hyperostosis and osteitis (SAPHO) syndrome [37]. Despite recent advances in the understanding of the epidemiologic, pathophysiologic, and immunogenic mechanisms involved in PPP, PAO and SAPHO syndrome, etiopathogenesis remains poorly understood. Researchers have found associations with PPP including smoking, infections, certain medications and genetics. *Propionibacterium acnes*, the microorganism associated with acne, has been recovered from bone biopsy in some patients with SAPHO syndrome, but the possible pathogenic role of an infectious agent in a genetically predisposed individual, resulting in exaggerated inflammatory response as "reactive osteitis," is a largely unproven hypothesis [38].

Low-dose and long-term oral macrolide therapy significantly improved refractory PPP which was unresponsive to topical corticosteroids in more than 75% of patients treated. A clinical effect was objectively recognized within 1–2 weeks after the start of the therapy and patients' evaluations were favorable after 4–12 weeks [13]. The authors concluded that 14-member macrolides down-regulated CXCL8 or Staphylococcal-superantigen in stimulated keratinocytes in refractory PPP. Several authors have also reported successful control of SAPHO syndrome with azithromycin [14–16]. Matzaroglou et al. [17] reported five patients with SAPHO syndrome, ages 27 to 44 years, with a beneficial response to macrolide, clindamycin, and the nonsteroidal anti-inflammatory drug, lornoxicam. All patients remained symptom-free for up to 4 years, after a 3–8-month course of treatment.

4 Psoriasis

Psoriasis is a chronic, systemic immune-mediated disease characterized by development of erythematous, indurated, scaly, pruritic plaques on the skin. Psoriatic immunopathogenesis is driven by circulating pro-inflammatory cytokines, including TNF-α, IL-17, IL-23 and type 1 and type 2 interferons (IFNs) including IFNα/β and IFNγ. These cytokines are produced by T-helper (Th) cells and activated dendritic cells (DCs) that infiltrate the skin and remain as memory T cells in lesional skin [39]; supporting the observation that psoriatic lesions generally recur in the same anatomical area [40]. Upregulation of these molecular pathways stimulates keratinocyte hyperproliferation and T cell-mediated inflammation [41]. Psoriasis is also characterized by the presence of neutrophil activation and overproduction of IL-6 and CXCL8 from keratinocytes [18]. It is now clear that macrolides inhibit the production of many proinflammatory chemokines and cytokines, perhaps by inhibiting ERK1/2 and suppressing nuclear transcription factors, and decreasing neutrophil activity [42]. Although in some studies it has been reported that antibiotics are not beneficial [43, 44], other studies have shown the efficacy of macrolides in psoriasis [18]. Because streptococcal throat infection is a primary trigger for psoriasis exacerbations, it is possible that streptococcal antigens may induce cross reactive T-cell responses against skin components [45, 46]. SEB (staphylococcal enterotoxin B) have also been associated with psoriatic disease [47]. Patients with psoriasis are at an increased risk for staphylococcal colonization compared with healthy individuals. Prospective studies on how bacterial loads correlate with disease activity can guide the clinical management of bacterial colonization while preventing the emergence of drug-resistant strains [19, 48]. Ten subjects with chronic plaque psoriasis were enrolled and took 150 mg of RXM orally twice a day. Six out of the ten patients had a decreased psoriasis area and severity index (PASI) score.

Macrolides, as a class, and azithromycin in particular, have a characteristic immunomodulatory potential, in addition to their main antibacterial action against streptococci. Azithromycin decreases levels of the chemokine CXCL8 in IFN-γ-treated keratinocytes as well as expression of MHC class II, secretion of IL-1 alpha, and superantigen presenting ability [49, 50]. Saxena and Dogra [20] used oral azithromycin in a single blind randomized case-control trial of 50 subjects with moderate-to-severe chronic plaque psoriasis. Of these, 30 subjects received azithromycin for 48 weeks as a single oral 500 mg daily dose for 4 days with a gap of 10 days. A significant improvement in PASI score was noted from 12 weeks most of the subjects in the azithromycin group. At the end of 48 weeks, 18 subjects (60%) showed excellent improvement, while 6 (20%) showed good improvement, and 4 (13.33%) showed mild improvement.

5 Adult-Onset Still's Disease (AOSD)

Adult-onset Still's Disease (AOSD) is a systemic inflammatory disorder characterized by prolonged fever, polyarthralgia, and an evanescent rash. The etiology is unknown but infections have been suggested to be a trigger in predisposed hosts and a role for dysregulation of innate immunity has been suggested. Based on this, it was suggested that macrolides may have induced a therapeutic response. Thanou-Stavraki et al. described a patient with AOSD complicated by calf fasciitis that serendipitously responded to clarithromycin administered for another indication [21]. Remarkable improvement followed rechallenges with clarithromycin for subsequent AOSD flares. Notably, other studies have reported therapeutic responses using clarithromycin in some patients with AOSD [21, 22].

6 Chronic Urticaria

Chronic urticaria is one of the most frequent skin diseases in medical practice. Urticaria is defined as acute if the wheal persists for less than 6 weeks and as chronic if it persists for longer. Chronic urticaria that lasts from several years to decades and significantly impairs the quality of life. There is evidence that *Helicobacter pylori* (HP) has a role in extragastric diseases such as chronic urticaria. A review suggested that antibiotics for HP eradication suppressed CSU (Chronic Spontaneous Urticaria) symptoms and improved remission with or without HP eradication [23]. In a subgroup analysis, high eradication rates of HP increased remission of CSU, while low eradication did not. Some antibiotics, such as clarithromycin, attenuate proinflammatory cytokine production during the innate immune response by inhibiting T2 cytokine secretion [24]. As well, the gut microbiome is a regulator in the gut–skin axis [51]. Antibiotics may alter microbiota, resulting in the reduction of systemic inflammation [52]. In addition, as HP itself induced the release of histamine by mast cells, HP eradication by antibiotics may have a favorable effect on the pathophysiology of CSU [53].

7 Pityriasis Rosea

Pityriasis rosea is a scaly, itchy rash that mainly affects young adults and lasts for 2 to 12 weeks. The effects of many available treatments are uncertain. Macrolides have anti-inflammatory and immunomodulating effects that might affect the course of Pityriasis Rosea or other cutaneous eruptions, independent of their antibacterial properties [54]. Several studies evaluated the use of macrolide antibiotics [55–59]. But none of these showed conclusive benefit on rash. Based on a single trial, EM is probably more beneficial in reducing the severity of itching than placebo. There is probably no difference between azithromycin and clarithromycin in resolution of itch [25].

8 Pityriasis Lichenoides Chronica

Pityriasis lichenoides (PL) represents a spectrum of inflammatory skin diseases comprising pityriasis lichenoides et varioliformis acuta (PLEVA) and pityriasis lichenoides chronica (PLC). PLEVA is an uncommon condition which presents acutely with papulo-vesicles that may develop necrotic, ulcerative, or hemorrhagic changes. This condition responses well to EM and ultraviolet light therapy. A systematic review was performed according to PRISMA guidelines for studies investigating PL treatment. A total of 441 papers were screened, and 37 original manuscripts meeting the inclusion and exclusion criteria were found, including12 case series, 18 reviews, four prospective studies, two comparative studies and a single randomized controlled study. Oral EM showed clearance rates ranging between 66% and 83%, whereas methotrexate up to 100% but in small but dated studies. Evidence for other treatments is scarce [26].

9 Bullous Pemphigoid

Bullous pemphigoid is the most common autoimmune-mediated bullous disease in men.

The treatment of localized or mild BP is mainly based on topical corticosteroids which can be combined with antibiotics [60]. Most patients with moderate-to-severe disease will require at least some oral corticosteroids. The aim of oral corticosteroids is to establish prompt remission and then wean to the lowest possible dose to maintain control with the aid of steroid-sparing adjuvants. Oral corticosteroids should then be tapered slowly to achieve a minimum effective dose for preventing new lesion formation. Tetracyclines and macrolides have been used as third-line options due to their immunomodulatory activity, and have shown efficacy as both monotherapy and adjuvant therapy [27].

10 Idiopathic Thrombocytopenic Purpura

Primary Idiopathic Thrombocytopenic Purpura (ITP) is an acquired immune disorder characterized by an isolated thrombocytopenia due to pathogenic anti-platelet autoantibodies, T cell-mediated platelet destruction, and impaired megakaryocyte function. Some studies have suggested that HP-positive ITP patients can be successfully treated by using a proton pump inhibitor, amoxicillin, and clarithromycin [28, 29]. It has been reported in some cases of ITP, such as HP-positive ITP, there are increased platelet counts with macrolide treatment [28, 61, 62]. Immunomodulatory effects from macrolides might be obtained by the eradication of bacteria or by modulation of the immune system involving the mucosa on which commensal bacteria reside [63].

11 Alopecia Areata

Campuzano-Maya described the case of a 43- year-old man with patchy alopecia areata and HP infection; the patient had hair regrowth after bacterial eradication [64]. RXM promotes hair growth and antagonizes catagen in patients with androgenic alopecia (AGA), presumably by inhibiting keratinocyte apoptosis [30]. While these hair effects could also derive from macrolide-induced immunomodulation, interestingly, in AGA the HF microbiome shows dysbiosis [65], characterized by an increased abundance of (RXM-susceptible) *Cutibacterium acnes*. Therefore, the effects of RXM on hair growth might also arise from microbiome changes. RXM also increased the percentage of HFs in the anagen phase [30].

12 Targeted Therapy and Chemotherapy Associated Skin Toxicities

Skin toxicities due to systemic cancer treatment are a significant problem for many patients and can greatly affect their quality of life. Preventing and managing skin-related toxicities can decrease treatment disruption and improve patient well-being. Treatments that cause skin toxicities are used to treat most cancers and affect a high percentage of patients. Adverse skin reactions can involve skin barrier function, hair, and nails. Epidermal growth factor receptor inhibitors (EGFRIs) are an important class of anticancer agents. Although these agents have a more favorable toxicity profile than other anticancer therapies, they have unique adverse events [66]. The primary toxicity associated with EGFRIs are an acneform rash that can occur in more than 80% of patients receiving these agents [67–69]. The rash associated with EGFRIs is mild in most cases, but it can lead to treatment cessation or dose modifications [70, 71]. Patients who experience an EGFRI rash experience negative effects on physical, functional, emotional, and social well-being [72]. Oral tetracyclines are effective in the treatment of papulopustular acne and rosacea [31]. Aside from the antibiotic properties of tetracyclines, these drugs have an anti-inflammatory effect, inhibiting matrix metalloproteinases and reducing neutrophil chemotaxis and the production of proinflammatory cytokines. They also have antiangiogenic properties and possibly affect immune modulation via reduced T-cell activation [73]. The use of either oral lymecycline or doxycycline is recommended, dependent on local availability, once or twice daily at the approved dose. However, lymecycline is preferred as a result of its slightly better adverse event profile, including the lesser risk of photosensitivity, compared with other tetracyclines. There is insufficient evidence for the usefulness of macrolide antibiotics. However, considering their immunomodulatory effects, they may be an alternative to tetracyclines in patients with tetracycline side effects.

13 Itch and Atopic Dermatitis

Tamaki investigated the antipruritic effects of macrolide antibiotics in several pruritic skin diseases and found that in most of the patients, the drug was effective. Macrolides may inhibit production of cytokines or neuropeptides that cause pruritus [32]. Seventeen subjects participated in an open trial of macrolides for treatment of psoriasis. Mean PASI scores dropped significantly, and itch was reduced in 11 subjects after therapy. Polat et al. reported that EM was more effective against pruritus than control therapy [33]. Six subjects with severe pruritus and six with moderate pruritus in the study group reported that itch disappeared completely after the treatment [18].

Chronic skin colonization by *Staphylococcus aureus (S. aureus)* can exacerbate atopic dermatitis (AD) and control of skin colonization using an antibiotic ointment might relieve AD-related skin inflammation. Topical treatment with josamycin improved the skin severity score in NC/Nga mice with AD-like skin lesions induced by *Dermatophagoides farinae* extract. This suppressive effect was associated with decreases in the *S. aureus* count on the lesional skin, scratching behavior of mice, and IL-31 mRNA expression in the skin. The severity of AD-like skin inflammation in NC/Nga mice correlated with the amount of *S. aureus* colonization and IL-31 production in the skin. Therefore, topical application of josamycin to AD lesions colonized by *S. aureus* may help control AD by eliminating skin *S. aureus* and by suppressing IL-31-induced scratching behavior [34].

14 Conclusion

There is strong evidence providing support to the benefit of using 14 or 15 member macrolides to treat some chronic skin disorders. The macrolides have some potentially useful immunomodulatory effects. Although additional studies are needed, macrolide therapy in some of chronic dermatoses has the potential of modifying the morbidity and possibly ameliorating the severity of some of these conditions.

Conflict of Interest Y. Ishiuji has received honoraria as a speaker from Maruho, Sanofi and AbbVie.

Ethics Compliance Statement Hereby, I consciously assure that for this manuscript the following is fulfilled:

- This material is the own original work, which has not been previously published elsewhere.
- The paper is not currently being considered for publication elsewhere.
- The paper reflects the own research and analysis in a truthful and complete manner.
- All sources used are properly disclosed (correct citation).
- I have been personally and actively involved in substantial work leading to the paper, and will take public responsibility for its content.

Acknowledgement I would like to express my sincere gratitude to Prof. Rubin and Prof. Shinkai for the special support of this article.

References

1. Ii JAW, Wilson WR, Fordyce D, Heilman R, Herrell WE, Wellman WE, et al. Erythromycin: a microbial and clinical perspective after 30 years of clinical use (first of two parts)*. Mayo Clin Proc. 1985;60:189–203. http://www.mayoclinicproceedings.org/article/S0025619612602195/fulltext
2. Healy DP. Macrolide immunomodulation of chronic respiratory diseases. Curr Infect Dis Rep. 2007;9:7–13.
3. López-Boado YS, Rubin BK. Macrolides as immunomodulatory medications for the therapy of chronic lung diseases. Curr Opin Pharmacol. 2008;8:286–91.
4. Shinkai M, Rubin BK. Macrolides and airway inflammation in children. Paediatr Respir Rev. 2005;6:227–35.
5. Brinkmeier T, Frosch PJ. Orale Antibiotika mit antiinflammatorischer/immunmodulatorischer wirkung für die therapie verschiedener dermatosen. Der Hautarzt. 2002;53:7.
6. Wu L, Zhang W, Tian L, Bao K, Li P, Lin J. Immunomodulatory effects of erythromycin and its derivatives on human T-lymphocyte in vitro. Immunopharmacol Immunotoxicol. 2008;29:587–96.
7. Labro MT. Anti-inflammatory activity of macrolides: a new therapeutic potential? J Antimicrob Chemother. 1998;41:37–46. https://academic.oup.com/jac/article/41/suppl_2/37/828013
8. Fernandez-Obregon A. Oral use of azithromycin for the treatment of acne rosacea. Arch Dermatol. 2004;140:489–90.

9. Modi S, Harting M, Rosen T. Azithromycin as an alternative rosacea therapy when tetracyclines prove problematic. J Drugs Dermatol. 2008;7:898–9.
10. Bakar Ö, Demirçay Z, Yuksel M, Haklar G, Sanisoglu Y. The effect of azithromycin on reactive oxygen species in rosacea. Clin Exp Dermatol. 2007;32:197–200.
11. Akhyani M, Ehsani AH, Ghiasi M, Jafari AK. Comparison of efficacy of azithromycin vs. doxycycline in the treatment of rosacea: a randomized open clinical trial. Int J Dermatol. 2008;47:284–8.
12. Kim JH, Oh YS, Choi EH. Oral azithromycin for treatment of intractable rosacea. J Korean Med Sci. 2011;26:694–6. https://doi.org/10.3346/jkms.2011.26.5.694.
13. Matsunaga Y, Bae S, Akiyama T, Kadota J, Katayama I. Low-dose and long-term 14-member macrolide therapy for palomoplantar pustulosis. Acta Med. Nagasaki. 45:25–31.
14. Schaeverbeke T, Lequen L, de Barbeyrac B, Labbe L, Marie Bebear C, Morrter Y, et al. Propionibacterium acnes isolated from synovial tissue and fluid in a patient with oligoarthritis associated with acne and pustulosis. Arthritis Rheum. 1998;41:1889–93.
15. Kirchhoff T, Merkesdal S, Rosenthal H, Prokop M, Chavan A, Wagner A, et al. Diagnostic management of patients with SAPHO syndrome: use of MR imaging to guide bone biopsy at CT for microbiological and histological work-up. Eur Radiol. 2003;13:2304–8.
16. Assmann G, Kueck O, Kirchhoff T, Rosenthal H, Voswinkel J, Pfreundschuh M, et al. Efficacy of antibiotic therapy for SAPHO syndrome is lost after its discontinuation: an interventional study. Arthritis Res Ther. 2009;11:1–8.
17. Matzaroglou C, Velissaris D, Karageorgos A, Marangos M, Panagiotopoulos E, Karanikolas M. SAPHO syndrome diagnosis and treatment: report of five cases and review of the literature. Open Orthop J. 2009;3:100.
18. Komine M, Tamaki K. An open trial of oral macrolide treatment for psoriasis vulgaris. J Dermatol. 2000;27:508–12.
19. Ohshima A, Takigawa M, Tokura Y. CD8+ cell changes in psoriasis associated with roxithromycin-induced clinical improvement. Eur J Dermatol. 2001;11:410–5. http://www.jle.com/fr/revues/ejd/e-docs/cd8_cell_changes_in_psoriasis_associated_with_roxithromycin_induced_clinical_improvement_100154/article.phtml?tab=texte
20. Saxena VN, Dogra J. Long-term oral azithromycin in chronic plaque psoriasis: a controlled trial. Eur J Dermatol. 2010;20:329–33. http://www.jle.com/fr/revues/ejd/e-docs/long_term_oral_azithromycin_in_chronic_plaque_psoriasis_a_controlled_trial_284638/article.phtml?tab=texte
21. Thanou-Stavraki A, Aberle T, Aksentijevich I, Bane BL, Harley JB. Clarithromycin in adult-onset still's disease: a potentially useful therapeutic. J Clin Rheumatol. 2011;17:373–6.
22. Saviola G, Benucci M, Abdi-Ali L, Baiardi P, Manfredi M, Bucci M, et al. Clarithromycin in adult-onset Still's disease: a study of 6 cases. Rheumatol Int. 2010;30:555–60.
23. Kim HJ, Kim YJ, Lee HJ, Hong JY, Park AY, Chung EH, et al. Systematic review and meta-analysis: effect of helicobacter pylori eradication on chronic spontaneous urticaria. Helicobacter. 2019;24:e12661. https://onlinelibrary.wiley.com/doi/full/10.1111/hel.12661
24. Tkalčević VI, Čužić S, Kramarić MD, Parnham MJ, Haber VE. Topical azithromycin and clarithromycin inhibit acute and chronic skin inflammation in sensitized mice, with apparent selectivity for Th2-mediated processes in delayed-type hypersensitivity. Inflammation. 2012;35:192–205. https://link.springer.com/article/10.1007/s10753-011-9305-9
25. Contreras-Ruiz J, Peternel S, Gutiérrez CJ, Culav-Koscak I, Reveiz L, de Silbermann-Reynoso ML. Interventions for pityriasis rosea. Cochrane Database Syst Rev. 2019;30(10):CD005068. https://doi.org/10.1002/14651858.CD005068.pub3.
26. Bellinato F, Maurelli M, Gisondi P, Girolomoni G. A systematic review of treatments for pityriasis lichenoides. J Eur Acad Dermatol Venereol. 2019;33:2039–49.
27. Jiang KW, Zhao CY, Lee KM, Cook DK. Bullous eruption on the limbs in an elderly patient. Aust J Gen Pract. 2022;51:338–9.

28. Ohe M, Shida H, Horita T, Furuya K, Hashino S. Successful treatment of primary immune thrombocytopenia accompanied by diabetes mellitus treated using clarithromycin followed by prednisolone. Drug Discov Ther. 2018;12:101–3.
29. Ohe M, Hashino S. Successful treatment with erythromycin for idiopathic thrombocytopenic purpura. Korean J Hematol. 2011;46:139.
30. Ito T, Fukamizu H, Ito N, Seo N, Yagi H, Takigawa M, et al. Roxithromycin antagonizes catagen induction in murine and human hair follicles: implication of topical roxithromycin as hair restoration reagent. Arch Dermatol Res. 2009;301:347–55. https://link.springer.com/article/10.1007/s00403-008-0899-1
31. Hayashi N, Akamatsu H, Iwatsuki K, Shimada-Omori R, Kaminaka C, Kurokawa I, et al. Japanese dermatological association guidelines: guidelines for the treatment of acne vulgaris 2017. J Dermatol. 2018;45:898–935. https://onlinelibrary.wiley.com/doi/full/10.1111/1346-8138.14355
32. Tamaki K. Antipruritic effect of macrolide antibiotics. J Dermatol. 2000;27:66–7.
33. Polat M, Lenk N, Yalcin B, Gür G, Tamer E, Artuz F, et al. Efficacy of erythromycin for psoriasis vulgaris. Clin Exp Dermatol. 2007;32:295–7.
34. Matsui K, Nakamura M, Obana N. Effects of josamycin on scratching behavior in NC/Nga mice with atopic dermatitis-like skin lesions. The Pharmaceutical Society of Japan. 2021;44:798–803.
35. Farshchian M, Daveluy S. Rosacea. In: StatPearls. Treasure Island (FL); 2022.
36. Humbert P, Treffel P, Chapuis JF, Buchet S, Derancourt C, Agache P. The tetracyclines in dermatology. J Am Acad Dermatol. 1991;25:691–7.
37. Chamot AM, Benhamou CL, Kahn MF, Beraneck L, Kaplan G, Prost A. Acne-pustulosis-hyperostosis-osteitis syndrome. Results of a national survey. 85 cases. Rev Rhum Mal Osteoartic. 1987;54:187–96. https://europepmc.org/article/med/2954204
38. Colina M, Monaco A, Khodeir M, Trotta F. Propionibacterium acnes and SAPHO syndrome: a case report and literature review. Clin Exp Rheumatol. 2007;25:457–60. https://www.clinexprheumatol.org/abstract.asp?a=3099
39. Hawkes JE, Chan TC, Krueger JG. Psoriasis pathogenesis and the development of novel, targeted immune therapies. J Allergy Clin Immunol. 2017;140:645.
40. Clark RA. Gone but not forgotten: Lesional memory in psoriatic skin. J Invest Dermatol. 2011;131:283.
41. Mahil SK, Capon F, Barker JN. Update on psoriasis immunopathogenesis and targeted immunotherapy. Seminars Immunopathol. 2015;38(1):11–27. https://link.springer.com/article/10.1007/s00281-015-0539-8
42. Tamaoki J, Kadota J, Takizawa H. Clinical implications of the immunomodulatory effects of macrolides. Am J Med Suppl. 2004;117:5–11.
43. Wilson JK, Al-Suwaidan SN, Krowchuk D, Feldman SR. Treatment of psoriasis in children: is there a role for antibiotic therapy and tonsillectomy? Pediatr Dermatol. 2003;20:11–5.
44. Owen CM, Chalmers RJG, O'Sullivan T, Griffiths CEM. A systematic review of antistreptococcal interventions for guttate and chronic plaque psoriasis. Br J Dermatol. 2001;145:886–90.
45. Valdimarsson H, Sigmundsdottir H, Jonsdottir I. Is psoriasis induced by streptococcal superantigens and maintained by M-protein-specific T cells that cross-react with keratin? Clin Exp Immunol. 1997;107(Suppl 1):21–4. https://europepmc.org/article/med/9020931
46. Prinz JC. Psoriasis vulgaris–a sterile antibacterial skin reaction mediated by cross-reactive T cells? An immunological view of the pathophysiology of psoriasis. Clin Exp Dermatol. 2001;26:326–32.
47. Balci DD, Duran N, Ozer B, Gunesacar R, Onlen Y, Yenin JZ. High prevalence of Staphylococcus aureus cultivation and superantigen production in patients with psoriasis. Eur J Dermatol. 2009;19:238–42. http://www.jle.com/fr/revues/ejd/e-docs/high_prevalence_of_staphylococcus_aureus_cultivation_and_superantigen_production_in_patients_with_psoriasis_280921/article.phtml?tab=texte

48. Ng CY, Huang YH, Chu CF, Wu TC, Liu SH. Risks for Staphylococcus aureus colonization in patients with psoriasis: a systematic review and meta-analysis. Br J Dermatol. 2017;177:967–77.
49. Konno S, Adachi M, Asano K, Okamoto K, Takahashi T. Inhibition of human T-lymphocyte activation by macrolide antibiotic, roxithromycin. Life Sci Pergamon. 1992;51:PL231–6.
50. Wakita H, Tokura Y, Furukawa F, Takigawa M. The macrolide antibiotic, roxithromycin suppresses IFN-gamma-mediated immunological functions of cultured normal human keratinocytes. Biol Pharm Bull. 1996;19:224–7.
51. Salem I, Ramser A, Isham N, Ghannoum MA. The gut microbiome as a major regulator of the gut-skin axis. Front Microbiol. 2018;10(9):1459. https://doi.org/10.3389/fmicb.2018.01459.
52. Rolig AS, Cech C, Ahler E, Carter JE, Ottemann KM. The degree of helicobacter pylori-triggered inflammation is manipulated by preinfection host microbiota. Infect Immun. 2013;81: 1382.
53. Tan RJ, Sun HQ, Zhang W, Yuan HM, Li B, Yan HT, et al. A 21–35 kDa mixed protein component from helicobacter pylori activates mast cells effectively in chronic spontaneous urticaria. Helicobacter. 2016;21:565–74. https://onlinelibrary.wiley.com/doi/full/10.1111/hel.12312
54. Chuh A, Lee A, Zawar V, Sciallis G, Kempf W. Pityriasis rosea–an update. Indian J Dermatol Venereol Leprol. 2005;71:311–5.
55. Ahmed N, Iftikhar N, Bashir U, Rizvi SDA, Sheikh ZI, Manzur A. Efficacy of clarithromycin in pityriasis rosea. J Coll Physicians Surg Pak. 2014;24:802–5. https://pubmed.ncbi.nlm.nih.gov/25404436/
56. Akhyani M, Mortazavi H, Izadi M, Ehsani A. The efficacy of oral erythromycin in the treatment of patients with pityriasis rosea: a randomized double-blind, placebo-controlled clinical trial. Iran J Dermatol. 2003;7:14–8. http://www.iranjd.ir/article_101095.html
57. Amer A, Fischer H, Li X. The natural history of pityriasis rosea in black American children: how correct is the "classic" description? Arch Pediatr Adolesc med. Arch Pediatr Adolesc Med. 2007;161:503–6.
58. Pandhi D, Singal A, Verma P, Sharma R. The efficacy of azithromycin in pityriasis rosea: a randomized, double-blind, placebo-controlled trial. Indian J Dermatol Venereol Leprol. 2014;80:36. https://ijdvl.com/the-efficacy-of-azithromycin-in-pityriasis-rosea-a-randomized-double-blind-placebo-controlled-trial/
59. Ehsani A, Esmaily N, Noormohammadpour P, Toosi S, Hosseinpour A, Hosseini M, et al. The comparison between the efficacy of high dose acyclovir and erythromycin on the period and signs of pitiriasis rosea. J Dermatol. 2010;55:246.
60. Cao P, Xu W, Zhang L, Hashimoto T, Kowalewski C, Mao X, et al. Rituximab, omalizumab, and dupilumab treatment cutcomes in bullous pemphigoid: a systematic review. Front Immunol. 2022;13:928621. https://doi.org/10.3389/fimmu.2022.928621.
61. Ohe M, Hashino S. Successful treatment of primary immune thrombocytopenia in aged patients using clarithromycin. J Formos Med Assoc. 2014;113:197–8.
62. Hashino S, Mori A, Suzuki S, Izumiyama K, Kahata K, Yonezumi M, et al. Platelet recovery in patients with idiopathic thrombocytopenic purpura after eradication of helicobacter pylori. Int J Hematol. 2003;77:188–91. https://pubmed.ncbi.nlm.nih.gov/12627857/
63. Tlaskalová-Hogenová H, Štěpánková R, Hudcovic T, Tučková L, Cukrowska B, Lodinová-Žádníková R, et al. Commensal bacteria (normal microflora), mucosal immunity and chronic inflammatory and autoimmune diseases. Immunol Lett. 2004;93:97–108.
64. Campuzano-Maya G. Cure of alopecia areata after eradication of helicobacter pylori: a new association? World J Gastroenterol. 2011;17:3165.
65. Bispo Lousada M, Edelkamp J, Lachnit T, Erdmann H, Paus R. Can antibiotic-induced changes in the composition of the hair follicle microbiome regulate human hair growth? Exp Dermatol. 2021;30:1440–1. https://onlinelibrary.wiley.com/doi/full/10.1111/exd.14364

66. Lucchini E, Pilotto S, Spada E, Melisi D, Bria E, Tortora G. Targeting the epidermal growth factor receptor in solid tumors: focus on safety. Expert Opin Drug Saf. 2014;13(5):535–49. https://doi.org/10.1517/14740338.2014.904283.
67. Lacouture ME, Anadkat M, Jatoi A, Garawin T, Bohac C, Mitchell E. Dermatologic toxicity occurring during anti-EGFR monoclonal inhibitor therapy in patients with metastatic colorectal cancer: a systematic review. Clin Colorectal Cancer. 2018;17:85–96.
68. Segaert S, van Cutsem E. Clinical signs, pathophysiology and management of skin toxicity during therapy with epidermal growth factor receptor inhibitors. Ann Oncol. 2005;16:1425–33. http://www.annalsofoncology.org/article/S0923753419549869/fulltext
69. Ocvirk J, Cencelj S. Management of cutaneous side-effects of cetuximab therapy in patients with metastatic colorectal cancer. J Am Acad Dermatol. 2010;24:453–9. https://onlinelibrary.wiley.com/doi/full/10.1111/j.1468-3083.2009.03446.x
70. Lacouture ME. The growing importance of skin toxicity in EGFR inhibitor therapy. Oncology. 2009;23(2):194.
71. Lacouture ME, Lai SE. The PRIDE (Papulopustules and/or paronychia, regulatory abnormalities of hair growth, itching, and dryness due to rpidermal growth factor receptor inhibitors) syndrome. Br J Dermatol. 2006;155:852–4.
72. Coleman S, Kovtun I, Nguyen PL, Pittelkow M, Jatoi A. A qualitative study of the ramifications of rash from epidermal growth factor receptor (EGFR) inhibitors. Psychooncology. 2011;20:1246.
73. Sapadin AN, Fleischmajer R. Tetracyclines: nonantibiotic properties and their clinical implications. J Am Acad Dermatol. 2006;54:258–65.

Macrolide Use in Preschool-Aged Children with Acute or Recurrent Respiratory Tract Illnesses with Wheezing

Lauren D. Benton and Fernando D. Martinez

Abstract Acute and recurrent lower respiratory tract illnesses with wheezing (WLRI) are a common problem among preschoolers and have high societal costs. Currently there are few options that are effective for either preventing or treating WLRI, especially in children without atopy. Macrolides may be a promising option for treating WLRI in preschool children, but there has been conflicting data on their efficacy. Their effect in WLRI may be due to their immunomodulatory or antimicrobial properties.

Keywords Macrolide · Azithromycin · Preschool · Children · Wheezing · Respiratory tract illness · Asthma · Bronchiolitis

1 Epidemiology of Lower Respiratory Tract Illnesses with Wheezing (WLRI)

Acute and recurrent WLRI are among the most common causes of morbidity in children, especially among preschoolers. Twenty percent of children will have a wheezing episode before 3 years of age and 50% will have one before 6 years of age [1, 2]. WLRI are the most frequent cause of emergency department visits and hospitalizations in this age group. Data from the National Hospital Ambulatory Medical Care Survey (NHAMCS) indicate that between 2010 and 2014, over 250,000 children aged 0–4 years visited an emergency department in the United States for "asthma" and of these, 28,000 were hospitalized [3]. These numbers may

L. D. Benton
Asthma and Airway Disease Research Center and Division of Pulmonary and Sleep Medicine, Department of Pediatrics, University of Arizona College of Medicine, Tucson, AZ, USA

University of Arizona Steele Children's Research Center, Tucson, AZ, USA

F. D. Martinez (✉)
Asthma and Airway Disease Research Center and Division of Pulmonary and Sleep Medicine, Department of Pediatrics, University of Arizona College of Medicine, Tucson, AZ, USA
e-mail: fdmartin@arizona.edu

B. K. Rubin, M. Shinkai (eds.), *Macrolides as Immunomodulatory Agents*, Progress in Inflammation Research 92, https://doi.org/10.1007/978-3-031-42859-3_14

underestimate the true incidence, because not all preschool children with WLRI are diagnosed with "asthma." A significant proportion of these children go on to develop persistent asthma, and WLRI are associated with deficits in lung function growth that may predispose for chronic obstructive pulmonary disease in adult life [4].

Despite the high burden and morbidity associated with WLRI, available treatments are often ineffective in reversing airway obstruction or preventing future acute episodes. Daily use of inhaled corticosteroids (ICS) or montelukast have proven to be effective in decreasing WLRI rates in asthmatic patients, but montelukast is inferior to ICS, and ICS is mostly effective in children with a T2 phenotype (i.e., associated with blood eosinophilia and/or allergic sensitization) [5]. Systemic corticosteroids are often used to treat acute WLRI episodes, but results have been mixed, with some studies showing no difference in hospitalization rates between oral corticosteroids versus placebo [6]. Short-acting beta agonists are also used in acute wheezing episodes for symptom treatment, but their effects are short lived [7]. There is the clear need for new approaches to the treatment of WLRI in preschool children, and especially among those who do not have evidence of a T2 phenotype.

Macrolide antibiotics such as azithromycin, erythromycin, clarithromycin, and roxithromycin have both antimicrobial and immunomodulatory effects and have been shown to be effective in the treatment of pulmonary diseases such as diffuse panbronchiolitis, cystic fibrosis, and severe nonatopic asthma in adults. This has led to an interest in using immunomodulatory macrolides for wheezy children to prevent worsening of WLRI and to shorten their course, thus decreasing the need for hospitalization.

2 Etiology of WLRI

Until recently, the established consensus regarding WLRI was that viruses were the most frequent triggers of these acute episodes of airway obstruction. However, in 2010, Bisgaard et al. showed that in children aged 4 months to 3 years, WLRI were associated with equally strong evidence of bacterial infection (mainly *H. influenzae, M. catarrhalis, and S. pneumoniae*) or viral infection [8]. Subsequently, Teo et al. reported that children whose nasopharynx was colonized with *S. pneumoniae* were more likely to have subsequent recurrent episodes of wheezing than those who were not [9]. More recently, Dumas et al. showed that children with increased proportions of *Haemophilus*-dominant or *Moraxella*-dominant nasopharyngeal microbiota profiles after an episode of bronchiolitis were more likely to have subsequent recurrent wheezing than those with other microbial profiles [10]. Finally, Kloepfer et al. reported that children 4–12 years old had twice the risk of having an asthma exacerbation if *S. pneumoniae* or *M. catarrhalis* were isolated from their nasal samples compared to children in whom neither *S. Pneumoniae* nor *M. catarrhalis* were isolated [11]. Taken together, these data suggest that bacteria may play a role in the pathogenesis of recurrent wheezing and seemed to provide support to the idea that antibiotics could be used to treat WLRI.

3 Biological Effects of Macrolides Relevant to WLRI

Macrolides are antibiotics with monolactone rings. In the United States of America commonly used macrolides include azithromycin, clarithromycin, and erythromycin. Macrolides have good respiratory penetration and can concentrate in inflammatory cells and mucus making them potential candidates to treat WLRI. Macrolides are bacteriostatic antibiotics that exhibit their effects by binding to the 50S ribosomal subunit stopping bacterial protein synthesis [12]. Apart from antimicrobial activity, some macrolides (azithromycin, clarithromycin, roxithromycin, erythromycin, dirithromycin, and troleandomycin) increase airway defense mechanisms, have immunomodulatory effects, and antiviral activity.

Macrolides have effects on host immune defense mechanisms. Airway epithelial cells form tight bonds that serve as a barrier. An intact epithelial barrier function is critical for respiratory health and is modulated by junctional complexes. Azithromycin, but not erythromycin, has been shown to increase epithelial barrier function independent of changes in bacterial colonization [13]. Mucus production and mucociliary clearance are an important part of the airways defense mechanism against pathogens. Goblet cells produce mucin, which creates a protective mucus layer that engulfs foreign particles, including viruses and bacteria; cilia beat these trapped particles up and out of the airway. In chronic inflammatory states, goblet cell hyperplasia can occur leading to greater mucus production. Clarithromycin, azithromycin, and erythromycin have been shown to decrease mucus production possibly by inhibiting MUC5A activation [14, 15].

Macrolides have immunomodulatory effects that may help protect against more severe respiratory infection and defend against viral respiratory infections. Neutrophils and macrophages migrate from the blood stream into the airway to help kill bacteria and viruses; however, these effects are nonspecific and can lead to the unintended consequence of injuring the airway. Viruses are known to induce neutrophilic inflammation and increase proinflammatory cytokines and chemokines such as IL-6, CXCL8, and IL-16 [16]. Atypical bacterial infections are also known to induce bronchial epithelial cell expression TNF-alpha, CXCL8, IFN-gamma, and nuclear factor kappa-beta, which in mice has been shown to induce bronchial hyper responsiveness [17]. Macrolides have been shown to alter these inflammatory pathways, leading to less secondary airway injury. Erythromycin inhibits neutrophil elastase and production of superoxide anions by neutrophils, which are both nonspecific inflammatory molecules that can damage the airway [18, 19]. Following initial stimulation of neutrophilic degranulation and oxidative burst, azithromycin has immunomodulatory effects via downregulating neutrophilic chemotactic factors such as CXCL8, reduction in oxidative burst by neutrophils, and upregulation of neutrophilic apoptosis [20–23]. Azithromycin also inhibits rhinovirus replication in airway epithelial cells and increases rhinovirus pattern recognition receptors, IFN, and IFN-stimulated gene mRNA levels [24]. Macrolides immunomodulatory effects may not be fully independent of their antimicrobial effects. In a study investigating clarithromycin's effects on cytokines and chemokines in children's nasal airways

Fonseca-Aten et al. found that clarithromycin decreased concentrations of TNF-α, IL-1β, and IL-10 [25] and that this effect attenuated in children with M pneumoniae and/or C pneumoniae. The relative role of antimicrobial, antiviral, and immunomodulatory effects of macrolides in their putative effects on WLRI prevention and treatment in currently unknown.

4 Use of Macrolides during Acute Wheezing Illnesses

Macrolide's efficacy in wheezing illnesses in children is debated and studies have shown conflicting data. A 2014 Cochrane review reported that antibiotics and, specifically, azithromycin use in children under 2 years old with bronchiolitis had no significant effect on length of hospitalization or duration of oxygen requirement and concluded that there was not sufficient evidence to support the use of antibiotics in bronchiolitis [26]. There have been a few meta-analyses investigating all macrolides that suggest they may be associated with less need for short-acting beta-agonist, lower risk of recurrent wheezing episodes, and shorter time to resolution of symptoms in children with asthma and wheezing [27–29]. However, these same meta-analyses have also shown little benefit of macrolide use in length of stay, need for oxygen, symptoms and signs of respiratory distress readmission rate, and rates of hospitalizations in these same children [27–29].

Studies investigating the efficacy of macrolides in WLRI have used mostly used azithromycin, which is the macrolide with the most consistent body of work completed. There have been fewer studies using clarithromycin or erythromycin [30]. Clarithromycin given at a dose of 15 mg/kg daily for 3 weeks to hospitalized patients with RSV bronchiolitis showed a reduction in length of stay and need for oxygen [30]. Since the 2014 Cochrane review, there have been additional randomized clinical trials investigating the use of azithromycin in preschool children with recurrent WLRI, and results have been mixed. A Danish study that recruited 1–3-year-old children with recurrent asthma-like illnesses from the Copenhagen Prospective Studies on Asthma in Childhood (COPSAC) 2010 Cohort randomized subjects with respiratory illnesses lasting longer than 3 days to either a 3-day course of 10 mg/kg azithromycin or a placebo. The study showed that the course of illness was shortened from 7.7 days in the placebo group to 3.4 days in the treatment group and that this effect was enhanced when azithromycin was given earlier in the course of illness. Also, treatment with azithromycin reduced the duration of short-acting beta agonist use [31]. Subsequently this same group assessed the hypopharyngeal microbiota during an acute WLRI in the children enrolled in this same trial [32]. They found that the composition of the airway microbiota was associated with the duration of the acute episode, and that the microbial richness of the sample before treatment increased the effect of azithromycin. These results suggested that the effects of azithromycin could be attributable to its antimicrobial and antiviral activity. Another study (the APRIL trial) recruited children 12 to 71 months of age from nine different US academic centers who had a history of recurrent severe WLRI but no impairment between episodes, and showed a positive effect of azithromycin when given early in the course of a respiratory illness [33]. In this study, the children's guardians were to start azithromycin (12 mg/kg once daily for 5 days) as soon as the child developed signs or symptoms of their "usual starting point before development of a severe lower respiratory tract illness." Children who received azithromycin had lower risk of progressing to a severe lower respiratory tract infection and those who did go on to develop a severe lower respiratory tract infection had fewer symptoms compared to those who received placebo. Azithromycin's effect was not modified by sex, asthma predictive index, viral detection, season of illness, or CXCL8 rs4073 genotype [33]. Although these studies showed a positive outcome when azithromycin was given to children with WLRI, a third study showed no positive effect. Mandhane et al. recruited children 12 to 60 months old who presented to Alberta Children's (Calgary) Stollery Children's (Edmonton) Hospital Emergency Departments in Canada with WLRI. Subjects were given azithromycin 10 mg/kg for 1 day and then 5 mg/kg for 4 days for a total course of 5 days of antibiotics or placebo. They found no significant difference in time to resolution of symptoms between the groups [34]. The difference in how these studies were conducted could possibly explain the reason for their different reports of benefit of use of azithromycin in respiratory tract illnesses. The Canadian investigators used a lower dosage and a shorter course of azithromycin in the treatment group, which may have led to less clinical benefit. They also recruited children who presented to the emergency department potentially later in their illness while the APRIL study, for example, recruited patients before the most severe phase of their illness, and this may have attenuated benefit. This is supported by the Danish study showing a greater effect when azithromycin was given earlier in the course of illness. Finally, the Canadian study enrolled all patients with a current wheezing illness, whereas both the US and Danish studies only enrolled patients with a previous history of wheezing. Of note, the Canadian study intended to enroll 440 participants and include approximately 400 in the primary analysis, but only 300 were finally randomized and 222 included in the primary analysis. It is unclear if these circumstances might have biased the results towards the null.

In summary, it is currently uncertain if azithromycin could be used to effectively treat WLRI among preschool children and if so, in which children. A limitation of all studies performed heretofore is that azithromycin was given to acutely ill children regardless of their microbial nasopharyngeal profile. Implicit in those studies' design is the assumption that efficacy of treatment with azithromycin would be attributable to nonantimicrobial effects of this antibiotic, but there is no definitive support for this assumption. To address this gap and provide definitive answers to this issue, one of us (FDM) co-leads an ongoing clinical trial called AZithromycin Therapy in Preschoolers With a Severe Wheezing Episode Diagnosed at the Emergency Department (AZ-SWED) (NCT04669288). Over 1500 preschool children will be randomized to either azithromycin (12 mg/kg/day for 5 days) or placebo, and the trial will be stratified by the presence or absence at the time of the acute illness of any one of the three taxa in the nasopharynx most frequently isolated in young children with WLRI (i.e., *H. influenzae, M. catarrhalis,* and *S. pneumoniae*). With this study design, the study will be able to determine if azithromycin is effective in preschool children with WLRI and if so, if it is specifically effective in those colonized with these pathogenic bacteria or if its effects are observed in all children regardless of bacterial colonization.

5 Azithromycin for Respiratory Syncytial Virus (RSV) Bronchiolitis to Prevent Future Wheezing Illnesses

Many infants who are hospitalized for acute bronchiolitis go on to have subsequent episodes of wheezing, and these recurrent episodes are associated with high morbidity and significant societal costs [35, 36]. There is some evidence that acute respiratory infections due to RSV are associated with a neutrophilic airway inflammation [37, 38], and this has suggested the possibility that, given azithromycin's anti-CXCL8 effects and associated attenuation of neutrophilic inflammation [39], it could play a role in the treatment of RSV bronchiolitis and in the subsequent development of recurrent wheezing.

Beigelman et al. studied otherwise healthy children hospitalized with RSV bronchiolitis. They were given either 14 days of placebo or azithromycin 10 mg/kg for 7 days and then 5 mg/kg for 7 days [40]. Infants treated with active drug had a greater decrease in nasal lavage fluid CXCL8 by day 15 and had a significantly prolonged time to the third WLRI episode post-RSV than those treated with placebo. They also had fewer days with respiratory symptoms (cough, wheeze, or shortness of breath) during a 50-week follow-up period. However, a subsequent, larger study by this same group of investigators did not confirm these results. They enrolled two hundred 1- to 18-month-old children hospitalized with RSV bronchiolitis in this single center and randomly assigned them to receive oral azithromycin (10 mg/kg daily for 7 days, followed by 5 mg/kg daily for 7 days) or placebo [41]. Azithromycin did not reduce the risk of post-RSV recurrent wheeze (47% in the azithromycin group vs. 36% in the placebo group; adjusted hazard ratio, $p = 0.11$). Azithromycin did have a biological effect, in that children in the active drug arm had lower levels of CXCL8 in nasal wash samples at 14 days postrandomization than those in the placebo group. Similarly, McCallum et al. investigated children 18 months or younger hospitalized for bronchiolitis [42]. In this study, children were given placebo or a single dose of 30 mg/kg of azithromycin. The azithromycin group did not have a difference in their rate of rehospitalization in 6 months of follow-up. These results thus suggest that azithromycin given to children hospitalized for bronchiolitis has no effect on the subsequent development of recurrent WLRI.

It is important to note here that most studies in which macrolides were shown to attenuate neutrophil dominant airway disease such as cystic fibrosis used long-term (i.e., 3 months or more) low-dose (e.g., thrice weekly) therapy. No such design has been attempted for the use of macrolide in the prevention of future WLRI in young children with RSV bronchiolitis.

6 Risks of Macrolide Use

The major side effect of macrolides is gastrointestinal issues and less commonly QT prolongation. Erythromycin can cause dose-dependent tinnitus and hearing loss. Erythromycin and clarithromycin may have interactions with drugs that use the cytochrome-P-450 system for metabolism. Many of the studies that use azithromycin report mild GI discomfort as the main side effect but in one of the clinic trials two people withdrew from the study due to side effects [34]. One subject had periorbital erythema and the other had diarrhea and vomiting [34]. Although the main side effect reported is GI discomfort there are concerns over widespread use of increasing macrolide resistance amongst bacteria, and gut dysbiosis.

Four studies have reported on the development of antibiotic resistance during trials in which azithromycin was tested; two of these trials were in adults and two in children. The AZISAST trial, which enrolled asthmatic patients 18 years or older, showed an increase in oropharyngeal carriage of azithromycin-resistant streptococci [43]. The AMAZES trial, which enrolled patients with asthma 18 years of age or older, did not report increased prevalence of azithromycin-resistant strains [44]. In the APRIL trial quoted earlier, assessment of nasopharyngeal samples from only one of the study centers showed an increase in azithromycin-resistant organisms in both the control and the treatment group, but the rates were higher in the azithromycin treated group, with *S aureus* being the most common resistant organism detected [33]. In a study of 5–15-year-old children with poorly controlled asthma, no azithromycin-resistant organisms were detected in the throat swabs collected. However, this was in only a small subset of their subjects due to COVID-19 not allowing collection of swabs in all subjects [45]. To provide more definitive answers regarding this issue and as part of a pre-established secondary outcome assessment, the AZ-SWED study is collecting nasopharyngeal swabs before and after administration of azithromycin to determine the development of resistance to the three bacterial taxa that have been implicated in the development WLRI.

The gut microbiota has commensal bacteria that may be altered by macrolides (or by any antibiotic). Dysbiosis could have negative consequences, since it has been shown that a healthy gut microbiome is important for protection against the development of asthma [46]. In the Beigelman et al. study quoted earlier, a post hoc analysis showed that children who had been treated with azithromycin during an RSV infection and were antibiotic naïve at the time of the acute episode had an increased risk of subsequent recurrent wheeze [41]. Why this effect was found in antibiotic-naïve children and not in those who had received antibiotics earlier is unknown. There have been previous studies and meta-analyses that show increased rates of asthma in children treated with antibiotics early in life; however, no causal relationship has been identified [47, 48]. Although perturbation of gut microbiome may be an adverse effect of macrolides, there have not been studies showing prolonged gut microbiome perturbations, and only short-term changes have been observed [49].

7 Conclusion

Whether macrolides are useful to prevent deterioration in acute wheezing episodes or prevent future wheezing episodes is yet to be determined. Studies looking at using macrolides in wheezing children have shown mixed results, but there is no fixed medication dosing or timing and many of the studies suffer from small sample sizes and very short study durations. Given that macrolides have both an antibiotic and immunomodulatory effects, they are likely to be helpful in subgroup of children with wheezing illnesses, and particularly, in those with non-T2-associated wheeze.

Compliance with Ethical Standards No human or animal studies were performed to complete this manuscript.

Conflict of Interest The authors have no conflicts of interest to disclose that are relevant to this article.

References

1. Martinez FD, Wright AL, Taussig LM, Holberg CJ, Halonen M, Morgan WJ. Asthma and wheezing in the first six years of life. The group health medical associates. N Engl J Med. 1995;332(3):133–8.
2. Bisgaard H, Hermansen MN, Buchvald F, Loland L, Halkjaer LB, Bonnelykke K, et al. Childhood asthma after bacterial colonization of the airway in neonates. N Engl J Med. 2007;357(15):1487–95.
3. Qin X, Zahran HS, Malilay J. Asthma-related emergency department (ED) visits and post-ED visit hospital and critical care admissions, National Hospital Ambulatory Medical Care Survey, 2010-2015. J Asthma. 2021;58(5):565–72.
4. Bisgaard H, Norgaard S, Sevelsted A, Chawes BL, Stokholm J, Mortensen EL, et al. Asthma-like symptoms in young children increase the risk of COPD. J Allergy Clin Immunol. 2021;147 (2):569–76 e9.
5. Fitzpatrick AM, Jackson DJ, Mauger DT, Boehmer SJ, Phipatanakul W, Sheehan WJ, et al. Individualized therapy for persistent asthma in young children. J Allergy Clin Immunol. 2016;138(6):1608–18.e12.
6. Castro-Rodriguez JA, Beckhaus AA, Forno E. Efficacy of oral corticosteroids in the treatment of acute wheezing episodes in asthmatic preschoolers: systematic review with meta-analysis. Pediatr Pulmonol. 2016;51(8):868–76.
7. Castro-Rodriguez JA, Rodrigo GJ, Rodríguez-Martínez CE. Principal findings of systematic reviews of acute asthma treatment in childhood. J Asthma. 2015;52(10):1038–45.
8. Bisgaard H, Hermansen MN, Bonnelykke K, Stokholm J, Baty F, Skytt NL, et al. Association of bacteria and viruses with wheezy episodes in young children: prospective birth cohort study. BMJ. 2010;341:c4978.
9. Teo SM, Mok D, Pham K, Kusel M, Serralha M, Troy N, et al. The infant nasopharyngeal microbiome impacts severity of lower respiratory infection and risk of asthma development. Cell Host Microbe. 2015;17(5):704–15.
10. Dumas O, Hasegawa K, Mansbach JM, Sullivan AF, Piedra PA, Camargo CA Jr. Severe bronchiolitis profiles and risk of recurrent wheeze by age 3 years. J Allergy Clin Immunol. 2019;143(4):1371–9 e7.

11. Kloepfer KM, Lee WM, Pappas TE, Kang TJ, Vrtis RF, Evans MD, et al. Detection of pathogenic bacteria during rhinovirus infection is associated with increased respiratory symptoms and asthma exacerbations. J Allergy Clin Immunol. 2014;133(5):1301–7. 7 e1–3
12. Nagel AA. Macrolide antibiotics. Chemistry, biology, and practice. Edited by Satoshi Ōmura. Academic Press, Inc., Orlando, FL 32887. 1984. 635 pp. J Pharm Sci. 1985;74(9):1023.
13. Asgrimsson V, Gudjonsson T, Gudmundsson GH, Baldursson O. Novel effects of azithromycin on tight junction proteins in human airway epithelia. Antimicrob Agents Chemother. 2006;50(5):1805–12.
14. Imamura Y, Yanagihara K, Mizuta Y, Seki M, Ohno H, Higashiyama Y, et al. Azithromycin inhibits MUC5AC production induced by the Pseudomonas aeruginosa autoinducer N-(3-Oxododecanoyl) homoserine lactone in NCI-H292 cells. Antimicrob Agents Chemother. 2004;48(9):3457–61.
15. Shimizu T, Shimizu S, Hattori R, Gabazza EC, Majima Y. In vivo and in vitro effects of macrolide antibiotics on mucus secretion in airway epithelial cells. Am J Respir Crit Care Med. 2003;168(5):581–7.
16. Papadopoulos NG, Papi A, Psarras S, Johnston SL. Mechanisms of rhinovirus-induced asthma. Paediatr Respir Rev. 2004;5(3):255–60.
17. Blasi F, Aliberti S, Allegra L, Piatti G, Tarsia P, Ossewaarde JM, et al. Chlamydophila pneumoniae induces a sustained airway hyperresponsiveness and inflammation in mice. Respir Res. 2007;8:83.
18. Mitsuyama T, Tanaka T, Hidaka K, Abe M, Hara N. Inhibition by erythromycin of superoxide anion production by human polymorphonuclear leukocytes through the action of cyclic AMP-dependent protein kinase. Respiration. 1995;62(5):269–73.
19. Gorrini M, Lupi A, Viglio S, Pamparana F, Cetta G, Iadarola P, et al. Inhibition of human neutrophil elastase by erythromycin and flurythromycin, two macrolide antibiotics. Am J Respir Cell Mol Biol. 2001;25(4):492–9.
20. Esterly NB, Furey NL, Flanagan LE. The effect of antimicrobial agents on leukocyte chemotaxis. J Invest Dermatol. 1978;70(1):51–5.
21. Miyachi Y, Yoshioka A, Imamura S, Niwa Y. Effect of antibiotics on the generation of reactive oxygen species. J Invest Dermatol. 1986;86(4):449–53.
22. Shinkai M, Foster GH, Rubin BK. Macrolide antibiotics modulate ERK phosphorylation and IL-8 and GM-CSF production by human bronchial epithelial cells. Am J Physiol Lung Cell Mol Physiol. 2006;290(1):L75–85.
23. Bosnar M, Cuzic S, Bosnjak B, Nujic K, Ergovic G, Marjanovic N, et al. Azithromycin inhibits macrophage interleukin-1beta production through inhibition of activator protein-1 in lipopolysaccharide-induced murine pulmonary neutrophilia. Int Immunopharmacol. 2011;11(4):424–34.
24. Schogler A, Kopf BS, Edwards MR, Johnston SL, Casaulta C, Kieninger E, et al. Novel antiviral properties of azithromycin in cystic fibrosis airway epithelial cells. Eur Respir J. 2015;45(2):428–39.
25. Fonseca-Aten M, Okada PJ, Bowlware KL, Chavez-Bueno S, Mejias A, Rios AM, et al. Effect of clarithromycin on cytokines and chemokines in children with an acute exacerbation of recurrent wheezing: a double-blind, randomized, placebo-controlled trial. Ann Allergy Asthma Immunol. 2006;97(4):457–63.
26. Farley R, Spurling GK, Eriksson L, Del Mar CB. Antibiotics for bronchiolitis in children under two years of age. Cochrane Database Syst Rev. 2014;10:CD005189.
27. Pincheira MA, Bacharier LB, Castro-Rodriguez JA. Efficacy of macrolides on acute asthma or wheezing exacerbations in children with recurrent wheezing: a systematic review and meta-analysis. Paediatr Drugs. 2020;22(2):217–28.
28. Lei WT, Lin HH, Tsai MC, Hung HH, Cheng YJ, Liu SJ, et al. The effects of macrolides in children with reactive airway disease: a systematic review and meta-analysis of randomized controlled trials. Drug Des Devel Ther. 2018;12:3825–45.

29. Lin CY, Yeh TL, Liu SJ, Lin HH, Cheng YJ, Hung HH, et al. Effects of macrolide treatment during the hospitalization of children with childhood wheezing disease: a systematic review and meta-analysis. J Clin Med. 2018;7(11)
30. Tahan F, Ozcan A, Koc N. Clarithromycin in the treatment of RSV bronchiolitis: a double-blind, randomised, placebo-controlled trial. Eur Respir J. 2007;29(1):91–7.
31. Stokholm J, Chawes BL, Vissing NH, Bjarnadottir E, Pedersen TM, Vinding RK, et al. Azithromycin for episodes with asthma-like symptoms in young children aged 1-3 years: a randomised, double-blind, placebo-controlled trial. Lancet Respir Med. 2016;4(1):19–26.
32. Thorsen J, Stokholm J, Rasmussen MA, Mortensen MS, Brejnrod AD, Hjelmso M, et al. The airway microbiota modulates effect of azithromycin treatment for episodes of recurrent asthma-like symptoms in preschool children: a randomized clinical trial. Am J Respir Crit Care Med. 2021;204(2):149–58.
33. Bacharier LB, Guilbert TW, Mauger DT, Boehmer S, Beigelman A, Fitzpatrick AM, et al. Early Administration of Azithromycin and Prevention of severe lower respiratory tract illnesses in preschool children with a history of such illnesses: a randomized clinical trial. JAMA. 2015;314 (19):2034–44.
34. Mandhane PJ, Zambrano P, de Silbernagel P, Aung YN, Williamson J, Lee BE, Spier S, et al. Treatment of preschool children presenting to the emergency department with wheeze with azithromycin: a placebo-controlled randomized trial. PLoS One. 2017;12(8):e0182411.
35. Zorc JJ, Hall CB. Bronchiolitis: recent evidence on diagnosis and management. Pediatrics. 2010;125(2):342–9.
36. Hall CB, Weinberg GA, Iwane MK, Blumkin AK, Edwards KM, Staat MA, et al. The burden of respiratory syncytial virus infection in young children. N Engl J Med. 2009;360(6):588–98.
37. Everard ML, Swarbrick A, Wrightham M, McIntyre J, Dunkley C, James PD, et al. Analysis of cells obtained by bronchial lavage of infants with respiratory syncytial virus infection. Arch Dis Child. 1994;71(5):428–32.
38. Pitrez PM, Pinto LA, Machado DC, Tsukazan MT, Jones MH, Stein RT. Upper airway cellular pattern in infants with acute bronchiolitis: neutrophils or eosinophils? J Pediatr. 2003;79(5): 443–8.
39. Beigelman A, Mikols CL, Gunsten SP, Cannon CL, Brody SL, Walter MJ. Azithromycin attenuates airway inflammation in a mouse model of viral bronchiolitis. Respir Res. 2010;11:90.
40. Beigelman A, Isaacson-Schmid M, Sajol G, Baty J, Rodriguez OM, Leege E, et al. Randomized trial to evaluate azithromycin's effects on serum and upper airway IL-8 levels and recurrent wheezing in infants with respiratory syncytial virus bronchiolitis. J Allergy Clin Immunol. 2015;135(5):1171–8.e1.
41. Beigelman A, Srinivasan M, Goss CW, Wang J, Zhou Y, True K, et al. Azithromycin to prevent recurrent wheeze following severe respiratory syncytial virus bronchiolitis. NEJM Evidence. 2022;1(4):EVIDoa2100069.
42. McCallum GB, Morris PS, Chatfield MD, Maclennan C, White AV, Sloots TP, et al. A single dose of azithromycin does not improve clinical outcomes of children hospitalised with bronchiolitis: a randomised, placebo-controlled trial. PLoS One. 2013;8(9):e74316.
43. Gibson PG, Yang IA, Upham JW, Reynolds PN, Hodge S, James AL, et al. Effect of azithromycin on asthma exacerbations and quality of life in adults with persistent uncontrolled asthma (AMAZES): a randomised, double-blind, placebo-controlled trial. Lancet. 2017;390 (10095):659–68.
44. Brusselle GG, Vanderstichele C, Jordens P, Deman R, Slabbynck H, Ringoet V, et al. Azithromycin for prevention of exacerbations in severe asthma (AZISAST): a multicentre randomised double-blind placebo-controlled trial. Thorax. 2013;68(4):322–9.
45. Ghimire JJ, Jat KR, Sankar J, Lodha R, Iyer VK, Gautam H, et al. Azithromycin for poorly controlled asthma in children: a randomized controlled trial. Chest. 2022;161(6):1456–64.
46. Depner M, Taft DH, Kirjavainen PV, Kalanetra KM, Karvonen AM, Peschel S, et al. Maturation of the gut microbiome during the first year of life contributes to the protective farm effect on childhood asthma. Nat Med. 2020;26(11):1766–75.

47. Chen IL, Huang HC, Chang YH, Huang HY, Yeh WJ, Wu TY, et al. Effect of antibiotic use for acute bronchiolitis on new-onset asthma in children. Sci Rep. 2018;8(1):6090.
48. Ahmadizar F, Vijverberg SJH, Arets HGM, de Boer A, Turner S, Devereux G, et al. Early life antibiotic use and the risk of asthma and asthma exacerbations in children. Pediatr Allergy Immunol. 2017;28(5):430–7.
49. Wei S, Mortensen MS, Stokholm J, Brejnrod AD, Thorsen J, Rasmussen MA, et al. Short- and long-term impacts of azithromycin treatment on the gut microbiota in children: a double-blind, randomized, placebo-controlled trial. EBioMedicine. 2018;38:265–72.

Macrolides and Immunomodulation: Today and the Future

Masaharu Shinkai

Abstract In this final chapter, we briefly summarized the contents of each chapter of the book and suggested thoughts for possible future directions and recommendations for future studies on macrolides as immunomodulators, including the development of new nonantimicrobial macrolides such as EP395.

Keywords macrolides · Immunomodulatory properties · Neutrophil-dominant (T17) inflammation · Nonantimicrobial macrolides · EM900 · EP395 · Solithromycin

Professor Rubin and I have been collaborators and friends for several decades, studying these unique immunomodulatory properties of the macrolide antibiotics [1], and leading to the clinical trials establishing their effectiveness in treating cystic fibrosis. This was summarized in the first edition of this book, published with Prof. Jun Tamaoki in 2005. It is clear that a great deal has happened since then and we are delighted to summarize this knowledge in this volume, organized in 15 chapters by experts on the mechanisms and clinical effects of macrolides as immunomodulators.

Prof. Rubin begins the Introductory Chapter, "A brief history of the macrolide antibiotics" with a history of the macrolide antibiotics with an emphasis on the discovery of their immunomodulatory properties. "Macrolides and Diseases Associated with Loss of Epithelial Barrier Integrity" discusses the diverse mechanisms of macrolide immunomodulatory action as well as the cytoprotective effects of macrolides on airway epithelial cells, and on skin and intestinal epithelium, and how these properties can be used to treat airway, skin, and intestinal diseases related to epithelial barrier disorders. "Macrolides and Inflammatory Cells, Signaling, and Mediators" continues to explore these diverse immunomodulatory mechanisms, including normalizing airway water and mucus secretion, inflammatory cytokines, chemokines, adhesion molecules, and inhibiting neutrophil infiltration through the involvement of transcription factors such as mitogen-activated protein kinase and NFκB. Additionally macrolides can affect the function of lysosomes, autophagy, and apoptosis, increasing affinity for cell membranes within and without the cell.

M. Shinkai (✉)
Tokyo Shinagawa Hospital, Tokyo, Japan

B. K. Rubin, M. Shinkai (eds.), *Macrolides as Immunomodulatory Agents*, Progress in Inflammation Research 92, https://doi.org/10.1007/978-3-031-42859-3_15

"Clinical Macrolide Use for DPB" then emphasizes that the first widespread use of macrolides as immunomodulators was in Japan, to treat diffuse panbronchiolitis (DPB). Macrolide therapy is most effective in the early stages of DPB, but the induction of clarithromycin resistance to *Mycobacterium avium* complex has been a problem, perhaps addressed by the clinical development of nonantimicrobial macrolides as discussed below. The use of macrolides, in particular azithromycin, to treat cystic fibrosis (CF) is reviewed in "Macrolides and Cystic Fibrosis" and non-CF bronchiectasis in "Non-CF Bronchiectasis". As noted in "Macrolide Use in Chronic Obstructive Pulmonary Disease", azithromycin therapy is now included in the Global Initiative for Chronic Obstructive Lung Disease (GOLD) guidelines as add-on therapy to decrease the frequency of acute exacerbations of chronic obstructive pulmonary disease (COPD) with a summary of these compelling data.

As early as the 1950s, and before their established use in DPB, troleandomycin, a 14-member macrolide antibiotic, was recommended as a "steroid-sparing" medication for patients with severe asthma. In "Macrolides and Asthma Therapy", the history of macrolide use for therapy of severe asthma, especially T17 dominant, nonallergic asthma is reviewed. This is now recommended for severe, difficult-to-treat asthma in both the NAEPP and GINA asthma guidelines. Furthermore, as discussed in "Macrolide Use in Preschool Aged Children with Acute or Recurrent Respiratory Tract Illnesses with Wheezing", macrolides may be a promising option for decreasing the occurrence of acute and recurrent lower respiratory illness with wheezing in preschool children.

In "Macrolides and Interstitial Lung Diseases", evidence is presented suggesting clinical benefits of add-on macrolide therapy for idiopathic pulmonary fibrosis, cryptogenic pneumonitis, and organizing pneumonitis when there is an incomplete response to antifibrotic or immunosuppressive agents. In the following 2 chapters, the effectiveness of macrolide antibiotics in calming the cytokine storm of acute respiratory distress syndrome (ARDS) and in ameliorating the risk of chronic lung allograft dysfunction (CLAD) and rejection in lung transplant recipients when administered early and before symptoms of CLAD is reviewed.

There are extensive data, largely from Drs. Suzaki's and Sakakura's otolaryngology research groups that macrolide antibiotics can be effective in treating both chronic rhinosinusitis and recalcitrant nasal polyposis. This again, appears to be especially true when there is neutrophil-dominant (T17) inflammation with prominent mucus hypersecretion and nasal discharge.

Chapter "Macrolides for Cancer" reviews the reported anticancer effects of the macrolide antibiotics. Macrolides inhibit ERK and this can impede the Raf to mitogen-activated protein kinase pathway, decreasing TGF-β activation, inducing apoptosis, enhancing antiangiogenic effects, and acting on autophagy. These drugs have also been reported to block resistance to anticancer drugs and/or to synergize with the use of other anticancer drugs. Clarithromycin significantly decreased mucosa-associated lymphoid tissue (MALT) lymphoma with *Helicobacter pylori* eradication. Clarithromycin has also been effective in treating multiple myeloma when used in combination with lenalidomide and dexamethasone. Finally, "Macrolides in Chronic Skin Disorders" reviews the use of macrolide antibiotics to tread inflammatory skin diseases, including rosacea, pustulosis palmoplantaris, psoriasis, pityriasis rosea, bullous pemphigoid, pityriasis lichenoides, alopecia areata, and atopic dermatitis.

Based on the accumulated data, macrolide therapy seems to be most effective for treating chronic neutrophilic epithelial inflammation that is poorly controlled with conventional therapy. Because of this, biomarkers of effectiveness might include tissue neutrophils and neutrophil-associated cytokines such as CXCL-8. Based upon extensive studies of DPB therapy from Japan, it is recommended that macrolide therapy should begin with erythromycin at low dose. Gastrointestinal side effects of erythromycin are generally minimal with low-dose therapy. Improvement in clinical symptoms such as cough and sputum is generally observed in 1–3 months, and improvement in pulmonary function testing and imaging findings is usually obvious by 6 months. At 6 months the clinical response should be evaluated to determine whether treatment with erythromycin should be continued or therapy changed to clarithromycin or azithromycin. Treatment should be continued for 1–2 years, and if the disease is stable, treatment can be discontinued at that time. If the disease relapses, it is appropriate to resume macrolide therapy as before. Although there are fewer studies addressing the duration of therapy in other epithelial inflammatory diseases, it is reasonable to extrapolate from the known affects when treating DPB.

Chronic and low-dose (sub-MIC90) macrolide therapy is well tolerated but carries the risk of inducing bacterial resistance. In East Asian countries where low-dose macrolide therapy is frequently used, macrolide-resistant *Streptococcus pneumoniae*, the most common causative agent of community acquired pneumonia, has become a major problem, with about 80% of isolates macrolide resistant [2]. Therefore, the Kitasato group aimed to develop nonantimicrobial macrolides with preserved immunomodulatory activity, focusing on the ability to promote the differentiation of monocytes into macrophages [3].

Exposing erythromycin A to weak acids forms intramolecular acetals, yielding EM201 [4]. When EM201 is placed under basic conditions, translactonization occurs, yielding EM701 with a 12-membered ring. Since EM701 is less stable to acids, its ethanol moiety can be reduced to obtain EM900, which is more stable to acids. After demethylation of EM900, a p-chlorobenzyl group is introduced to obtain EM905. EM900 administration in a guinea pig model of cigarette smoke-induced airway disease, deceased airway resistance, residual air volume, and alveolar dilatation and suppressed endotoxin shock. EM905, with no antimicrobial activity, induced monocyte differentiation into macrophages 30-fold more than that erythromycin A. It further had a marked anti-inflammatory effect in a rat model of refractory colitis.

EP395 [5], EpiEndo Pharmaceutical's lead compound is a new class of macrolide named "barriolds." EP395 has anti-inflammatory activity in lipopolysaccharide and respiratory syncytial virus induced lung disease in mice. EP395 dose-dependently inhibited neutrophil infiltration with ED50 of 3.7 ($n = 10$) and 14 μmol/kg/week ($n = 8$), respectively. Concentrations of the proinflammatory cytokines TNFα and IL-6 were significantly reduced by 2 weeks of pretreatment with EP395, comparable to that seen with azithromycin and roflumilast. These data support the potential of

EP395 to treat diseases such as COPD that involve neutrophil infiltration and epithelial barrier dysfunction. A randomized, double-blind, placebo-controlled, multicenter trial is underway to evaluate EP395 in patients with COPD [6]. Patients will receive EP395 or placebo as oral capsules once daily for 12 weeks. Safety, tolerability, lung function, lung inflammation, systemic inflammation, patient symptoms, and quality of life will be evaluated.

Telithromycin is a ketolide agent with a ketone group introduced at the 8th position of the 14-membered ring to decrease bacterial macrolide resistance. It has strong antibacterial activity against macrolide-resistant *Streptococcus pneumoniae*. The introduction of ketone groups and modification of the side-chain structure increases acid stability and enhances its binding to the bacterial ribosome. It also has antibacterial activity against Gram-negative respiratory pathogens such as *Haemophilus influenzae* and *Moraxella catarrhalis*. However, it is not used clinically due to reports of serious liver damage, syncope, and loss of consciousness in patients treated with telithromycin. A modification of this ketolide is solithromycin. Solithromycin is a novel fluoroketolide antibiotic that is reported to avoid the syncope that was a problem with telithromycin. Oral solithromycin was found to be noninferior to oral moxifloxacin in the treatment of community-acquired pneumonia [7]. Kobayashi et al. [8] showed that solithromycin suppressed TNFα/CXCL8 production and phorbol 12-myristate 13-acetate-induced matrix metalloproteinase 9 (MMP9) activity in macrophage-like U937 cells and peripheral blood mononuclear cells from COPD patients, about tenfold more potently than erythromycin, clarithromycin, azithromycin, and telithromycin under oxidative stress conditions. Furthermore, oxidative stress induced activation of NFκB was completely suppressed by solithromycin. It shows a better anti-inflammatory profile compared to currently used macrolide antimicrobials while preserving antimicrobial activity even in macrolide-resistant bacteria. We also showed that solithromycin inhibits IL-13-induced goblet cell hyperplasia and MUC5AC by suppressing the expression of chloride channel accessory 1 (CLCA1) and anoctamin-1 (ANO-1) [9].

Macrolides are classic examples of drug repurposing. Drugs, like the macrolides, that affect multiple target molecules can be extremely effective even when the effects on individual pathways are weak. Macrolides have many effects on the inflammatory cascade that have been reported, although the mechanisms underlying these effects are still being determined. Future research can be directed toward the development of topical macrolide therapies, such as aerosols for pulmonary diseases and creams/lotion for skin diseases as well as more potent immunomodulatory macrolides without antimicrobial properties.

Conflict of Interest Statement Masaharu Shinkai participated in a clinical trial of solithromycin at FUJIFILM Toyama Chemical Co., Ltd.

Ethics Compliance Statement There are no ethical concerns.

References

1. Shinkai M, Henke MO, Rubin BK. Macrolide antibiotics as immunomodulatory medications: proposed mechanisms of action. Pharmacol Ther. 2008;117(3):393–405.
2. Feldman D, Reinert RR, Hirakata Y, Rodloff A. Increasing prevalence of antimicrobial resistance among isolates of Streptococcus pneumoniae from the PROTEKT surveillance study, and comparative in vitro activity of the ketolide, telithromycin. J Antimicrob Chemother. 2002;50 (Suppl S1):25–37.
3. Keicho N, Kudoh S, Yotsumoto H, Akagawa KS. Erythromycin promotes monocyte to macrophage differentiation. J Antibiot (Tokyo). 1994;47(1):80–9.
4. Sugawara A, Sueki A, Hirose T, Nagai K, Gouda H, Hirono S, et al. Novel 12-membered non-antibiotic macrolides from erythromycin a; EM900 series as novel leads for anti-inflammatory and/or immunomodulatory agents. Bioorg Med Chem Lett. 2011;21(11):3373–6.
5. Kricker J, Gardarsson F, Lehmann F, Bech M, Gudjonsson T, Page C, et al. Inhibition of neutrophilic inflammation by targeting the airway epithelial barrier with EP395. Eur Respir J. 2022;60:312.
6. Parnham MJ, Norris V, Kricker JA, Gudjonsson T, Page CP. Prospects for macrolide therapy of asthma and COPD. Adv Pharmacol. 2023; in press
7. Barrera CM, Mykietiuk A, Metev H, Nitu MF, Karimjee N, Doreski PA, et al. Efficacy and safety of Oral solithromycin versus oral moxifloxacin for treatment of community-acquired bacterial pneumonia: a global, double-blind, multicenter, randomized active-controlled, non-inferiority trial (SOLITAIRE-ORAL). Lancet Infect Dis. 2016;16(4):421–30.
8. Kobayashi Y, Wada H, Rossios C, Takagi D, Higaki M, Mikura S, et al. A novel macrolide solithromycin exerts superior anti-inflammatory effect via NF-κB inhibition. J Pharmacol Exp Ther. 2013;345(1):76–84.
9. Kimura Y, Shinoda M, Shinkai M, Kaneko T. Solithromycin inhibits IL-13-induced goblet cell hyperplasia and MUC5AC, CLCA1, and ANO1 in human bronchial epithelial cells. PeerJ. 2023;11:e14695.

GPSR Compliance

The European Union's (EU) General Product Safety Regulation (GPSR) is a set of rules that requires consumer products to be safe and our obligations to ensure this.

If you have any concerns about our products, you can contact us on ProductSafety@springernature.com

In case Publisher is established outside the EU, the EU authorized representative is:

Springer Nature Customer Service Center GmbH
Europaplatz 3
69115 Heidelberg, Germany

Batch number: 10732044

Printed by Printforce, the Netherlands